QW
568
C997
1988
v.2

LIBRARY
UNIVERSITY OF TEXAS
SOUTHWESTERN MEDICAL SCHOOL
DALLAS, TEXAS

SOUTHWESTERN MEDICAL SCHOOL
DALLAS, TEXAS

Cytolytic Lymphocytes and Complement: Effectors of the Immune System

Volume II

Editor

Eckhard R. Podack, M.D.
Professor of Microbiology and Immunology
and
Professor of Medicine
New York Medical College
Valhalla, New York

Current address:
Professor
Department of Microbiology and Immunology
University of Miami School of Medicine
Miami, Florida

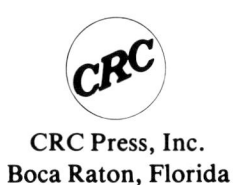

CRC Press, Inc.
Boca Raton, Florida

Library of Congress Cataloging-in-Publication Data

Cytolytic lymphocytes and complement

  Includes bibliographies and index.
  1. T cells. 2. Killer cells. 3. Complement
(Immunology) I. Podack, Eckhard R. [DNLM: 1. Complement
--immunology. 2. Cytotoxicity, Immunologic. 3. Killer
Cells, Natural--immunology. 4. T Lymphocytes,
Cytotoxic--immunology. QW 568 C997]
QR185.8.T2C98 1988   616.07′9   87-22431

ISBN 0-8493-6968-1 (v. 1)
ISBN 0-8493-6969-X (v. 2)

  This book represents information obtained from authentic and highly regarded sources. Reprinted material is quoted with permission, and sources are indicated. A wide variety of references are listed. Every reasonable effort has been made to give reliable data and information, but the author and the publisher cannot assume responsibility for the validity of all materials or for the consequences of their use.

  All rights reserved. This book, or any parts thereof, may not be reproduced in any form without written consent from the publisher.

  Direct all inquiries to CRC Press, Inc., 2000 Corporate Blvd., N.W., Boca Raton, Florida, 33431.

© 1988 by CRC Press, Inc.

International Standard Book Number 0-8493-6968-1 (Volume I)
International Standard Book Number 0-8493-6969-X (Volume II)
Library of Congress Card Number 87-22431
Printed in the United States

Dedication

To my father, Dr. med. Waldemar W. Podack, in gratitude for stimulating my interest in science.

INTRODUCTION

These volumes, *Cytolytic Lymphocytes and Complement: Effectors of the Immune System,* originate from the realization that pathways of recognition and killing of foreign targets follow similar routes in the humoral and cellular part of the immune system. In particular, the homology of immunoglobulins with the T-cell-MHC-antigen receptor at the beginning of the recognition sequence and the homology of complement component C9 with lymphocyte perforin 1 (P1) as pore formers at the end of the effector sequence are striking examples.

From my own point of view, the catalyst for suspecting mechanistically similar pathways in the effector systems of complement and cytolytic lymphocytes derived from the discovery of the polymerization of C9 to the circular structure of poly C9 (see Figure 1), which is responsible for the well-known ultrastructural complement lesions described originally in 1964. This simple finding immediately clarified conceptually the mechanisms for the formation of transmembrane pores both by complement and by cytolytic T- and NK-cells.

The motivation to assemble these volumes through the contributions of outstanding investigators in complement and lymphocyte research thus was, and is, to increase the awareness that mechanisms and molecular models studied in one system may well be of relevance to the other. Since complement has been studied in detail in all of its aspects, including activation, host protection, cytolysis, and repair mechanisms, it can serve as a guiding model system for the investigator of cellular mechanisms.

Effector cells, on the other hand, have the facility to interact with targets through surface membrane receptors allowing them an additional degree of complexity compared to humoral systems. This complexity, combined with the subcellular organization of cells (for example, the sequestration of cytolytic proteins in granules), offers alternatives for the mediation and regulation of cellular pathways that can be quite different from the humoral pathway.

Owing to these differences, the approaches to the use of the two effector systems for immune therapy are quite distinct. However, both are being explored at this time, and only future work will tell which combination of immune therapy will be most effective.

It is one of the most fascinating aspects of research to experience the development of common concepts with the attendant simplifications and understanding at the molecular level of previously poorly understood phenomena. It is hoped that this book will contribute to this process.

E. R. Podack

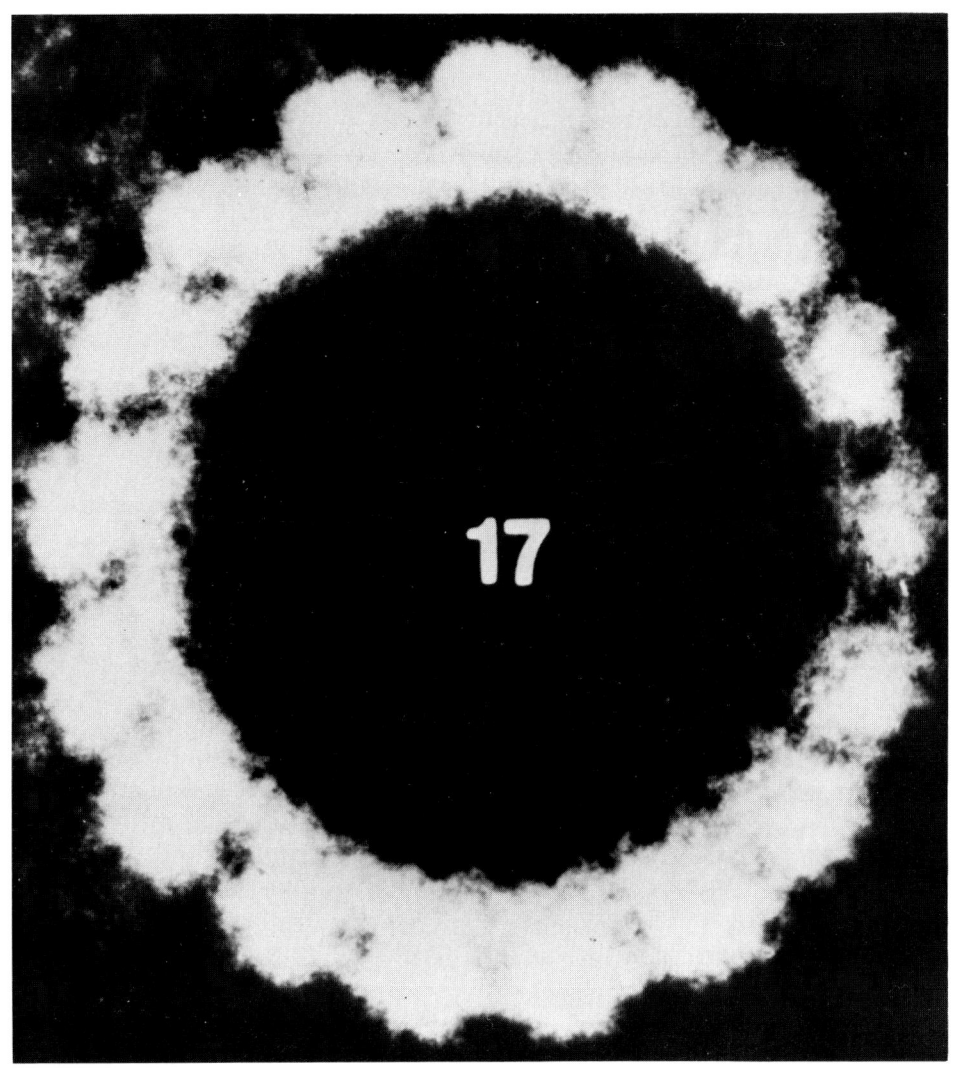

FIGURE 1. Poly C9.

THE EDITOR

Eckhard R. Podack, M. D., was appointed Full Professor of Microbiology and Immunology at the University of Miami School of Medicine in 1987. Prior to this appointment, he had been Professor of Medicine, Microbiology, and Immunology at the New York Medical College in Valhalla, New York, since 1984. From 1974 to 1984, he was associated with the Department of Immunology at the Research Institute of Scripps Clinic in La Jolla, California.

Dr. Podack holds the M.D. from Johann-Wolfgang-Goethe University in Frankfurt, Germany, and wrote his dissertation in Biochemistry at the Georg August University of Göttingen in Germany. His research thesis was honored with the Annual Award by the German Diabetes Society in 1973. Post-doctoral fellowship training was completed in the Department of Biochemistry at the University of Göttingen before he moved to this country in 1974. In biochemistry and immunology, Dr. Podack is internationally recognized and is a frequent invited lecturer to universities in Europe and the United States.

After collaborating with Hans Müller-Eberhard at the Scripps Research Foundation from 1974 to 1978 on complement components and activation, he spent the next six to eight years studying independently the molecular biology of molecules that cytotoxic lymphocytes use to kill their targets.

Dr. Podack is the recipient of two National Institutes of Health grants, an American Cancer Society grant, two Fellowship grants for his Post-Doctoral fellows, and a proposal of studies from private industry.

Dr. Podack is Associate Editor of the *Journal of Immunology* and Ad Hoc Reviewer for nine additional scientific journals. He reviews grant applications for the Veterans Administration, the National Science Foundation, the Fogarty International Fellowship Center, and the National Institutes of Health.

CONTRIBUTORS, VOLUME I

M. Amin Arnaout
Department of Pediatrics
Children's Hospital
Boston, Massachusetts

Barbara A. Benson
Research Service
VA Medical Center
Minneapolis, Minnesota

Gideon Berke
Department of Cell Biology
Weizmann Institute of Science
Rehovot, Israel

Steven J. Burakoff
Department of Pediatrics
Dana-Farber Cancer Institute
Boston, Massachusetts

David F. Carney
Department of Pathology
University of Maryland
Baltimore, Maryland

Zanvil A. Cohn
The Rockefeller University
New York, New York

Neil R. Cooper
Department of Molecular Immunology
Scripps Clinic and Research Foundation
La Jolla, Callifornia

Agustin P. Dalmasso
Laboratory Service
VA Medical Center
Minneapolis, Minnesota

Gunther Dennert
Department of Microbiology
University of Southern California
Los Angeles, California

Julia L. Greenstein
Department of Pediatric Oncology
Dana-Farber Cancer Institute
Boston, Massachusetts

Zvi Keren
Department of Cell Biology
Weizmann Institute of Science
Rehovot, Israel

M. Edward Medof
Department of Pathology and Medicine
Case Western Reserve University
Cleveland, Ohio

Steven J. Mentzer
Department of Pediatric Oncology
Dana-Farber Cancer Institute
Boston, Massachusetts

Michael K. Pangburn
Department of Biochemistry
University of Texas Health Center
Tyler, Texas

Eckhard R. Podack
Department of Microbiology
 and Immunology
University of Miami
 School of Medicine
Miami, Florida

David H. Raulet
Center for Cancer Research and
 Department of Biology
Massachusetts Institute of Technology
Cambridge, Massachusetts

Verne N. Schumaker
Molecular Biology Institute
University of California, Los Angeles
Los Angeles, California

Moon L. Shin
Department of Pathology
University of Maryland
Baltimore, Maryland

Jürg Tschopp
Institute of Biochemistry
University of Lausanne
Epalinges-sur-Lausanne, Switzerland

John Ding-E. Young
Cell Physiology and Immunology
  Laboratory
Rockefeller University
New York, New York

Robert J. Ziccardi
Department of Molecular Immunology
Scripps Clinic and Research Foundation
La Jolla, California

CONTRIBUTORS, VOLUME II

Bharat B. Aggarwal
Department of Molecular Biology
  and Immunology
Genentech, Inc.
South San Francisco, California

Ramani A. Aiyer
Department of Molecular Biology
  and Immunology
Genentech, Inc.
South San Francisco, California

Michael J. Bevan
Department of Immunology
Scripps Clinic and Research Foundation
La Jolla, California

Benjamin Bonavida
Department of Microbiology and
  Immunology
School of Medicine
University of California, Los Angeles
Los Angeles, California

Thomas J. Braciale
Department of Pathology
Washington University School of
  Medicine
St. Louis, Missouri

Vivian Lam Braciale
Department of Pathology
Washington University
  School of Medicine
St. Louis, Missouri

Jen W. Chiao
Department of Medicine
New York Medical College
Valhalla, New York

John J. Cohen
Department of Microbiology and
  Immunology
University of Colorado Medical School
Denver, Colorado

Zanvil A. Cohn
The Rockefeller University
New York, New York

Gunther Dennert
Department of Microbiology
University of Southern California
Los Angeles, California

Richard C. Duke
Department of Microbiology
  and Immunology
University of Colorado Medical School
Denver, Colorado

Brett T. Gemlo
Department of Surgery
University of California
San Francisco, California

Elizabeth Ann Grimm
Departments of Tumor Biology
  and General Surgery
University of Texas System Cancer
  Center
M. D. Anderson Hospital
Houston, Texas

Hans Hengartner
Department of Experimental Pathology
Institute of Pathology
Zurich, Switzerland

Frederick C. Kull, Jr.
Wellcome Research Laboratories
Research Triangle Park
North Carolina

Lewis L. Lanier
Research and Development Department
B.D. Monoclonal Center
Mountain View, California

Leo Lefrancois
Department of Immunology
Scripps Clinic and Research Foundation
La Jolla, California

Ben-Yao Lin
Department of Microbiology
New York Medical College
Valhalla, New York

Aron Lukacher
Department of Pathology
Washington University School of
 Medicine
St. Louis, Missouri

Abraham Mittelman
Division of Neoplastic Disease
New York Medical College
Valhalla, New York

Warren W. Myers
Department of Research
Becton Dickinson
Mt. View, California

Carl F. Nathan
Cornell Medical College
New York Hospital
New York, New York

Kristin Penichet
Department of Microbiology and
 Immunology
New York Medical College
Valhalla, New York

Joseph H. Phillips
Department of Research and Development
Becton Dickinson
Mt. View, California

Eckhard R. Podack
Department of Microbiology
 and Immunology
University of Miami
 School of Medicine
Miami, Florida

Anthony A. Rayner
Department of Surgery
University of California
San Francisco, California

Nancy H. Ruddle
Department of Epidemiology
 and Public Health
Yale University Medical School
New Haven, Connecticut

Donald Scott Schmid
Division of Viral Diseases
Centers for Disease Control
Atlanta, Georgia

Uwe D. Staerz
Basel Institute for Immunology
Basel Switzerland

Marianne T. Sweetser
Department of Pathology
Washington University School of
 Medicine
St. Louis, Missouri

Carl-Wilhelm Vogel
Department of Biochemistry and
 Medicine, and Vincent T. Lombardi
 Cancer Center
Georgetown University
Washington, D.C.

Susan C. Wright
Department of Microbiology and
 Immunology
UCLA School of Medicine
Los Angeles, California

John Ding-E. Young
Cell Physiology and Immunology
 Laboratory
Rockefeller University
New York, New York

TABLE OF CONTENTS, VOLUME I

Section I.A: Recognition — Complement

Chapter 1
C1 Structure and Antibody Recognition 3
V. N. Schumaker

Chapter 2
Activation of C1 and the Classical Pathway of Complement 21
R. J. Ziccardi and N. R. Cooper

Chapter 3
Initiation and Activation of the Alternative Pathway of Complement.................... 41
M. K. Pangburn

Chapter 4
Decay Accelerating Factor and the Defect of Paroxysmal Nocturnal
Hemoglobinuria 57
M. Edward Medof

Section I.B: Recognition — Killer Lymphocytes

Chapter 5
T Cell Specificity and the T Cell Receptor α, β, and γ Chains 89
D. H. Raulet

Chapter 6
Structure and Function of a Family of Leukocyte Adhesion Molecules (LEU-CAM)
Involved in T Cell Killing and Complement Mediated Phagocytosis 109
M. A. Arnaout

Chapter 7
The Role of Accessory Molecules in T Cell Recognition.............................. 127
J. L. Greenstein, S. J. Mentzer, and S. J. Burakoff

Chapter 8
Toward Understanding Target Binding and Lysis by Natural Killer Cells 143
G. Dennert

Chapter 9
The Homology between Specific- and Nonspecific-Lectin or Oxidation Dependent
CTL/Target Interactions 155
G. Berke and Z. Keren

Section II.A: Cytolytic Mechanism — Complement

Chapter 10
Assembly and Structure of the Membrane Attack (MAC) of Complement 173
E. R. Podack

Chapter 11
Structure and Function of C9 and Poly C9 185
J. Tschopp and E. R. Podack

Chapter 12
Pore Size of Lesions Induced by Complement on Red Cell Membranes and Its
Relation to C5b-8, C5b-9, and Poly C9 207
A. P. Dalmasso and B. A. Benson

Chapter 13
Pore Size and Functional Properties of Defined MAC and Poly C9 Complexes:
Reconstitution into Model Lipid Membranes 221
J. Ding-E Young, Z. A. Cohn, and E. R. Podack

Chapter 14
Mechanisms of the Cellular Defense Response of Nucleated Cells to Membrane
Attack by Complement 229
M. L. Shin and D. F. Carney

Index 253

TABLE OF CONTENTS, VOLUME II

Section II.B: Cytolytic Mechanism — Killer Lymphocytes

Chapter 15
Properties and Function of Cytolytic Lymphocyte Granules 3
E. R. Podack

Chapter 16
Properties of Transmembrane Channels Induced by Cytolytic Lymphocytes............. 19
J. Ding-E. Young, E. R. Podack, C. Nathan, H. Hengartner, and Z. A. Cohn

Chapter 17
The Role of Nuclear Damage in Lysis of Target Cells by Cytotoxic T
Lymphocytes 35
R. C. Duke and J. J. Cohen

Section II.C: Soluble Cytotoxic Factors Produced by Lymphocytes

Chapter 18
Production and Function of Lymphotoxin Secreted by Cytolytic T Cells 61
D. S. Schmid and N. H. Ruddle

Chapter 19
Tumor Necrosis Factor/Cachectin 75
F. C. Kull, Jr.

Chapter 20
Natural Killer Cytotoxic Factor (NKCF) as Mediator in the Lytic Pathway of NK
Cell Mediated Cytoxicity..91
B. Bonavida and S. C. Wright

Chapter 21
Tumor Necrosis Factors 105
R. A. Aiyer and B. B. Aggarwal

Section III. Therapeutic Applications

Chapter 22
Antibody Conjugates with Cobra Venom Factor as Selective Agents for Tumor Cell
Killing..135
C.-W. Vogel

Chapter 23
A Function for NK Cells in Acute Bone Marrow Allograft Rejection 153
G. Dennert

Chapter 24
Cytolytic T Lymphocyte Clones in Anti-Viral Immunity: Effector Function In Vivo
and Mechanism of Action 161
T. J. Braciale, A. E. Lukacher, M. T. Sweetser, and V. L. Braciale

Chapter 25
Interleukin-2 Activated Cytoxic Lymphocytes (LAK cells) as Antigen Nonspecific
Amplifiers of the Immune Response: General Characteristics and Considerations for
Cancer Therapy 175
E. A. Grimm

Chapter 26
The Contribution of Natural Killer and T-Cells to the Lymphokine Activated Killer
Cell Phenomenon..193
J. H. Phillips, B. T. Gemlo, W. W. Myers, A. A. Rayner, and L. L. Lanier

Chapter 27
Targeting for T-Lymphocyte-Mediated Lysis by Hybrid Antibodies.....................205
U. D. Staerz, L. Lefrancois, and M. J. Bevan

Chapter 28
Longterm Growth and Expansion of Il2 Activated NK-Cells for Cancer
Therapy 219
E. R. Podack, K. O. Penichet, B. Y. Lin, J. W. Chiao, and A. Mittelman

Index 227

Section II.B: Cytolytic Mechanism — Killer Lymphocytes

Chapter 15

PROPERTIES AND FUNCTION OF CYTOLYTIC LYMPHOCYTE GRANULES

Eckhard R. Podack

I.	Introduction	4
II.	The Role of Granules in Cell-Mediated Cytolysis	4
III.	Composition of Cytolytic Granules	4
	A. Perforin 1	6
	B. Homology of Perforin 1 and Complement Component C9	8
	C. Perforin 2	9
	D. Granule-Associated Esterases	10
	E. Granule-Associated Factors Mediating P1 Independent L-Cell Killing	11
	F. Granule-Associated Factors Responsible for DNA Degradation in Target Cells	12
	G. Granule-Associated Proteoglycans	12
	H. Chemotactic, Granule-Associated Factors	13
IV.	Summary and Perspectives	14
References		16

I. INTRODUCTION

The last few years have witnessed rapid advances in our understanding of the molecular events in lymphocyte mediated cytotoxicity. This rapid development was triggered mainly by two findings. First, the demonstration by Dourmashkin and collaborators[1] of membrane lesions formed by lympocytes attacking target cells that are detectable by electron microscopy suggested complement-like killing mechanisms. Second, the purification of isolated granules from cytolytic T-cells and NK-cells and the demonstration of their potent Ca-dependent cytolytic and pore forming activity[2,3] allowed the purification of granule-associated factors believed to be the effector molecules in lympocyte-mediated cytolysis.

Even though the author believes that cytolytic granules are an essential compartment for the delivery of the lethal hit of cytolytic lymphocytes, it is emphasized that the issue as to whether granules constitute the major killing mechanism or play only a minor part in cell-mediated cytolysis remains to be resolved. With the recent introduction of cytolytic lymphocytes as immunotherapeutic agents for the treatment of cancer[4,5] in combination with Interleukin 2, the question of the molecular mechanism of tumor cell lysis by lymphocytes becomes ever more urgent.

II. THE ROLE OF GRANULES IN CELL-MEDIATED CYTOLYSIS

Cloned lymphocytes of T- or NK-origin, as well as lymphokine-activated killer cells, are large granular lymphocytes (e.g., see Reference 6). The cytoplasmic granules can be isolated by conventional cell fractionation procedures in relatively homogenous forms. Isolated granules when incubated with nucleated target cells or with erythrocytes mediate potent, Ca- and temperature-dependent cytolysis. Granule-mediated lysis in the presence of Ca at 37° is extremely rapid and virtually complete within 2 min.[2] The lysis is unspecific with regard to the target cell membrane. Virtually all target cells tested are susceptible to lysis by isolated granules independent of their MHC-type and species of origin.[7,8] In addition, granules isolated from various cloned and unclonal CTL or NK-cells show identical protein composition, functional activity, and immunological cross-reactivity. Thus the granules, in contrast to the cells from which they are derived, show no clonal specificity (Figure 1). This finding indicates that the killer cell specificity is a function of plasma membrane receptors of the killer cell, whereas the killing step *per se* is unspecific and triggered through the specific membrane receptor interaction of the cell from which they are derived.

Based on these findings, both Henkart's laboratory[8] and our group[9] proposed that cytolysis by lymphocytes is a secretory phenomenon (Figure 2). Upon killer target cell interaction, the killer cell is rapidly polarized in a Ca-dependent reaction to reorient its secretory apparatus (microtubule organizing center and Golgi complex)[10,11] as well as its cytolytic granules[9] towards the contact area. Subsequently, the contents of cytolytic granules are released into the contact area, where the granule components initiate the cytolytic attack on target membrane, as described below. The reorientation and release of granules can be directly observed by phase contrast microscopy, as shown in Figure 3, or fluorescence microscopy.[9] This model of cell-mediated tumor lysis is consistent with a large body of earlier studies implicating secretory phenomena in lymphocyte-mediated cytolysis (for review see Reference 8).

III. COMPOSITION OF CYTOLYTIC GRANULES

Isolated cytolytic granules have relatively complex protein banding patterns on SDS-gels, including six major bands and several minor components ranging in mol wt from 75 kDalton to about 10 to 14 kDalton.[2,3] This complexity suggests that granules are endowed with various factors that may participate in cytolysis. We are just now beginning to understand the

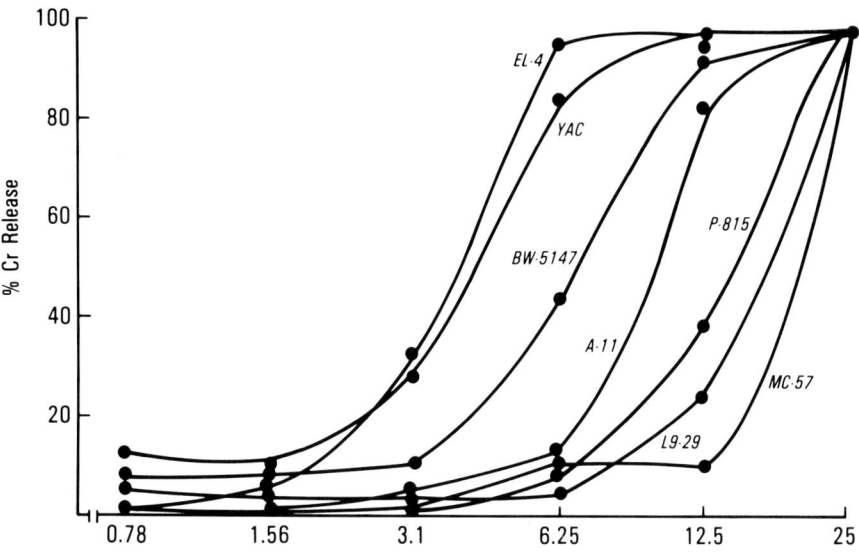

FIGURE 1. Activity of cytolytic granules isolated from cloned cytolytic lymphocytes. All targets tested are susceptible to granule mediated cytolysis in the presence of Ca. Granules, isolated by Percoll density gradient centrifugation, were used.

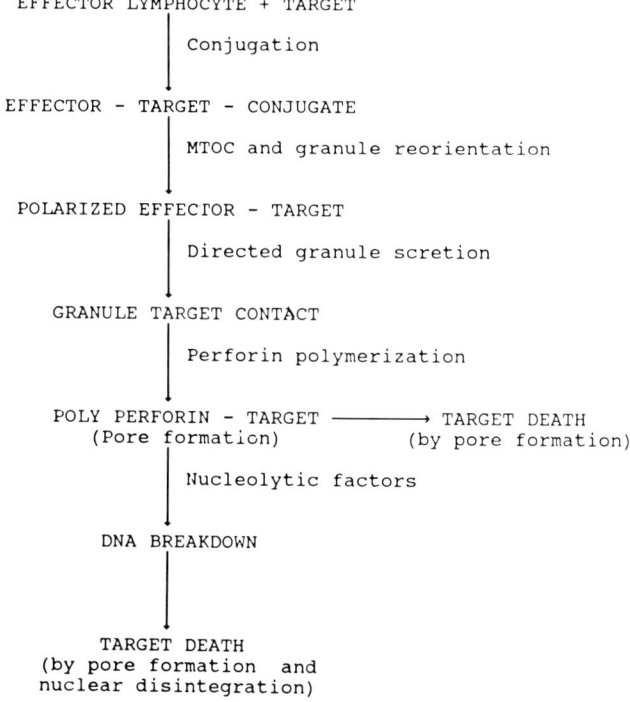

FIGURE 2. Schematic representation of steps in lymphocyte mediated cytolysis.

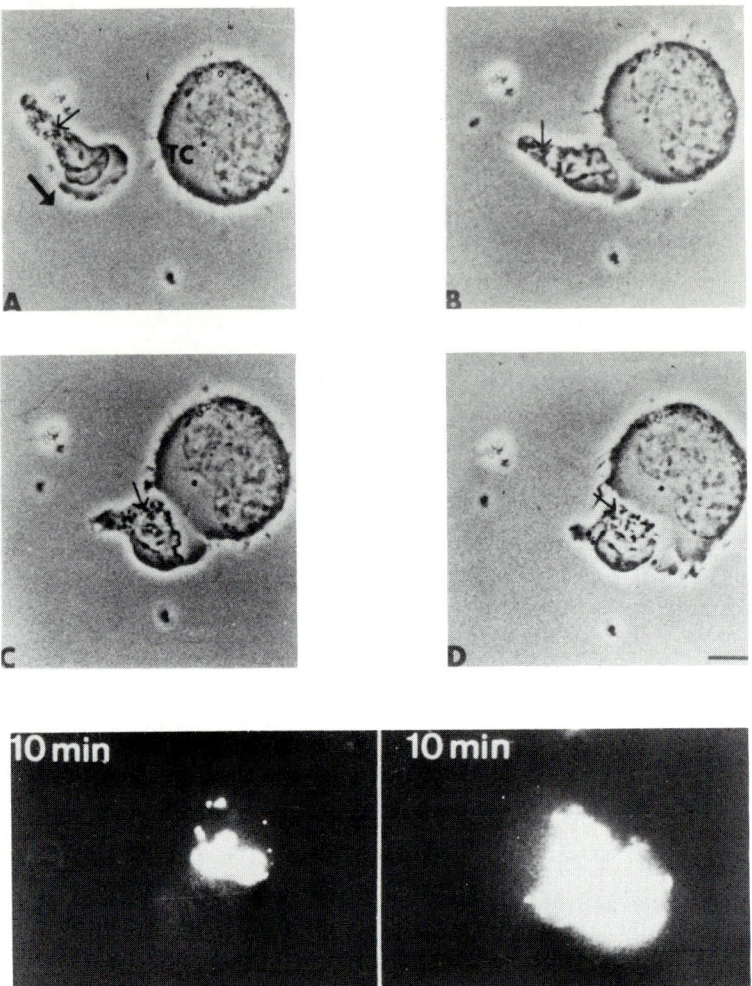

FIGURE 3. Phase contrast micrographs taken from 16 mm film of a thin preparation of CTL-target cell (TC) interaction. A CTL is shown interacting with a target cell that it can kill. The small arrows indicate CTL granule position at various times. Before contact, Panel A, the large arrow indicates the direction of CTL movement. In Panel B, the CTL has made contact with the target cell. Panel C shows 2 min after initial contact. The CTL has begun to round up and initiate granule reorientation. Panel D shows 10 min after initial contact. The CTL granules occupy a position in the zone of CTL-target cell contact. Bar = 10 μm. (Panels A to D From Yanelli, J. R. et al., *J. Immunol.*, 136, 377, 1986.) Lower panels: Demonstration of granule release by CTL by fluorescence microscopy using granule specific antibodies. Killer-target conjugates after 10 min incubation were fixed on slides and stained with antibody and fluoresceinated second antibody. Left panel: target at 7 O'clock. Right panel: target at 10 O'clock. The bright staining granules are in the contact area and seem to be secreted.

properties of some of the granule components and their putative functions. The list of granule factors enumerated below is not complete because not all granule components have been isolated in homogenous form. Is is therefore probable that additional granule-associated cytolytic factors will be described and isolated that may contribute to cytolysis.

A. Perforin 1 (P1)

Perforin 1 (P1 or cytolysin) is the pore-forming protein of cytolytic granules. P1 migrates as a 70 to 75 kDalton protein upon SDS-polyacrylamide gel electrophoresis under reducing conditions. Unreduced, its apparent mol wt is about 60 kDalton.[13,14] Isolated P1 mediates

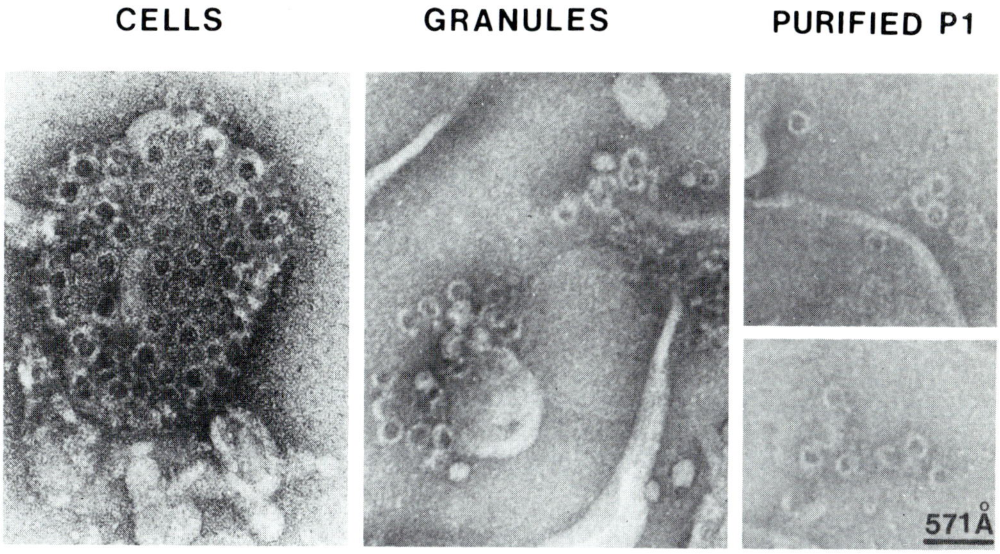

CELLS   **GRANULES**   **PURIFIED P1**

FIGURE 4. Poly P1 lesions assembled by intact killer lymphocytes, by isolated granules and by purified P1 on target membranes.

Ca-dependent lysis of erythrocytes and nucleated target cells. P1 thus is the protein responsible for the Ca-dependent cytolytic activity of isolated granules. Cytolysis by isolated perforin is accompanied by the formation of membrane lesions on target cells that are identical in size[2,13,14,15,16] to those formed by intact cells or by granules (Figure 4). Upon incubation with Ca, isolated P1 polymerizes to tubular complexes (poly P1) of 160 Å length and 160 Å internal diameter (Figure 4). This reaction is analogous to the polymerization of complement component C9 (see Volume I, chapter 11). In the presence of target membranes P1 inserts, polymerization proceeds within the membranes and results in the formation of large, stable transmembrane channels.[17] If polymerization of P1 is induced by Ca in the absence of membranes, the cytolytic activity is lost. Apparently, already polymerized P1 cannot insert into membranes. For activity of P1 to be expressed the polymerization reaction has to proceed in the target membrane.

The channel-forming activity of P1 is independent of membrane proteins and has been demonstrated in artificial bilayer membranes.[17,18] Similar to complement component C9 (see Volume I, Chapter 11) P1 upon polymerization in the presence of Ca apparently undergoes a restricted unfolding, exposing hydrophobic domains, previously internal within the molecule, enabling it to insert and polymerize in target membranes (Figure 5). Lysis by poly P1, in analogy to complement lysis, then may proceed by colloid osmotic imbalance of the target cell and by disassembly of bilayer membranes.

It is important to emphasize that even smaller oligomers of poly P1 that have no ring structure in the electron miscroscope (center panel in Figures 4 and 5) are cytolytically active. In analogy to non-circularly polymerized C9 (see Volume I, Chapter 11), this effect may be due to the formation of a membrane pore that is only partly walled by protein. The hydrophilic, luminal face of inserted P1-oligomers, in all probability, repels the hydrophobic lipid chains of the bilayer, possibly creating micellar domains. In this situation, the transmembrane pore caused by oligo P1 is composed, in part, of reoriented lipid that may be described as a *leaky patch*. The pores created by oligo-P1 and circular poly P1 are believed to be responsible for the heterogeneity of the pore size created by polymerizing P1 in the membrane.[17]

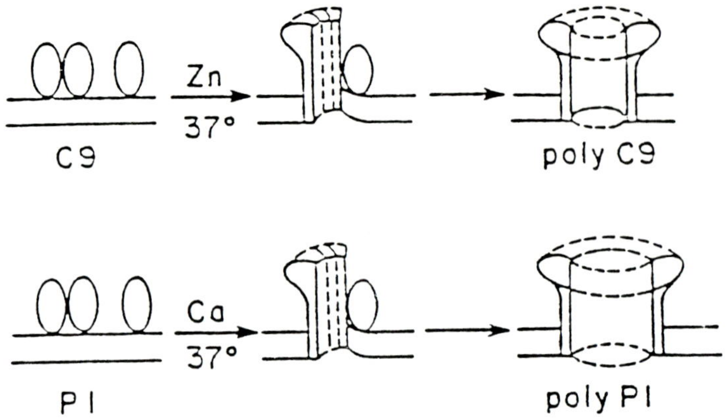

FIGURE 5. Analogy of restricted unfolding, tubular polymerization, and transmembrane channel formation of C9 of complement and perforin 1 (P1) of cytolytic T-cells and NK-cells.

Circularly polymerized P1, in contrast to oligo P1, is resistant to dissociation by boiling in SDS and migrates as a complex exceeding 10^6 kDalton. (Figure 6). It is estimated that approximately 20 perforin monomers comprise a poly P1 tubule. The property of SDS resistance of poly P1 is analogous to poly C9, which requires 6 M guanidine thiocyante for dissociation into C9 monomers[19] (Volume I, Chapter 11). Similarly, poly P1, like poly C9, is resistant to degradation by proteases.[1,15,16,19] This resistance of poly P1 to degradation by proteases and dissociation by detergents is believed to be an important property of cytolytic complexes in order to resist defense mechanisms by target cells.

B. Homology of Perforin 1 and Complement Component C9

The above-described properties of P1 already showed many functional and structural similarities of P1 of cytolytic lymphocytes with C9 of complement. Independently, Tschopp et al.[20] and our laboratory[21] discovered antigenic cross-reactivity of these two proteins, which was subsequently confirmed by Zalman.[22] The antigenic sites shared by murine P1 and human C9 are exposed only after disulfide bond reduction. C9 and P1 thus may contain cystein-rich domains similar to those found in the N-terminal and C-terminal part of C9.[23,24] These cystein-rich domains are also present in the LDL-receptor.[25] The antiserum recognizing both reduced C9 and reduced P1 in fact also recognizes the reduced LDL-receptor.[26] Figure 7 shows the sequence comparison of the C-terminal portion of human C9 with that of murine P1 (Lowrey et al., unpublished). The homology is approximately 26% and includes the C-terminal cysteine-rich domains of C9 homologous to the EGF-precursor.

One important difference between P1 and C9, however, must be emphasized. Whereas C9 under physiological conditions is not cytolytic in the absence of the C5b-8 complex even when it polymerizes in the presence of Zn, perforin 1 has potent activity without additional proteins. The only cofactor required is Ca. Thus P1 is distinguished form C9 by its ability to insert *and* polymerize in target membranes without the aid of a receptor complex like C5b-8. The inhibition of P1 activity by phospholipids has led Henkart's laboratory to propose that P1 may recognize the phospholipid head groups of lipid bilayer membranes followed by insertion and Ca-induced polymerization.[27]

The above-summarized results on the properties of perforin 1 indicate that this protein is the major pore-forming protein of cytolytic lymphocytes. It is highly probable, although conclusive evidence is not yet at hand, that granule-associated perforin 1, upon oligomerization or formation of circular polymers, plays a major functional role in lymphocyte-mediated cytolysis.

FIGURE 6. Resistance of poly P1 to dissociation by SDS. P1 was polymerized in Ca and analyzed on 2 to 10% polyacrylamide gradient gels. The upper band migrates with an apparent molecular weight of approximately 1.5×10^6.

C. Perforin 2

Electron miscroscopical analysis of membranes lysed by isolated granules or by intact killer cells showed the presence of a second pore-forming complex named poly P2.[15,16] The complex had an inner diameter of 50 to 70 Å and was morphologically distinct from poly P1. Masson and Tschoppp,[14] using isolated P1, showed that upon polymerization, complexes with the morphology of both poly P1 and poly P2 were assembled. It is possible therefore that polymerizing P1 can give rise two types of complexes. It is, on the other hand, also possible that poly P2 is assembled from a distinct component or from an altered P1 molecule, such as a proteolytic cleavage product of P1. Which of these alternatives is correct has to await further investigation. It is clear, however, that the Ca-dependent cytolytic activity of

(412) R K Y A F E L K E K L L R G T V I D V T D F V N N - A S S I N D A P V L I S
.... L ..... L L ... G .... F .... N .. A S - .... P .. L ...

..... Q K L S P I Y N L V P V K M K N A H L K K Q N L E R - A I E D Y I N E F S V
.... L .. P ..... L .... - - N . - - K ..... L .. R .. A I .... Y I ....

..... R K - C H T - C Q N G G V T I L M D G K C L C A C P F - K F E G I A C E I S
.... C ..... C .... G .... D ... - C .. C .. C ...... K .... C .... -

..... K Q K I S E G L P A L E T P N E K STOP
.... Q ....

FIGURE 7. Sequence homology of human C9 and murine P1. An Eco R1 fragment of a cDNA clone obtained from a CTL-expression library was sequenced. One open reading frame showed the homology to C9 as depicted.

granules resides in P1, because the activity coisolates with this protein during the purification procedure.

D. Granule-Associated Esterases

Pasternack and Eisen[28] found that cytolytic lymphocyte clones contain esterolytic activity cleaving the synthetic sybstrate N$^\alpha$-benzyloxycarbonyl-1-lysine-thiobenzylester (BLT). This activity is blocked by serine esterase inhibitors. The mol wt of the esterase was determined to be 28,000 by affinity labeling with radiolabeled diisoproplyfluorophosphoridate (DFP).

More recently, cDNA clones specific for cytolytic lymphocytes were obtained and the protein sequence derived from the nucleotide sequence.[29,30] The protein sequence predicts a protease that may be related to the rat mast cell protease type III. The predicted mol wt of this protease is 25,700, close to the mol wt mentioned above.[28] A second related T-cell specific protease whose full sequence is not yet fully established was described by Lobe et al.[30]

Even though the complete identification has not yet been achieved, it appears highly probable that the esterases described above are located in cytolytic T- or NK-cell granules. Isolated granules contain esterolytic activity cleaving BLT (Figure 8), and granule peptides can be labeled with radiolabeled DFP. The granule esterases have the following properties:

Esterase 1 — Esterase 1 (granzyme 1) is a 60 kDalton protein that, upon reduction and SDS-polyacrylamide gel electrophoresis, contains 2 subunits with apparent mol wt of about 30 kDalton. Esterase 1 cleaves the synthetic substrate BLT. Esterase levels strongly increase during induction of cytolytic T-Cells in mixed lymphocyte reactions or after concanvalin A stimulation, suggesting a role in the cytolytic reaction. The enzyme is inhibited by the esterase inhibitions PMSF and DFP. The natural substrate is not known.

Esterase 2 — Esterase 2 (granzyme 2) is a 28 to 30 kDalton esterase based on its incoproration of radiolabeled DFP. The 28 to 30 kDalton esterase 2 has no esterolytic activity on any of the protein or synthetic substrates tested.

The function of these two granule-associated esterases in the cytolytic sequence is not known. PMSF and DFP treatment of granules does not block their cytolytic activity.

Thus, the role of esterases in cytolysis is speculative at the present time. Several possible mechanisms for their action are discussed below.

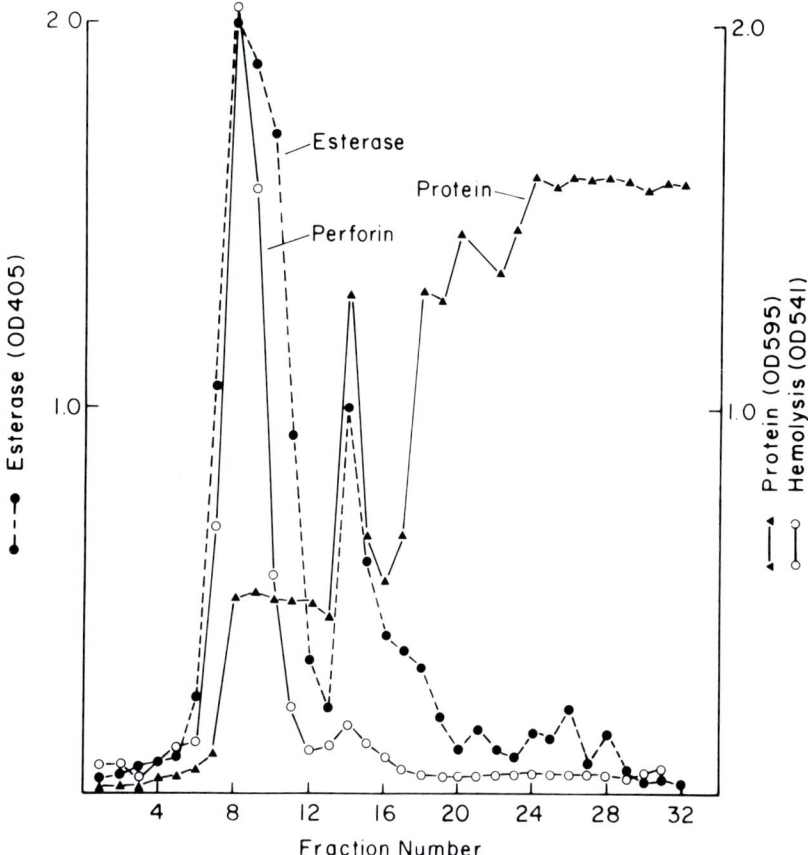

FIGURE 8. Codistribution of granule esterase and granule perforin in Percoll gradients. Sedimentation is to the left.

1. The esterases may activate granule-associated proteins from inactive precursors upon granule secretion, possibly mediated by Ca.
2. The esterases may be important for the digestion of target-membrane-associated proteins to facilitate target-membrane perforation by polymerizing P1.
3. The esterases may gain entry into the target cell, mediated directly or indirectly by poly P1 pores and effect internal target destruction.
4. The esterases may facilitate killer cell recycling by cleaving adhesion proteins required for the initial killer-target-cell conjugation.
5. The esterases may digest matrix proteins to facilitate killer cell spreading.

Which of these functions is mediated by esterase 1 or 2 or other esterases remains to be established.

E. Granule-Associated Factors Mediating P1 Independent L-cell Killing

L-cells (a mouse fibroblast line) are the classical target for lymphotoxin and tumor necrosis factor. (The structure and function of lymphotoxin (LT) and tumor necrosis factor (TNF) are described in Chapters 18, 19, and 21). As biological assay for these cytolytic cytokines, the lysis of L-cells is generally used in a 24- to 48-hr assay.

Isolated granules contain a factor or factors that lyse L-cells. This activity is independent of P1 according to the following evidence.[31] P1 can be inactivated by polymerization upon preincubation of granules in the presence of Ca. Granules treated in this way are hemolytically inactive, yet they kill L-cells in a dose-dependent reaction within 24 to 48 hr. In contrast to the P1-dependent rapid killing (2 min 37°) of L-cells[7] the P1-independent killing is slow and requires 24 to 48 hr. This slow killing of L-cells is similar to the kinetics observed with LT or TNF. In contrast to LT and TNF, the granule factor(s) also lyse TNF and LT resistant L-cells. This observation could suggest that the granule factors resposible for L-cell lysis are distinct from LT and TNF. Alternatively, other granule factors could induce uptake of granule components by endocytosis, thus providing an entry mechanism for these molecules (see Figure 10).

Antibody inhibition studies using anti LT and anti TNF resulted in only 20 to 40% neutralization of P1-independent granule-associated L-cell killing activity.[31] Since the molecular nature of the granule factors responsible for L-cell killing has not yet been established, it is not possible to decide whether they are identical to TNF or LT, related to these proteins, or completely independent entities.

F. Granule-Associated Factors Responsible for DNA Degradation in Target Cells

Evidence that cytolytic granules mediate DNA degradation in target cells is still preliminary at the present time (for a detailed discussion of DNA degradation refer to Chapter 17). The difficulty with this system is that granules due to the presence of P1, very rapidly lyse target cells (within 2 min at 37°). This rapid lysis of plasma membrane and the consequent leakage of cellular components may prevent the triggering of the target-associated pathway, leading to DNA-breakdown.[32,33,34] If, on the other hand, P1 is inactivated, the killing process by P1-independent granule factors is very slow (24 to 48 hr), which makes the analysis of specific DNA release more difficult.

Incubation of ^{125}I UdR labeled E14 target cells with P1-inactivated granules results in the slow release of labeled DNA, reaching a maximum after 18 hr incubation. Analysis of the released DNA upon phenol extraction and ethanol precipitation by agarose gel electrophoresis shows that the DNA is released as fragments of 200 base pairs and multiples thereof. In control cells exposed to heat-inactivated granules, DNA is not released and remains intact.[31]

These experiments provide evidence that granules contain factors responsible for DNA degradation and nuclear breakdown of target cells killed by CTL, as first described by Russel et al.[32] and reviewed in Chapter 17.

The molecular nature of this putative factor and its relation to the lymphotoxin-like killing activity described in the previous paragraph is under investigation. It should be noted at this point that authentic lymphotoxin has been proposed to mediate its cytolytic activity, at least in part, via triggering the DNA-degrading pathway in target cells[35] (and see Chapter 18). Similarly, TNF may function through this mechanism (N. H. Ruddle, personal communication). It is tempting, therefore, to speculate that the granule-associated L-cell killing activity also mediates DNA-degradation.

G. Granule-Associated Proteoglycans

Secretory granules in many cells have been shown to contain proteoglycans.[36] The function of proteoglycans is believed to allow the condensation and packaging of various granule-associated proteins in the granule compartment at high concentrations. In the case of NK-cells, chondroitinsulfate A was shown to be the major granule-associated proteoglycan.[37] Chondroitinsulfate A is a 200 kDalton proteoglycan with a protein core and many highly sulfated carbohydrate side chains. It is not stained by Comassie blue and therefore not detectable on SDS-polyacrylamide gels of granules stained in this way. As shown by Schmidt et al.[37] NK-cells, concurrent with mediating cytolytic activity, release S^{35}-labeled chondroitinsulfate. This observation is the first direct evidence of the secretion of granule-associated components during lymphocyte-mediated target cell lysis. There is considerable circumstantial evidence that P1 and possibly other components may be associated with

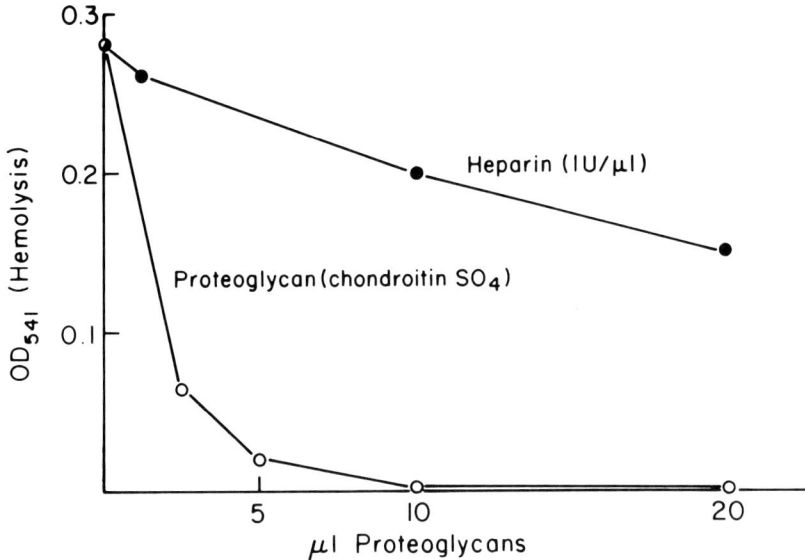

FIGURE 9. Inhibition of P1 by proteoglycan. The high molecular weight proteoglycan of granules in comparison to heparin.

proteoglycans, presumably through polar interaction with the negatively charged sulfate groups as outlined below:

1. Perforin 1 binds to Heparin-Sepharose. Although Heparin is a different proteoglycan than chondroitinsulfate, it shares with it the highly sulfated carbohydrate side chains.
2. Chondroitinsulfate inhibits P1 activity (Figure 9), presumably by association with P1 and inhibition of its polymerization. Proteoglycans thus may bind P1 within granules and keep it unpolymerized until released. They may also protect the killer cell from attack by their own cytolytic proteins (Figure 10).
3. Granule-associated P1 can be most easily solubilized by high concentration phosphate buffers. PO_4-ions are highly negatively charged and may compete with the sulfate side chains of proteoglycans for P1 binding.

What is the role of proteoglycans in cell mediated cytolysis? It may be two-fold. In the intact granule, proteoglycans probably serve to package and stabilize the granule-associated proteins at high local concentrations. Upon release of the granule upon killer-target conjugate formation, the proteoglycan may protect the killer cells from its own cytolytic factors. The granule membrane may be coated with a lining of proteoglycan. The highly negatively charged sulfate groups inhibit the cytolytic action of perforin should it attempt to attack the granule membrane itself and thus neutralize its activity. The proteoglycans may thus indirectly confer directionality to the killing process towards the target cell. How perforin and possibly other granule associated proteins are released from granule proteoglycans or whether they are secreted together with non-granule-membrane-bound proteoglycans as a "multi-warhead missile" remains to be established.

H. Chemotactic, Granule-Associated Factors

Greenberg et al.[38] have described chemotactic factors secreted by large granular lymphocytes that attract monocytes, macrophages, and granulocytes and stimulate intracellular bactericidal action. Recently, these authors have found this factor to be located in granules

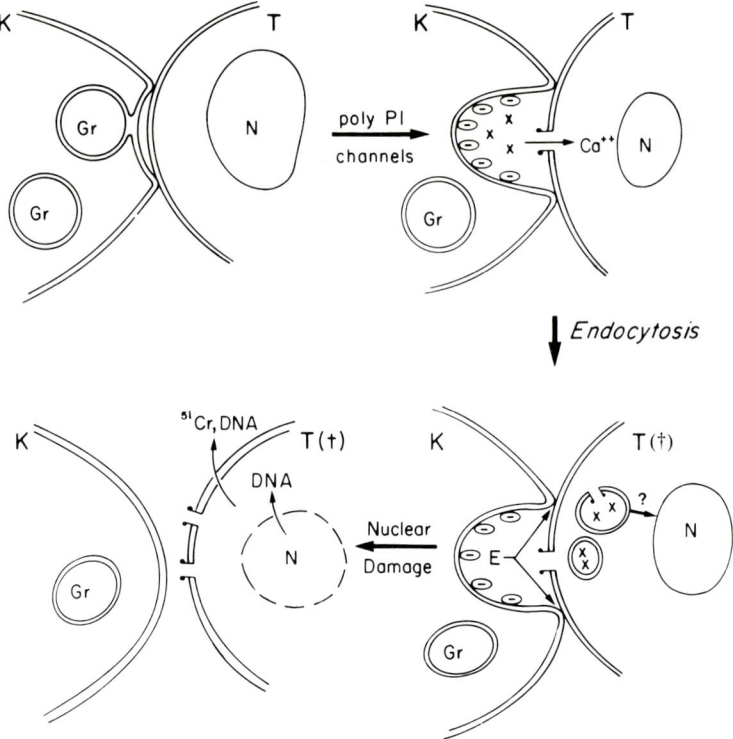

FIGURE 10. Hypothetical scheme for the function of granule components in target lysis. K, killer cell; T, Target cell: G, granule; N, nucleus; −, proteoglycan; E, esterase; X, granule components; †, dead target. In this scheme, granule components (⊖) protect the killer cell (proteoglycan), cause channel formation (P1), are endocytosed (X) and mediate DNA degradation, and facilitate detaching and recycling of killer cell (E).

of the rat NK-like lymphoma isolated by Reynolds et al.[39] The molecular nature of this chemotatic factor has not as yet been identified.

IV. SUMMARY AND PERSPECTIVES

As summarized above, cytolytic granules contain numerous proteins whose known properties are consistent with an important function of granules in cell-mediated cytolysis. These proteins comprise:

1. Poreforming proteins
2. Esterases and proteases
3. Lymphototoxin-like factors
4. Proteoglycans
5. Chemotatic factors

In Table I the properties of known granule associated proteins are summarized.

It is likely that this list of granule-associated proteins will continue to grow as additional granule proteins are identified and purified. Viewing the heterogenous properties of these proteins with regard to structure and function, it is possible to postulate a specific function for each of these factors in the cytolytic sequence following conjugate formation and triggering of granule secretion (Figure 10).

Table 1
COMPOSITION OF CYTOLYTIC GRANULES

Component	Mol Wt (kDalton)	Chain structure	Putative function	Remarks
Perforin 1	70—75	Single chain	Transmembrane channel	C9-like
Chondroitin-SO$_4$	~200	Peptide core, multiple CHO-side chains	Packaging, protection of K-cell?	Released during attack
Esterase 1	60	Two, 30 kDalton, S-S linked	?	Substrate: BLT, binds DFP
Esterase 2	28	Single chain	?	No known substrate, bind DFP
Nucleolytic factor	?	?	DNA-damage	Can act independently of P1
Monocyte-macrophage chemotactic factor	?	?	Attraction of phagocytic cells	—

According to the scheme in Figure 10, the sequence of events may proceed as follows: After conjugate formation, the granule membrane fuses with the plasma membrane. Granule contents are released into the interstitial space. If, as appears likely, the contact zone of the killer-target membrane adjacent to the granule is sealed, the granule-associated proteins come into contact only with the granule membrane and with an area of the target membrane. This reaction may, of course, occur at several sites over the entire killer-target contact area. Ca enters into the fused granule space (by an unknown mechanism) and activates P1 and possibly other granule-associated proteins. Transmembrane pores on the target cell are generated by polymerization of P1 and formation of complete poly P1 tubules or incomplete P1-oligomers. The *killer* cell membrane at the contact site is formed by the granule membrane in this area and may be protected from P1 attack by its negative charge, conferred to it by granule membrane associated proteoglycans. Granule factors such as esterases and/or lymphotoxin-like factors (x,x in Figure 10) may enter the target cell through the pore shown in the upper right panel or, perhaps more likely, through endocytotic mechanisms (lower right panel). The internalized factors then may trigger the target cell specific pathway for nuclear disintegration and DNA degradation and initiate the killer cell independent target cell lysis. The killer cell then detaches from the target, presumably by proteolytic cleavage of the adhesion receptors by one of the granule enzymes (E in Figure 7) and recycles, killing additional target cells.

In this scheme poly P1 or oligo P1 may have two functions: first it may cause target death directly by perforation of the membrane. Second, poly P1 or oligo P1 may cause the delivery of toxic granule-associated molecules into the target cell by an indirect mechanism. The pore of poly P1 or oligo P1 allows the entry into the target cell of Ca ions. Ca ions are a strong stimulus for endocytosis (see Volume I, Chapter 14). Endocytosis in this particular situation would concomitantly internalize granule-associated factors previously secreted into the interstitial space. The endocytotic vesicles thus formed contain granule-associated proteins (and possibly poly perforins). They are probably analogues to vesicles formed by receptor-mediated endocytosis and will be processed by the cell in the usual way. Thus, the endocytosed granule-associated factors could mediate the same activity as soluble toxic factors internalized through receptor-mediated entry (e.g., TNF or LT), even on cells not containing receptors for these molecules.

Evidence for secretory events and the importance of P1 in CTL-mediated cytolysis is already at hand in the experiment described in Chapter 27 by Staerz, Lefrancois, and Bevan. These authors were able to show that CTL will lyse erythrocytes when a heteroconjugate of antibodies to the red cell membrane and the T-cell receptor provides for contact and triggering of the T-cell. The fact that the target red cell is lysed in this situation provides direct evidence for the involvement of secreted granules and secreted Perforin 1, since these are the only T-cell components that are known to be able to lyse erythrocytes.

REFERENCES

1. **Dourmashkin, R. R., Deteix, P., Simone, C. B., and Henkart, P. A.**, Electron microscipic demonstration of lesions on target cell membranes associated with antibody dependent cytotoxicity, *Clin. Immunol.*, 43, 554, 1980.
2. **Podack, E. R. and Konigsberg, P. J.**, Cytolytic T-cell Granules: Isolation Structural, Biochemical and Functional Characterization, *J. Exp. Med.*, 160, 695, 1984.
3. **Millard, P. J., Henkart, M. P., Reynolds, C. W., and Henkart, P. A.**, Purification and properties of cytoplasmic granules from cytotoxic rat LGL-tumors, *J. Immunol.*, 132, 3197, 1984.
4. **Rosenberg, S. A., Lotze, M. T., Muul, L. M., Leitman, S., Chang, A. E., Ettinghausen, S. E., Matory, Y. L., Skibber, J. M., Shilom, E., Vetto, J. T., Seipp, C. A., Simpson, C., and Reichert, C. M.**, Observations on the systemic administration of autologous lymphokine-activated killer cells and recombinant interleukin 2 to patients with metastatic cancer, *N. Engl. J. Med.*, 313, 1485, 1985.
5. **Podack, E. R. and Mittelman, A.**, Geration of interleukin 2 activated killer cells for tumor therapy in patients with metastatic cancer, unpublished observations.
6. **Acha-Orbea, H., Groscurth, P., Lang, R., Stitz, L., and Hengartner, H**, Characterization of cloned cytotoxic lymphocytes with NK activity, *J. Immunol.*, 130, 1952, 1983.
7. **Podack, E. R., Konigsberg, P. J., Acha-Orbea, H., Pircher, H., and Hengartner, H**, Cytolytic T-cell granules biochemical properties and functional specificity, in *Mechanisms of Cell Mediated Cytotoxicity*, Vol. II, Henkart, P. A. and Mark, E., Eds., Plenum Publishing, New York, 1985, 99.
8. **Henkart, P. A.** Mechanism of lymphocyte mediated cytotoxicity, *Ann. Rev. Immunol.*, 3, 31, 1985.
9. **Podack, E. R.**, The molecular mechanism of lymphocyte mediated tumor cell lysis, *Immunol. Today*, 6, 21, 1985.
10. **Geiger, B., Rosen, D., and Berke, G.**, Spatial Relationships of microtubular organizing center and the contact area of cytotoxic T-lymphocytes and target cells, *J. Cell Biol.*, 95, 137, 1982.
11. **Kupfer, A. A., Dennert, G., and Singer, S. J.**, Polarization of the microtubule-organizing center within cloned natural killer cells bound to their targets, *Proc. Natl. Acad. Sci. USA*, 80, 7224, 1983.
12. **Yanelli, J. R., Sullivan, J. A., Mandell, G. L., and Engellhard, V. H.**, Reorientation and fusion of cytotoxic lymphocyte granules after interaction with target cells as determined by high resolution cinemicrography, *J. Immunol.*, 136, 377, 1986.
13. **Podack, E. R., Young, J. D. E., and Cohn, E. A.**, Isolation and biochemical and functional characterization of perforin 1 from cytolytic T-cell granules, *Proc. Natl. Acad. Sci. USA*, 82, 8629, 1985.
14. **Masson, D. and Tschopp, J.**, Isolation of a lytic, pore forming protein (perforin) from cytolytic T-lymphocytes, *J. Biol. Chem.*, 260, 9069, 1985.
15. **Podack, E. R. and Dennert, G.**, Assembly of two types of tubules with putative cytolytic function by cloned natural killer cells, *Nature (London)*, 302, 5907, 1983.
16. **Dennert, G. and Podack, E. R.**, Cytolysis by H-2-specific T-killer cells, Assembly of tubular complexes on target membranes, *J. Exp. Med.*, 157, 1483, 1983.
17. **Young, J. D. E., Nathan, C. F., Podack, E. R., Palladino, M. A., and Cohn, Z. A.**, Functional channel formation associated with cytotoxic T-cell granules, *Proc. Natl. Acad. Sci. USA*, 83, 150, 1986.
18. **Blumenthal, R., Millard, P. J., Henkart, M. P., Reynolds, C. W., and Henkart, P. A.**, Liposomes as targets for granule cytolysin from cytotoxic large granular lymphocyte tumors, *Proc. Natl. Acad. Sci. USA*, 81, 5551, 1984.
19. **Podack, E. R. and Tschopp, J.**, Circular polymerization of the ninth component of complement. Ring closure of the tubular complex confers resistance to detergent dissociation and to proteolytic degradation, *J. Biol. Chem.*, 257, 15204, 1982.
20. **Tschopp, J. and Mollnes, T. E.**, Antigenic homology of C8 and C9, *Complement*, 2, 230, 1985.
21. **Podack, E. R., Young, J. D. E., Weeks-Levy, C., Lowrey, D., and Cohn, Z. A.**, Isolation and characterization of perforin 1, a cytolytic T-cell granule protein with homology to C9, *Complement*, 2, 63, 1985.
22. **Zalman, L. S., Brothers, M. A., Chin, F. J., and Muller-Eberhard, H. J.**, Anti C9 reactive proteins in the granules of large granular human lymphocytes, *Complement*, 2, 90, 1985.

23. **DiScipio, R. G., Gehring, M. R., Podack, E. R., Kan, C. C., Hugli, T. E., and Fey, G. J.**, Nucleotide sequence of cDNA and derived amino acid sequence of human complement component C9, *Proc. Natl. Acad. Sci. USA*, 81, 7298, 1984.
24. **Stanley, K. K., Kocher, H. P., Lucio, G. P., Jackson, P., and Tschopp, J.**, The sequence and topology of human complement component C9, *EMBO J.*, 4, 375, 1985.
25. **Yamamoto, T., Davis, C. G., Brown, M. S., Schneider, W. J., Casey, M. L., Goldstein, J. L., and Russet, D. W.**, The human LDL-receptor, a cysteine rich protein with multiple Alu-Sequences in its mRNA, *Cell*, 39, 27, 1984.
26. **Podack, E. R.**, Perforins, A new family of pore forming proteins in immune cytolysis, *Proceedings of the UCLA Symposium on Membrane Medicated Cytotoxicity*, Collier, R. J. and Bonavida, B., Eds., Alan R. Liss, New York, 1987, 329.
27. **Yue, C. C., Kenny, J. J. K., Cerney, J., and Henkart, P. A.**, Evidence for choline recognition by granule cytolysin of cytotoxic lymphocytes: cross-reaction with anti TEPC-15 anti-idiotypic antibodies, *J. Cell. Biochem.*, (Suppl.), 10B, 95, 1986.
28. **Pasternack, M. S. and Eisen, H. N.**, A novel serine esterase expressed by cytotoxic T lymphocytes, *Nature*, 314, 743, 1985.
29. **Gershenfeld, H. K. and Weissman, I. L.**, Cloning of a cDNA for a T-cell-specific serine protease from a cytotoxic T lymphocyte, *Science*, 232, 854, 1986.
30. **Lobe, C. G., Finlay, B. B., Parachych, W., Paetkau, V. H., and Bleackley, R. C.**, Novel serine proteases encoded by two cytotoxic T lymphocyte-specific genes, *Science*, 323, 858, 1986.
31. **Konigsberg, P. J. and Podack, E. R.**, DNA damage of target cells by cytolytic T-cell granules, *J. Cell. Biochem.*, (Suppl.), 10B, 85, 1986.
32. **Russel, J. H., Masakowski, V. B., and Dobos, C. B.**, Mechanism of immune lysis, I Physiological distinction between target cell death mediated by cytotoxic T-Lymphocytes and antibody plus complement, *J. Immunol.*, 124, 1100, 1980.
33. **Duke, R. C., Chervenak, R., and Cohen, J. J.**, Endogenous endo-nuclease-induced DNA fragmentation: an early event in cell mediated cytolysis, *Proc. Natl. Acad. Sci. USA*, 80, 6363, 1983.
34. **Gromkowsky, S. H., Brown, T. C., Cerutti P.A., and Cerottini, J. C.**, DNA of human Raji target cells is damaged upon lymphocyte-mediated lysis, *J. Immunol.*, 136, 752, 1986.
35. **Scott-Schmid, D., Tite, J. P., and Ruddle, N. H.**, DNA fragmentation: manifestation of target cell destruction mediated by cytotoxic T-cell lines, lymphotoxin secreting helper T-cell clones, and cell free lymphotixin-containing supermatants, *Proc. Natl. Acad. Sci. USA*, 83, 1881, 1986.
36. **Ruoslahti, E., Hayman, G. E., and Pierschbader, M. D.**, Extracellular matrices and cell adhesion, *Arteriosclerosis*, 5, 581, 1985.
37. **Schmidt, R. E., MacDermott, R. P., Bartley, G., Bertovich, M., Amato, D. A., Austen, K. F., Schlossman, S. F., Stevens, R. L., and Ritz, J.**, Specific release of proteoglycans from human natural killer cells during target lysis, *Nature*, 318, 289, 1985.
38. **Greenberg, A. H., Khalil, N., Pohajdak, B., Talgory, M., Henkart, P., and Orr, F. W.**, NK-leukocyte chemotactic factor (NK-LCF) a large granular lymphocyte (LGL) granule-associated chemotactic factor, *J. Immunol.*, in press.
39. **Reynolds, C. W., Bere, E. W., Jr., and Ward, J. M.**, Natural killer activity in the rat, III, Characterization of transplantable large granular lymphocyte (LGL) leukemias in F344 rat, *J. Immunol.*, 132, 534, 1984.

Chapter 16

PROPERTIES OF TRANSMEMBRANE CHANNELS INDUCED BY CYTOLYTIC LYMPHOCYTES

John Ding-E Young, Eckhard R. Podack, Carl F. Nathan, Hans Hengartner, and Zanvil A. Cohn

TABLE OF CONTENTS

I.	Introduction	20
II.	Functional Assays Used to Study Pore-Formation Mediated by Effector Cells	20
III.	Lytic Granules Isolated From Effector Cells	21
IV.	Functional and Structural Lesions Produced by Isolated Granules	22
	A. Structural Lesions	22
	B. Functional Lesions	22
V.	Properties of the Pore-Forming Protein (PFP) Isolated From Granules	25
	A. Isolation of Putative Pore-Former	25
	B. Polymerization of the PFP	25
	C. Functional Lesions Produced by PFP/Perforin: Effect on Cells	27
	D. Functional Lesions Produced by PFP/Perforin: Effect on Lipid Vesicles	28
	E. Functional Lesions Produced by PFP/Perforin: Effect on Planar Bilayers	28
	F. PFP/Perforin Mediates Lysis of Tumor Cells	28
	G. Immunological Cross-Reactivity Between C9 and PFP/Perforin	28
	H. PFP/Perforin is a Secretory Protein	30
	I. PFP/Perforin in Other Cell Types	30
VI.	Conclusion	30
Acknowledgments		31
References		32

I. INTRODUCTION

Cytotoxic T lymphocytes (CTL) and natural killer (NK) cells lyse tumor cells by a contact-dependent mechanism (for reviews, see References 1 to 5). Henkart and Blumenthal first demonstrated that a permeability increase in the target membrane occurs in association with its interaction with effector cells.[6] The involvement of pore-formation in target membrane damage, particularly in the antibody-dependent cell cytotoxicity (ADCC) was further substantiated by ultrastructural studies demonstrating that tubular lesions were formed on target membranes that had an internal diameter of 15 nm.[7] These observations were later extended by Podack and Dennert to cloned CTL[8] and NK cells.[9]

Functional studies carried out by several investigators have suggested an active role for pore-formation in CTL and NK cell killing:

1. The dose-response curve of killing is consistent with a one-hit mechanism.[10]
2. The release of small molecular weight markers always precedes the release of large molecular weight contents.[11]
3. The addition of extracellular macromolecules blocks T cell killing, suggesting the involvement of either an osmotic or diffusion-limiting protective mechanism.[12]
4. After initial effector-target cell contact, the killing is programmed to reach completion even in the subsequent absence of effector cells, as they leave to kill other cells.[13,14]
5. Estimates of the size of the lesion produced by lymphocytes are comparable to those estimated for complement-induced lesions.[15,16]

Recently, cloned cell lines with high cytotoxic activity have become available.[17-23] It has now become possible to grow large numbers of homogeneous populations of cells for biochemical and biophysical studies. This feature has recently allowed work on lymphocyte and NK cell cytolysis to be extended to subcellular levels and to purified protein. Here, we review the cytolytic properties associated with the cytoplasmic granules isolated from these cells and with the protein responsible for the tubular lesions produced on target cell membranes.

II. FUNCTIONAL ASSAYS USED TO STUDY PORE-FORMATION MEDIATED BY EFFECTOR CELLS

As pointed out, because of the feasibility of growing cytotoxic T cell lines to large numbers, we have used these cells as a source of lytic material in our experiments. Our aim was to isolate an active principle from CTL and NK cells that could explain the mechanism of the cytolysis observed with intact cells. Towards this end, we needed to design functional assays that could be used to screen for the membrane lytic activity.

A pore-forming protein (PFP) produced by killer cells and presumably used to lyse target cells would be expected to change the transmembrane electrolyte balance in a drastic way. This phenomenon could be investigated at several levels of cellular organization. First, at the intact cell level, PFPs should be able to lyse anucleated red blood cells and to depolarize the resting membrane potential of nucleated cells. Hemolysis should occur because of the transmembrane equilibration of salts, water, and macromolecules and because of an apparent lack of significant membrane repair mechanism in erythroyctes. Hemolysis can be used as a convenient assay for the lytic material.[24-28] A simple hemolysis microassay to screen for large numbers of fractions in a relatively short time has also been designed.[29,30] To measure membrane potential changes, voltage-sensitive probes,[27-29] direct microelectrode impalement of target cells,[29,31] and whole cell patch-clamp[32] have all been used.

Putative PFPs can also be assayed and examined in greater detail by using lipid vesicles as model target membranes.[27-29,32,33] The lipid vesicles may be labeled with fluorescent

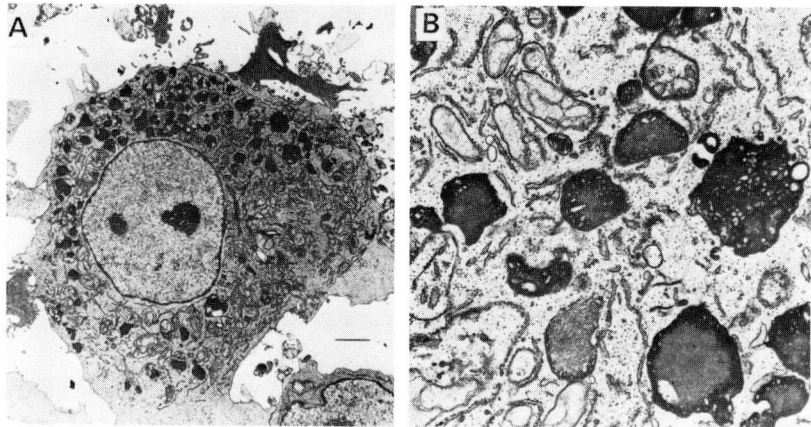

FIGURE 1. (A) morphology of Hy 3-Ag 3 killer cell line, showing numerous electron-dense granules in the cytoplasm. (B) An enlarged view of a selected region of the cytoplasm containing granules. Note the amorphous matrix of granules surrounded by the more electron-dense vesicular membranes. Scale bar corresponds to 3.5 μm in (A) and 657 nm in (B). (From Young, J. D.-E. et al., *Cell*, 44, 849, 1986. Copyright Cell Press. With permission.)

markers[33] or voltage-sensitive probes[27-29] and assayed to verify the extent of membrane leakiness induced by pore-forming material derived from effector cells.

Perhaps the most sensitive functional assay for pore-formation is direct single-channel recording using planar lipid bilayers[27-32] and patch clamped membranes (unpublished observations) as target membranes. Because of the high impedance of bilayers studied by these techniques, even very small current fluctuations induced by individual functional molecules of PFPs can be assayed at high resolution. These techniques also allow direct examination of some molecular sieving and biophysical properties of PFPs that would not be obtained by using any other procedures.

Because the effector cells studied here have been shown to induce the formation of tubular lesions on target membranes,[7-9] any putative PFP should also be able to assemble tubular lesions under appropriate conditions, and moreover the tubular lesions should resemble structurally the lesions formed by intact cells.

Finally, the purified PFP should be able to bypass the need for intact cells or any other subcellular compartment in mediating lysis of tumor cells. Standard functional cytotoxicity assays, such as ^{51}Cr labeling and release from target cells, can be used to assess this possibility.[24-26,32]

III. LYTIC GRANULES ISOLATED FROM EFFECTOR CELLS

Killing by CTL and NK cells appears to involve a secretory phenomenon, with the lytic apparatus of these cells localized in a cytoplasmic granule population.[24-33] So far all these studies have been carried out with mouse cytotoxic T cell and NK-like lines and rat large granular lymphocyte lines (LGL),[24-29] all of which have yielded comparable results. The LGL appear to correspond morphologically and functionally to NK cells.[30,31] CTL and NK cell clones usually contain numerous large cytoplasmic granules (Figure 1). Ultrastructural examination of the granules reveals a fine amorphous material in the center, surrounded by more electron-dense vesicular material (Figure 1B).

Granules from these effector cells have been isolated by centrifugation of cytoplasmic material through continuous and discontinuous Percoll gradients[24-29] (Figure 2). The different subcellular fractions have been assayed for enzymatic, hemolytic, and pore-forming activity

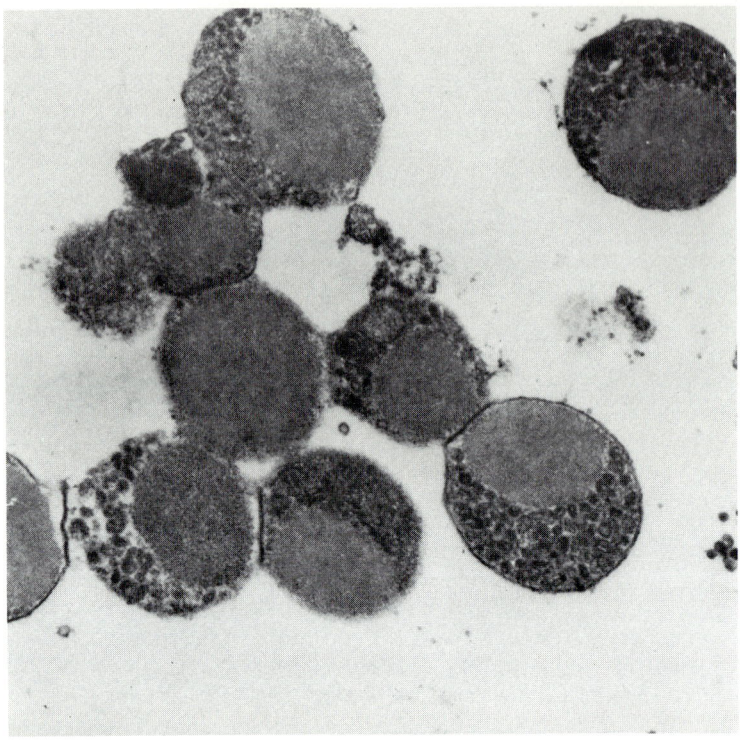

FIGURE 2. Ultrastructure and homogeneity of granules isolated by Percoll gradient from CTLL All cells. Scale bar: 270 nm. (From Young, J. D.-E. et al., *Proc. Natl. Acad. Sci. U.S.A.*, 83, 150, 1986. With permission.)

in model lipid bilayers. The active fractions have been shown to be lysosomal in nature, containing high B-glucuronidase activity.[24-29] Morphologically, the active fractions correspond to the cytoplasmic granule population[24-29] (Figure 2). This fraction has been shown to migrate with a density ranging 1.06 to 1.09 for mouse cytotoxic T cells.[26,29] The lytic activity has also been found in a small vacuolar compartment that does not migrate with the main granule fraction (unpublished observations).

IV. FUNCTIONAL AND STRUCTURAL LESIONS PRODUCED BY ISOLATED GRANULES

A. Structural Lesions

The isolated granules are capable of assembling membrane lesions when incubated at 37°C, in the presence of Ca^{2+}.[24-29] Tubular structures of approximately 160 Å are observed for granules isolated from mouse cytolytic cell lines[24-29] (Figure 3). In addition to complete rings, partially assembled tubules and linear polymers have also been frequently observed (Figure 3). It seems, therefore, that isolated granules are capable of producing structural lesions resembling those formed by intact killer cells.

B. Functional Lesions

As noted, granules from CTL and NK-like cells are highly hemolytic in the presence of millimolar amounts of Ca^{2+}.[24-33] The kinetics of hemolysis can be measured simply as a decrease of turbidity of an erythrocyte suspension at 700 nm[28,29] (Figure 4). Such kinetic studies show the rapid hemolysis induced by the granules and promoted by Ca^{2+} can be

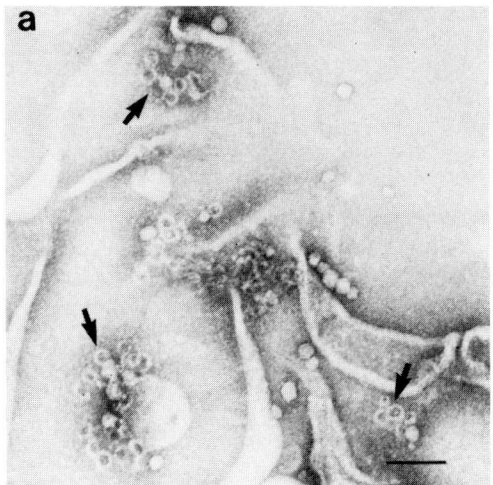 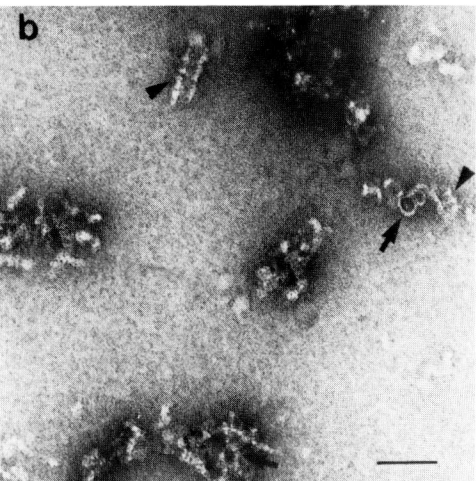

FIGURE 3. Ultrastructure of ring lesions produced by granules and granule-derived proteins. (a) Membrane lesions produced by incubation of SRBC with isolated granules. Scale bar: 70 nm. (b) Granules from CTLL All were extracted with ammonium acetate. The high-speed centrifugation supernatant was supplemented with 0.5% deoxycholate and dialyzed against detergent-free buffer for 48 hr at 37°C. Scale: 60 nm. Arrows point to cross sections of circular lesions. Arrowheads correspond to a longitudinal view of the tubular lesion. (From Young, J. D.-E. et al., *Proc. Natl. Acad. Sci. U.S.A.*, 83, 150, 1986. With permission.)

effectively blocked by EGTA, even after hemolysis has been initiated (Figure 4). The hemolysis can be effectively restored by addition of Ca^{2+}.[28]

The isolated granules depolarize the membrane potential of nucleated cells,[27-29] induce marker release and ion fluxes across membranes of lipid vesicles,[27-29,33] and result in the formation of functional channels in high-resistance planar lipid bilayers.[27-29]

Figure 5 illustrates a typical planar bilayer experiment. A planar bilayer, prepared by the technique of Montal and Mueller,[34] is exposed to granular material derived from mouse CTL. An immediate rise in membrane current is observed, which typically occurs as a summation of discrete steps, often progressing until the membrane breaks down (Figure 5). The sizes of channels are heterogeneous, ranging 0.4 to 6 nS per channel in 0.1 M NaCl (1 S = 1 A/1 V). The current change associated with the granule material is suggestive of incorporation of discrete channels into the bilayer which results in an ion flow of more than 10^8 ions per unit per sec, a rate that would be much faster than that achieved by a carrier or active-transport mechanism. This rate is also faster than the rise time that can be resolved by our instrumentation, therefore explaining the nature of the discrete current events observed here.

The granule-derived channels show a number of remarkable and distinct electrical features. These channels are highly resistant to closing by an increase in the transmembrane electrical field, with most channels persisting in the open state (Figure 6). A significant amount of channel closing can be induced only at voltages that exceed 70 mV (Figure 6A). The current-voltage plot for granule-derived channels shows a linear curve, with only some deviation from linearity occurring at voltages exceeding 70 mV (Figure 6B). This behavior indicates that the channels studied here are large, stable and voltage-resistant, which are all attributes that would favor an active role for these channels in cytolysis.

Because channels persist in the open state most of the time, single channel fluctuations are rare and can be observed only by imposing high transmembrane potentials.[27-29]

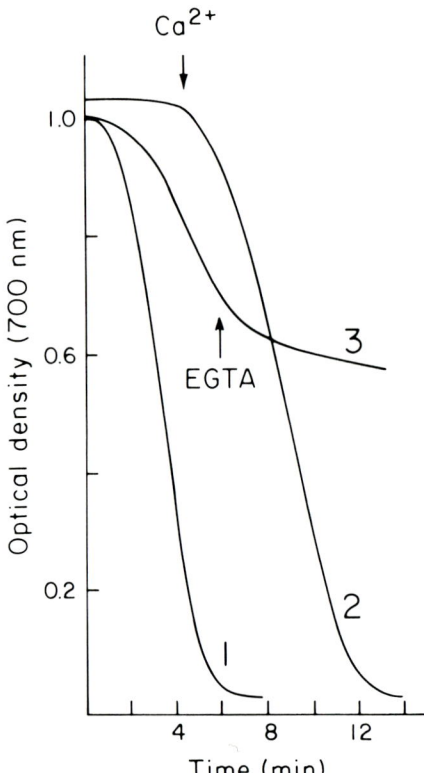

FIGURE 4. Hemolytic activity associated with granules of Hy 3-Ag 3 killer cells. Sheep red blood cells were resuspended in buffer containing 1 mM Ca^{2+} (curve 1), 0.1 mM Ca^{2+} (curve 3) and no Ca^{2+} (curve 2). Granules were added to the granule suspension at time 0 to a final protein concentration of 6 μg/mℓ. In curve 2, 1 mM Ca^{2+} was added where indicated. In curve 3, EGTA was added to a final concentration of 5 mM (*arrow*). The temperature of all experiments was 37°C. CTL1 A11 cells. (From Young, J. D.-E. et al., *Cell,* 44, 849, 1986. Copyright Cell Press. With permission.)

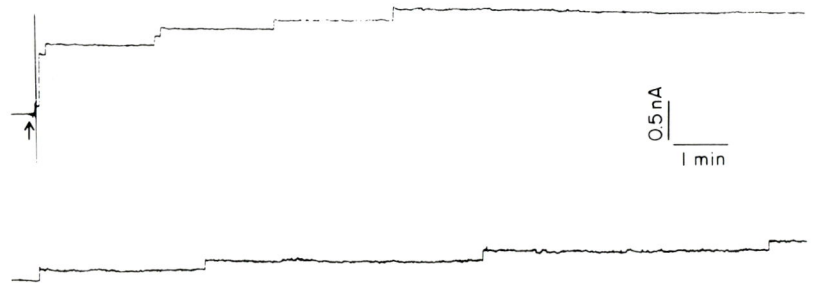

FIGURE 5. Effect of granule-derived material on bilayer conductance. Planar bilayer was made in 0.1 M NaCl and clamped at 30 mV. Granule proteins from CTLL A2 were introduced into the *cis* compartment; current was considered positive when flowing from *cis* to *trans* side. Note the increase of membrane current in discrete steps; current trace (top, right) is continued at the bottom (left). (From Young, J. D.-E. et al., *Proc. Natl. Acad. Sci. U.S.A.,* 83, 150, 1986. With permission.)

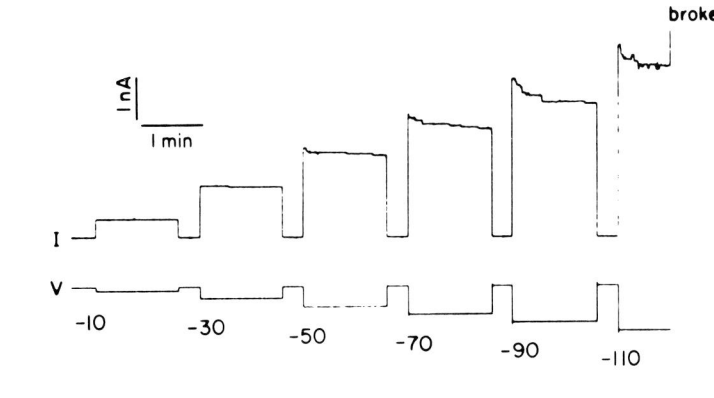

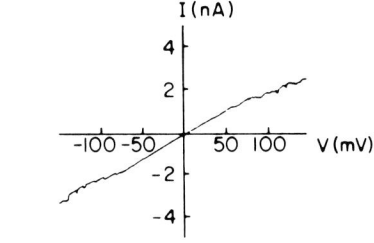

FIGURE 6. (a) Steady-state membrane current (I) as a function of membrane voltage (V). Bilayer exposed to granule proteins was exposed to increments of voltage. (b) Current-voltage plot generated by passing a continuous voltage ramp from −150 to +150 mV in 1 s to a bilayer exposed to granule proteins. (From Young, J. D.-E. et al., *Proc. Natl. Acad. Sci. U.S.A.*, 83, 150, 1986. With permission.)

V. PROPERTIES OF THE PORE-FORMING PROTEIN (PFP) ISOLATED FROM GRANULES

A. Isolation of Putative Pore-Former

The putative pore-former from the cytolytic T cell granules has been named cytolysin[24,25,33] and perforin.[26,32] The PFPs (cytolysin, perforin) from mouse cytotoxic T cells and NK-like lymphocytes have recently been purified.[29-32,35] In our laboratories, we have used a combination of molecular sieving and ion exchange chromatography. We have also recently purified this protein by affinity chromatography, using affinity purified antibodies directed against the mouse PFP and coupled to gel matrix as the immunoabsorbent.[36] The eluted fractions from the columns are assayed for hemolytic and pore-forming activity.

The monomeric protein migrates with a M_r of 66 to 68 kDalton[35] and 70 to 75 kDalton[29-32] when analyzed by SDS-polyacrylamide gel electrophoresis under reducing conditions (Figure 7B). The nonreduced form migrates with an apparent M_r of 60 to 66 kDalton, as observed by gel electrophoresis and by molecular sieving chromatography (Figure 7A). The independent size estimate obtained by HPLC[29,30] rules out the possibility that the active species might be related to the closely comigrating albumin or with some other minor species not identified by gel electrophoresis.

B. Polymerization of the PFP

The purified protein polymerizes in the presence of Ca^{2+} at 37°C, resulting in the formation of a polymeric species of M_r greater than 1 million Daltons that resists partially dissociation by SDS and reducing agents (Figure 8). In the absence of Ca^{2+}, polymerization is not

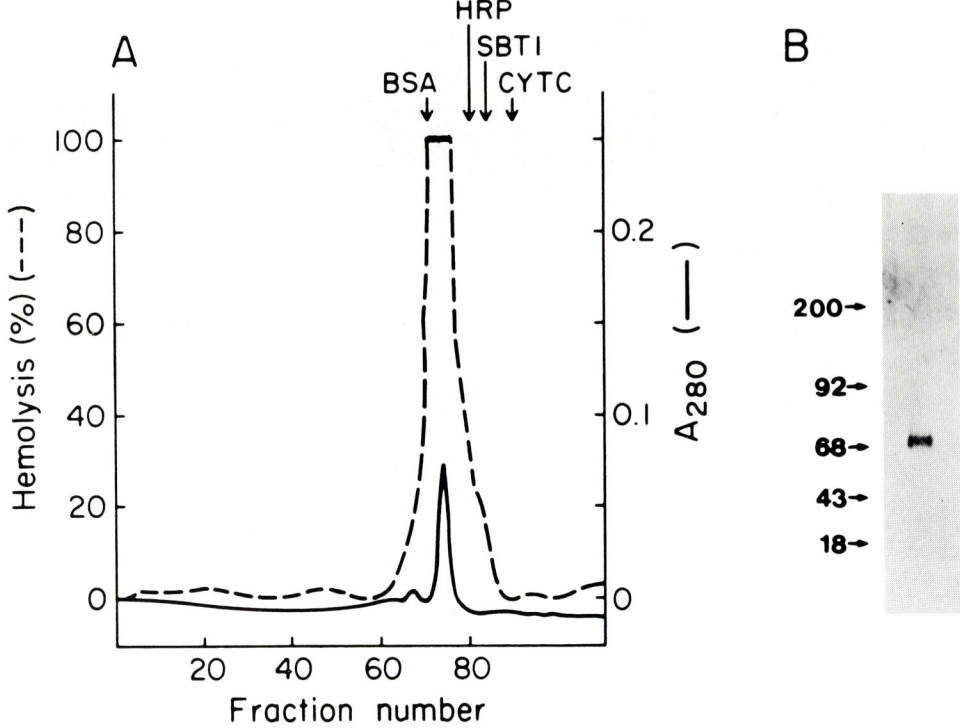

FIGURE 7. Purification of PFP by HPLC. (A) Hemolysis (A_{690}) and protein (A_{280}) determinations in HPLC fractions containing eluted PFP from CTLL A11. The injected sample was previously purified by Sephacryl S-200 and Mono Q columns. (B) SDS-PAGE profile of peak-hemolytic fraction from (A). (From Young, J. D.-E. et al., *Anal. Biochem.*, 154, 649, 1986. With permission.)

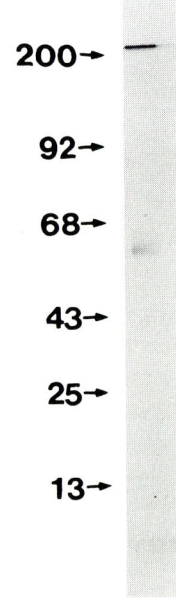

FIGURE 8. Polymerization of lymphocyte PFP (CTLL A11) in the presence of Ca^{2+}. 10 µg of PFP from TSK G3000 column was incubated at 37°C, 48 hr, with 1 mM $CaCl_2$, 0.1% deoxycholate, 0.5 mM PMSF, 0.1 U/mℓ of aprotinin and applied to a gel slab (4 to 11% gradient) under reducing conditions.

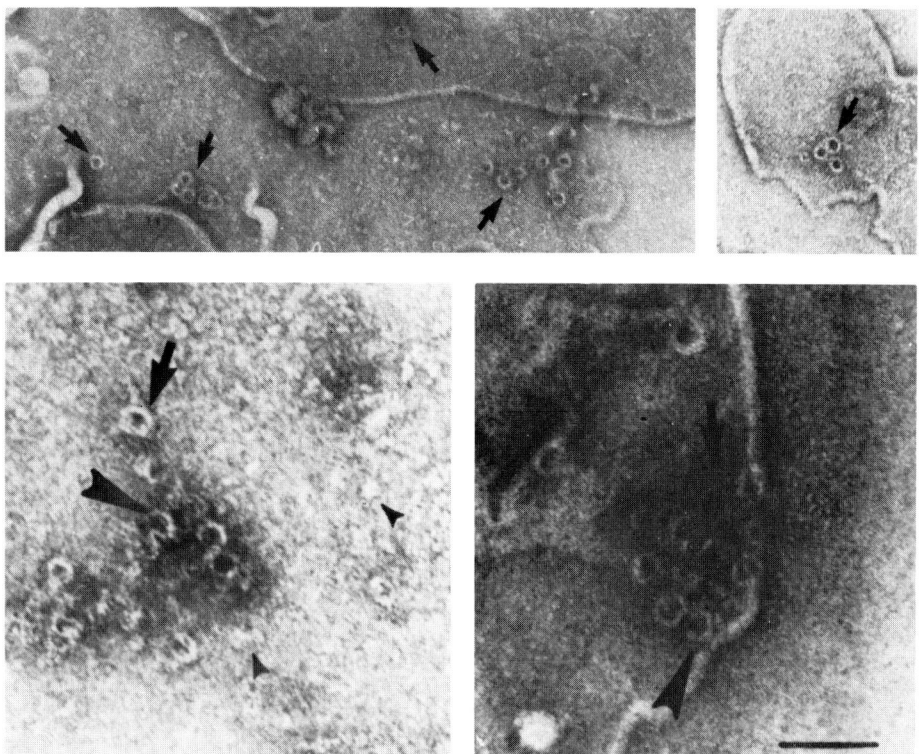

FIGURE 9. Selected images of PFP polymerized on SRBC membranes. Typical tubules of 160 Å internal diameter are observed. Complete rings (arrows) and incompletely polymerized (arrowheads) tubules are observed. Scale bar: upper panels, 250 nm: lower panels, 85 nm. (From Young, J. D.-E. et al., *J. Exp. Med.*, 164, 144, 1986. Copyright The Rockefeller University Press. With permission.)

observed.[29-32] The polymerization of the monomeric species can also be demonstrated by chromatography. Following incubation with Ca^{2+} at 37°C and elution through Sephacryl S-200 column, most of the protein elutes in the void volume (unpublished).

The purified protein assembles tubular lesions on erythrocyte membranes, similar to those produced by intact cells and granules[29,31,32] (Figure 9). Tubular lesions averaging 160 Å in diameter are observed.

C. Functional Lesions Produced by PFP/Perforin: Effect on Cells

The purified protein shows potent hemolytic activity (Figure 7A). One ng of protein is sufficient to lyse completely 10^8 sheep red blood cells.[30] Assuming a M_r of 70 kDalton, this number would correspond to 86 molecules/cell. PFP/perforin does not bind to membranes and appears to require Ca^{2+} for both membrane attachment and polymerization.[29]

PFP/perforin depolarizes rapidly the membrane potential of a number of cell types.[29,31,32] Chicken embryo myoblasts, impaled with microelectrodes, rapidly depolarize following exposure to the protein (Figure 10). Ca^{2+} is required for depolarization, and PFP that had been previously incubated at 37°C no longer remains cell active (presumably polymerized and inactivated) (Figure 10).

Patch clamp recording of target cell, in the whole cell configuration, shows insertion of current steps into the bilayer that occurs effectively only in the presence of Ca^{2+} (Figure 11).[32] The current steps probably correspond to a progressive incorporation of ion channels.

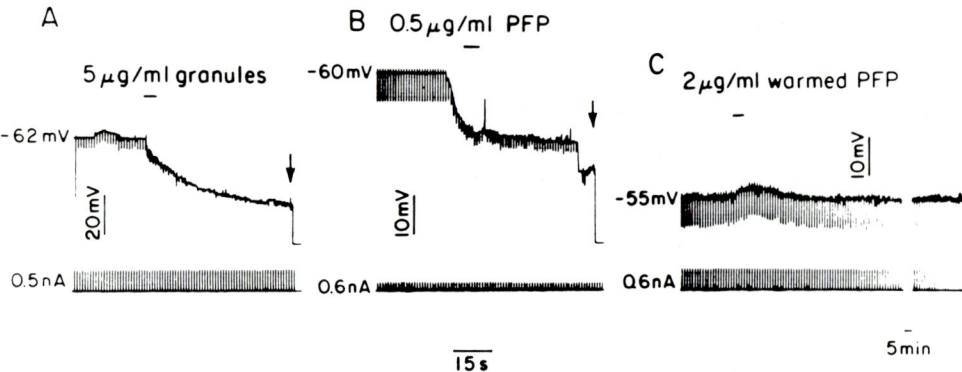

FIGURE 10. Depolarization of cultured chicken muscle cells by PFP. Cells were exposed to Hy 3-Ag3 granules (A) and PFP (B) (addition indicated by bars). Arrows indicate withdrawal of microelectrode. (C) PFP was incubated at 37°C, 4 hr, in the presence of 1 mM Ca^{2+} prior to addition to cells. The lower traces show the applied current pulses. (From Young, J. D.-E. et al., *Cell*, in press. Copyright Cell Press. With permission.)

D. Functional Lesions Produced by PFP/Perforin: Effect on Lipid Vesicles

Lipid vesicles that had been exposed to the monomeric species become leaky to monovalent (Na$^+$, K$^+$, Li$^+$, Cl$^-$, I$^-$) and divalent ions (Ca^{2+}, Mg^{2+}, Ba^{2+}, Zn^{2+}) and to large macromolecules like sucrose (mol. wt. 342) and lucifer yellow (mol. wt. 457).

E. Functional Lesions Produced by PFP/Perforin: Effect on Planar Bilayers

PFP induces step-wise conductance changes in planar bilayers similar to those produced by solubilized granule contents.[29,31] Similar voltage-current relationships and ion selectivity ratios are observed for the purified protein. The channels produced by PFP have large conductance steps and are voltage-resistant to closing. Bilayers treated with the protein become leaky to glucosamine (with Stokes diameter of 8 Å), Tris, and EGTA, implying a large functional diameter for the assembled pores. Single-channel recordings obtained with PFP/perforin show two populations of channel sizes. The soluble protein inserts spontaneously into lipid bilayers to produce single units of 400 pS in 0.1 M NaCl[29,31] (Figure 12). The protein that has been polymerized in lipid vesicles and transferred to planar bilayers by a vesicle-bilayer fusion protocol produces much larger single units, in the range of 1 to 6 nS.[31] These results indicate that PFP/perforin may polymerize into multiple sizes, corresponding to complete and incomplete rings, all of which may be functionally active in the bilayer. It is conceivable that PFP may produce effective membrane damage without undergoing complete polymerization to form the large EM-visible tubular lesions.

F. PFP/Perforin Mediates Lysis of Tumor Cells

The purified protein is lytic to a number of cell lines.[31] Interestingly, the amount of protein required to attain cytolysis is always several-fold higher than that required for hemolysis or channel formation.

G. Immunological Cross-Reactivity Between C9 and PFP/Perforin

The poly C9 channel (as described in this volume) closely resembles the PFP/perforin in a number of functional features. The possibility that these two molecules might also share homologous amino acid domains was recently assessed by using polyclonal antibodies raised against purified C9 and lymphocyte perforin to check for immunological cross-reactivity.[36,43,44] The homology is limited to a domain that is only exposed when the two molecules are chemically reduced.[36,44]

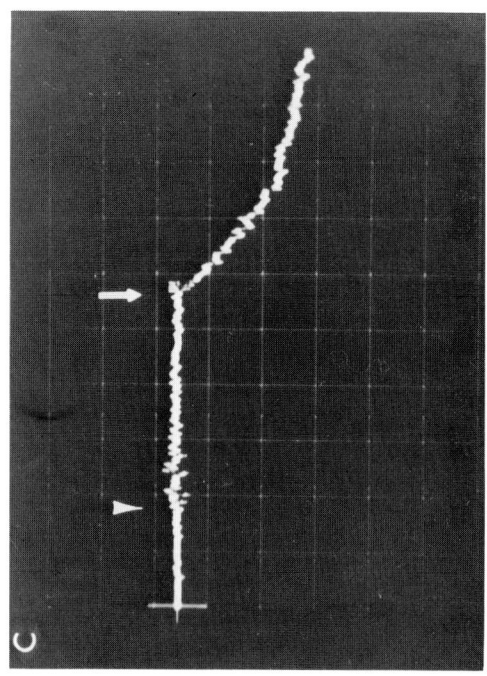
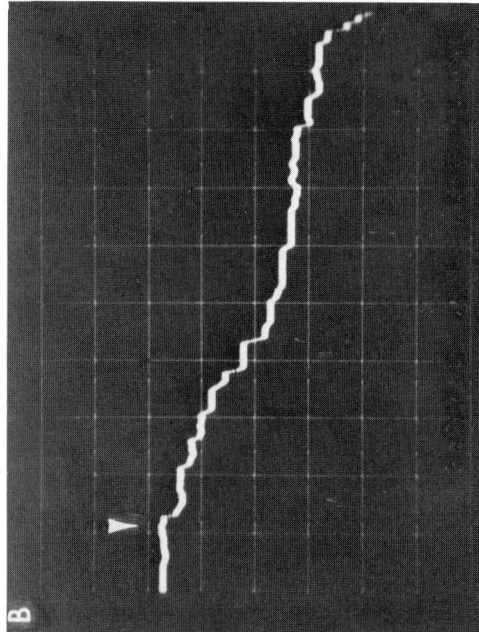
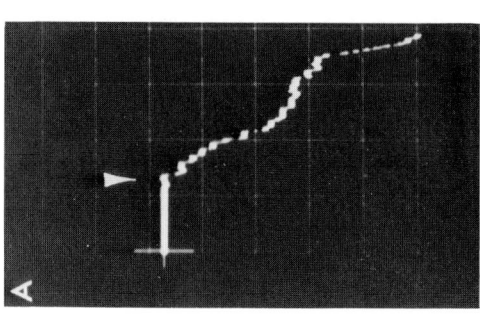

FIGURE 11. Patch-clamp of S49.1 cells, in the whole-cell configuration. Cells were clamped at −60 mV during PFP application. PFP (to 0.1 µg/mℓ, from Hy 3-Ag3 cells) was added from a second micropipette at a distance of about 100 µm from the cell (arrowheads point to beginning of perfusion). Scales per box: vertical, 200 pA; horizontal, 5 s. (B) Horizontal expansion of A, 4 ×. (C) Cell bathed in Ca^{2+}-free medium. Ca^{2+} was subsequently added from a third pipette to a final concentration of 0.5 mM (arrow). Same scale as in A. Downward deflections represent inward currents. (From Podack, E. R. et al., *Proc. Natl. Acad. Sci. U.S.A.*, 82, 8629, 1985. With permission.)

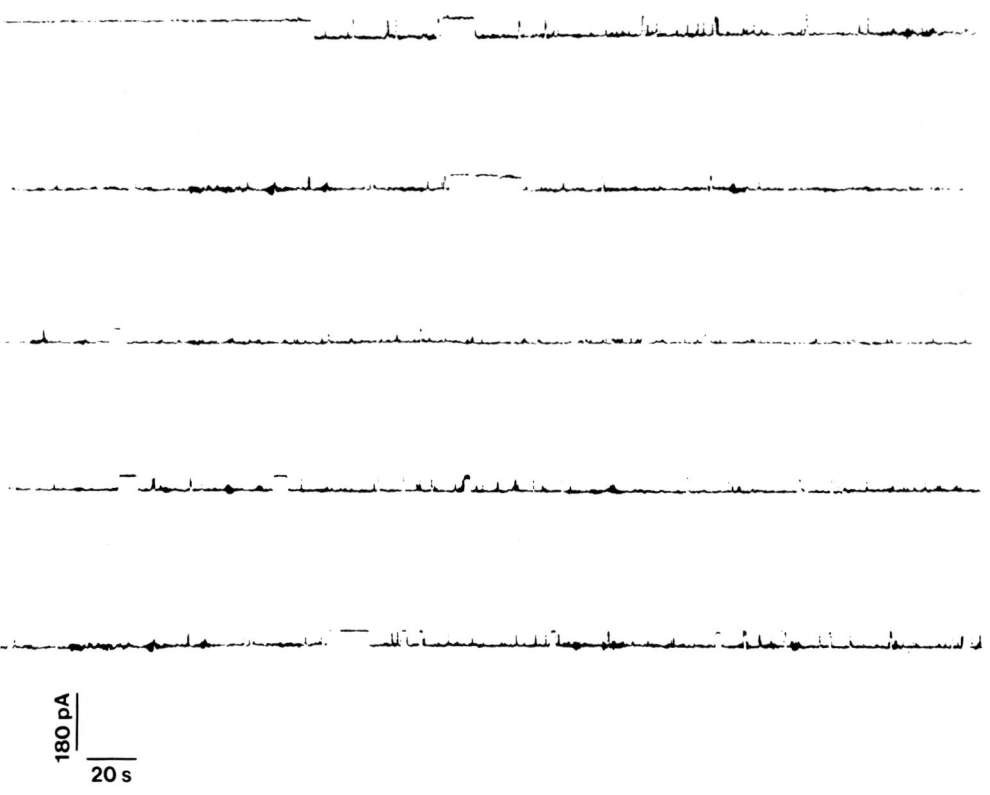

FIGURE 12. Continuous single channel trace produced by 1 ng PFP of Hy 3-Ag3 cells in 0.1 M NaCl. The bilayer was clamped at +120 mV. Note the incorporation of one single channel in the beginning of the record (top left). Downward deflection corresponds to channel opening. Note that the channel stays preferentially in the open state. Temperature: 23°C; resolution: 1 ms. (From Young, J. D.-E. et al., *Cell*, 44, 849, 1986. Copyright Cell Press. With permission.)

H. PFP/Perforin is a Secretory Protein

The monomeric species is actively secreted into the extracellular medium following cell stimulation with A23187, a Ca^{2+} ionophore.[45] Release of PFP is accompanied simultaneously by cell degranulation.[45] The protein released by mouse cytolytic T cells assembles into tubular lesions, binds to lipids, and has been positively identified as perforin using specific polyclonal antibodies as immunoprecipitation reagents. We are presently investigating the release of PFP by NK cell clones following incubation of cells with immunocomplexes. The release of the pore-former via the Fc mechanism (i.e., binding to the surface Fc receptors) would be expected to occur during the antibody-dependent, contact-mediated killing by NK cells.

I. PFP/Perforin in Other Cell Types

Recent work has also identified this protein in human peripheral blood lymphocytes and human NK cell clones. The molecular weight of the protein found in human killer cells resembles that of mouse PFP/perforin and also cross-reacts with specific antibodies directed against human C9.[46,47]

VI. CONCLUSION

The killing of tumor cells mediated by CTL and NK cells appears to involve pore-formation. The cytolytic protein localized in the granules is released into the intercellular space following the effector-target cell contact. The released protein then assembles into tubular complexes on the target membrane in the presence of Ca^{2+}. The strategic localization of this pore-forming protein in the effector cell granules avoids the possibility of self-inflicted injury (the amount of Ca^{2+} in the granules presumed to be much lower than that required for tubular assembly) and allows the cell to produce a directed and localized membrane injury on the target by directing the fusion of cytoplasmic granules with the plasma membrane (or degranulation) only at the site of contact or surface stimuli. The polarization of the cytoplasmic organelles towards the target cell during killing has recently been demonstrated by immunofluorescence studies.[37] In this regard, it should also be pointed out that Ca^{2+} appears to be required for both degranulation and the assembly of the PFP/perforin, and the requirements for Ca^{2+} for these two events are clearly different.[29,45] The fusion of isolated granules with target membranes prior to lysis has recently been demonstrated by morphological studies (unpublished observations).

Pore-formation has long been accepted as an efficient way of mediating cell lysis. In the past, pore-formation has been described for a number of bacterial toxins and antibiotics.[38,39] Recently, PFPs have also been identified in the protozoan parasite *Entamoeba histolytica*.[40,41] The eosinophil cationic protein, a major protein of human eosinophil granules, is also a pore-former.[42] Pore-formation may therefore represent a common mechanism of killing shared by a variety of different professional killer cells. It is conceivable that the different immune cell types differ mainly in the mechanism of recognition of the appropriate targets. Once triggered, the killing event (involving secretion of PFPs) may develop in a similar fashion for the different effector cells. It still remains to be resolved how the effector cell protects itself from injury once PFPs have been released into the extracellular space. The observation that even certain distantly related pathogenic protozoan parasites have proteins with similar function substantiates further our view that these effector molecules must play an important role during cell killing.

It is intriguing that the poly C9 and PFP/perforin channels may share so many similar functional and structural features. It is entirely possible that the two molecules originated from the same ancestral protein and only diverged later during evolution in order to carry out the specialized functions of cellular and humoral responses.

Other proteins localized in the granules may also play a vital role in cell killing. It is conceivable, for example, that the size of the protein channels described here could allow the free permeation of other toxic molecules from the granules into the target cell, which would potentiate the membrane damage mediated only by the pore-former.

Although the molecular structure and gene expression of these various PFPs still need to be elucidated for our complete appreciation of their role in cell killing, it is tempting to suggest here a crucial role for these proteins in the contact-dependent cytotoxicity mediated by CTL and NK cells.

ACKNOWLEDGMENTS

We thank the generous assistance and advice from Dr. M. A. Palladino during the early phase of this work and the excellent technical assistance of S. S. Ko, M. A. DiNome, L. G. Leong, A. Damiano, and R. Lang. We thank Dr. P. Groscurth for his contribution to the electron microscopy studies. J. D.-E. Young is a Lucille P. Markey Scholar. Carl F. Nathan is a Scholar of the Rita Allen Foundation. This work was supported in part by grants from the Lucille P. Markey Charitable Trust and the Cancer Research Institute to J. D.-E. Young; by USPHS grants AI18525 and CA34524, and American Cancer Society grant IM396 to Eckhard R. Podack; by grant 3.329-0.82 from the Swiss Nationalfonds to Hans Hengartner; by USPHS grant CA22090 to Carl F. Nathan; and by USPHS grants CA30198 and AI07012 to Z. A. Cohn.

REFERENCES

1. **Berke, G.,** Cytotoxic lymphocytes-T. How do they function? *Immunol. Rev.,* 72, 5, 1983.
2. **Martz, E.,** Mechanism of specific tumor cell lysis by alloimmune T-lymphocytes: resolution and characterization of discrete steps in cellular interaction, *Contemp. Top. Immunobiol.,* 7, 301, 1977.
3. **Henney, C. S.,** T cell-mediated cytolysis: an overview of some current issues, *Contemp. Top. Immunobiol.,* 7, 245, 1977.
4. **Herberman, R. B., Djeu, J. Y., and Kay, H. D.,** Natural killer cells: characteristics and regulation of activity, *Immunol. Rev.,* 44, 43, 1979.
5. **Trinchieri, G. and Perussia, B.,** Human natural killer cells: biologic and pathologic aspects, *Lab. Invest.,* 50, 489, 1984.
6. **Henkart, P. and Blumenthal, R.,** Interaction of lymphocytes with lipid bilayer membranes: a model for lymphocyte-mediated lysis of target cells, *Proc. Natl. Acad. Sci. U.S.A.,* 72, 2789, 1975.
7. **Dourmashkin, R. R., Deteix, P., Simone, C. B., and Henkart, P.,** Electron microscopic demonstration of lesions on target cell membranes associated with antibody-dependent cellular cytotoxicity, *Clin. Exp. Immunol.,* 42, 554, 1980.
8. **Dennert, G. and Podack, E. R.,** Cytolysis by H-2 specific T killer cells. Assembly of tubular complexes on target membranes, *J. Exp. Med.,* 157, 1483, 1983.
9. **Podack, E. R. and Dennert, G.,** Assembly of two types of tubules with putative cytolytic function in cloned natural killer cells, *Nature,* 302, 442, 1983.
10. **Henney, C. S.,** Studies on the mechanism of lymphocyte-mediated cytolysis. II. The use of various target cell markers to study cytolytic events, *J. Immunol.,* 110, 73, 1973.
11. **Ziegler, H. K. and Henney, C. S.,** Antibody-dependent cytolytically active human leukocytes: an analysis of inactivation following in vitro interaction with antibody-coated target cells, *J. Immunol.,* 115, 1500, 1975.
12. **Ferluga, J. and Allison, A. C.,** Observations on the mechanism by which T-lymphocytes exert cytotoxic effects, *Nature,* 250, 673, 1974.
13. **Golstein, P. and Smith, E.,** Mechanism of T cell-mediated cytolysis: the lethal hit stage, *Contemp. Top. Immunobiol.,* 7, 273, 1977.
14. **Koren, H. S., Ax, W., and Freund-Moelbert, E.,** Morphological observations on the contact-induced lysis of target cells, *Eur. J. Immunol.,* 3, 32, 1973.
15. **Simone, C. B. and Henkart, P. A.,** Permeability changes induced in erythrocyte ghost targets by antibody-dependent cytotoxic effector cells: evidence for membrane pores, *J. Immunol.,* 124, 954, 1980.
16. **Giavedoni, E. B., Chow, Y. M., and Dalmasso, A. P.,** The functional size of the primary complement lesion in resealed erythrocyte membrane ghosts, *J. Immunol.,* 122, 240, 1979.
17. **Dennert, G.,** Cloned cell lines of natural killer cells, *Nature,* 287, 47, 1980.
18. **Dennert, G., Yogeeswaran, G., and Yamagata, S.,** Cloned cell lines with natural killer activity, *J. Exp. Med.,* 153, 545, 1981.
19. **Nabel, G., Bucalo, L. R., Allard, J., Wigzell, H., and Cantor, H.,** Multiple activities of a cloned line mediating killer cell function, *J. Exp. Med.,* 153, 1582, 1981.
20. **Brooks, C. G., Kuribayashi, K., Sale, G. E., and Henney, C. S.,** Characterization of five cloned murine cell lines showing high cytolytic activity against YAC-1 cells, *J. Immunol.,* 128, 2326, 1982.
21. **Sagamura, K., Tanaka, Y., and Hiruma, Y.,** Two distinct human cloned T cell lines that exhibit natural killer-like and anti-human effector activities, *J. Immunol.,* 128, 1749, 1982.
22. **Kornbluth, J. and Dupont, B.,** Cloning and functional characterization of primary alloreactive human T lymphocytes, *J. Exp. Med.,* 152, 1645, 1980.
23. **Acha-Orbea, H., Groscurth, P., Lang, R., Stitz, L., and Hengartner, H.,** Characterization of cloned cytotoxic lymphocytes with NK-like activity, *J. Immunol.,* 130, 2952, 1983.
24. **Henkart, P. A., Millard, P. J., Reynolds, C. W., and Henkart, M. P.,** Cytolytic activity of purified cytoplasmic granules from cytotoxic rat large granular lymphocyte tumors, *J. Exp. Med.,* 160, 75, 1984.
25. **Millard, P. J., Henkart, M. P., Reynolds, C. W., and Henkart, M. P.,** Purification and properties of cytoplasmic granules from cytotoxic rat LGL tumors, *J. Immunol.,* 132, 3197, 1984.
26. **Podack, E. R. and Konigsberg, P. J.,** Cytolytic T cell granules. Isolation, structural, biochemical and functional characterization, *J. Exp. Med.,* 160, 695, 1984.
27. **Young, J. D.-E., Nathan, C. F., and Cohn, Z. A.,** Interaction of immune cells with target cell membranes: is there a common mechanism of killing? *J. Cell. Biochem.,* 9A, 161, 1985.
28. **Young, J. D.-E., Nathan, C. F., Podack, E. R., Palladino, M. A., and Cohn, Z. A.,** Functional channel formation associated with cytotoxic T-cell granules, *Proc. Natl. Acad. Sci. U.S.A.,* 83, 150, 1986.
29. **Young, J. D.-E., Hengartner, H., Podack, E. R., and Cohn, Z. A.,** Purification and characterization of a cytolytic pore-forming protein from granules of cloned lymphocytes with natural killer activity, *Cell,* 44, 849, 1986.

30. **Young, J. D.-E., Leong, L. G., DiNome, M. A., and Cohn, Z. A.,** A semi-automated hemolysis microassay for membrane lytic proteins, *Anal. Biochem.,* 154, 649, 1986.
31. **Young, J. D.-E., Podack, E. R., and Cohn, Z. A.,** Properties of a purified pore-forming protein from cytotoxic T cell granules, *J. Exp. Med.,* 164, 144, 1986.
32. **Podack, E. R., Young, J. D.-E., and Cohn, Z. A.,** Isolation, biochemical and functional characterization of perforin 1 from cytolytic T-cell granules, *Proc. Natl. Acad. Sci. U.S.A.,* 82, 8629, 1985.
33. **Blumenthal, R., Millard, P. J., Henkart, M. P., Reynolds, C. W., and Henkart, P. A.,** Liposomes as targets for granule cytolysin from cytotoxic large granular lymphocyte tumors, *Proc. Natl. Acad. Sci. U.S.A.,* 81, 5551, 1984.
34. **Montal, M. and Mueller, P.,** Formation of bimolecular membranes from lipid monolayers and a study of their electrical properties, *Proc. Natl. Acad. Sci. U.S.A.,* 69, 3561, 1972.
35. **Masson, D. and Tschopp, J.,** Isolation of a lytic, pore-formation protein (perforin) from cytolytic T-lymphocytes, *J. Biol. Chem.,* 260, 9069, 1985.
36. **Young, J. D.-E., Cohn, Z. A., and Podack, E. R.,** The ninth component of complement and the pore-forming protein (perforin 1) from cytotoxic T cells: structural, immunological and functional similarities, *Science,* 233, 184, 1986.
37. **Kupfer, A. and Dennert, G.,** Reorientation of the microtubule-organizing center and the golgi apparatus in cloned cytotoxic lymphocytes triggered by binding to lysable target cells, *J. Immunol.,* 133, 2762, 1984.
38. **Latorre, R. and Alvarez, O.,** Voltage-dependent channels in planar bilayer membranes, *Physiol. Rev.,* 61, 77, 1981.
39. **Schein, S. J., Kagan, B. L., and Finkelstein, A.,** Colicin K acts by forming voltage-dependent channels in phospholipid bilayer membranes, *Nature,* 276, 159, 1978.
40. **Lynch, E. C., Rosenberg, I. M., and Gitler, C.,** An ion-channel forming protein produced by *Entamoeba histolytica, EMBO J.,* 1, 801, 1982.
41. **Young, J. D.-E., Young, T. M., Lu, L. P., Unkeless, J. C., and Cohn, Z. A.,** Characterization of a membrane pore-forming protein from *Entamoeba histolytica, J. Exp. Med.,* 156, 1677, 1982.
42. **Young, J. D.-E., Peterson, C. G. B., Venge, P., and Cohn, Z. A.,** Mechanism of membrane damage mediated by human eosinophil cationic protein, *Nature,* 321, 613, 1986.
43. **Tschopp, J., Masson, D., and Stanley, K. K.,** Structural/functional similarity between proteins involved in complement- and cytotoxic T-lymphocyte-mediated cytolysis, *Nature,* 322, 831, 1986.
44. **Young, J. D.-E, Liu, C.-C., Leong, L. G., and Cohn, Z. A.,** The pore-forming protein (perforin) of cytolytic T lymphocytes is immunologically related to the components of membrane attack complex of complement through cysteine-rich domains, *J. Exp. Med.,* 164, 2077, 1986.
45. **Young, J. D.-E., Leong, L. G., Liu, C.-C., and Cohn, Z. A.,** Extracellular release of lymphocyte pore-forming protein (perforin) after ionophore stimulation, *Proc. Natl. Acad. Sci. U.S.A.,* 83, 5668, 1986.
46. **Zalman, L. S., Brothers, M. A., Chiu, F. J., and Müller-Eberhard, H. J.,** Mechanism of cytotoxicity of human large granular lymphocytes: relationship of the cytotoxic lymphocyte protein to the ninth component (C9) of human complement, *Proc. Natl. Acad. Sci. U.S.A.,* 83, 5262, 1986.
47. **Liu, C.-C., Perussia, B., Cohn, Z. A., and Young, J. D.-E.,** Identification and characterization of a pore-forming protein of human peripheral blood natural killer cells, *J. Exp. Med.,* 164, 2061, 1986.

Chapter 17

THE ROLE OF NUCLEAR DAMAGE IN LYSIS OF TARGET CELLS BY CYTOTOXIC T LYMPHOCYTES

Richard C. Duke and J. John Cohen

TABLE OF CONTENTS

I.	Introduction: Mechanism of Cytotoxic T Lymphocyte-Mediated Cytolysis	36
II.	Characteristics of CTLMC	36
	A. The Lytic Process is Unidirectional	36
	B. Effector Cell-Dependent and Independent Phases of CTLMC	37
	C. Differences Between CTL- and Complement-Mediated Cytolysis: Colloid Osmotic Lysis	37
	D. Changes in Nuclear Structure	38
III.	DNA Fragmentation Induced During CTLMC	39
	A. DNA Fragmentation Assay	39
	B. Induction of DNA Fragmentation in Target Cells by CTL	40
	1. DNA Fragmentation is an Early Event in CTL-Mediated Cytolysis	41
	2. DNA Fragmentation is Characterized by Production of Oligonucleosomes	41
	3. Breakdown of DNA-Nucleoprotein Interactions in Target Cells is an Early Event in CTLMC	43
IV.	The Relationship Between DNA Fragmentation and Target Cell Lysis	44
	A. Testable Models	44
	B. The Induction of DNA Fragmentation and Target Cell Lysis Require Extracellular Calcium	45
	C. Only Target Cells Which Have Already Been Induced to Fragment Their DNA Lyse During the Killer Cell-Independent Phase of CTLMC	45
	D. The Effects of Various Inhibitors on DNA Fragmentation and ^{51}Cr Release During CTLMC	46
	E. Does DNA Fragmentation Inevitably Lead to Lysis?	47
V.	A Model of CTLMC Involving Synergy Between External and Internal Damage Induced in the Target Cell by CTL	49
VI.	What is the Mechanism of Induction of DNA Fragmentation and Target Cell Lysis?	50
	A. The Consequences of CTL-Target Cell Binding and Delivery of the Lethal Hit	50
	B. Activation of a Cell Death Program Intrinsic to the Target Cell	51
	C. The Lack of Double-Stranded DNA Fragmentation in Human Target Cells Supports an Intrinsic Cell Death Program	52
VII.	Conclusions	52
Addendum		53
Acknowledgment		53
References		53

I. INTRODUCTION: MECHANISM OF CYTOTOXIC T LYMPHOCYTE-MEDIATED CYTOLYSIS

Cytotoxicity mediated by T lymphocytes represents the most specific weapon available to the immune system. CTL can recognize virally infected or chemically modified cells and eliminate them without damaging normal cells. The way in which cytotoxic T lymphocytes (CTL) destroy target cells has provoked a considerable amount of research. These studies, while leading to important discoveries concerning the nature of T cell recognition and binding, have not yet elucidated the nature of the lytic mechanism itself.

Two general types of models have been developed to explain CTL-mediated cytolysis (CTLMC). In these models, target cell death, as measured by loss of membrane integrity (lysis), occurs as the result of one of two fundamentally different mechanisms:

1. Lysis is the result of direct membrane damage, similar to that observed during complement-mediated lysis: the target cell is a passive victim of external attack.
2. Lysis is the indirect result of internal damage, similar to that observed during apoptosis, in which the target actively participates in its own destruction.

In either type of model, the primary damage, whether internal or external, is induced by the CTL. Both external and internal damage lead to target cell lysis; however, the mechanisms by which damage and/or lysis are induced can be imagined to be quite different.

Models of CTLMC involving external damage have been discussed in detail elsewhere in this volume. Models of CTLMC favoring internal damage emphasize the differences in the morphological and biochemical changes induced in the target cell during CTL-mediated vs. complement mediated cytolysis.[1-4] In this review, we will discuss data which suggest that the CTL induces internal damage in the target cell. The relationship of the internal damage, which is observed as disruption of target cell nuclear structures, to lysis will be discussed. In addition, the effect of CTL-induced external damage on target cell lysis will be incorporated into a general model of CTL-mediated cytolysis.

II. CHARACTERISTICS OF CTLMC

Before discussing the biochemistry of CTL-mediated cytolysis, it is necessary to review certain characteristics of CTL killing. any model which hopes to describe CTL-mediated cytolysis satisfactorily must take these observations into account.

A. The Lytic Process is Unidirectional

Cytotoxic T lymphocytes bind to target cells via highly specific receptor-ligand interactions. CTL generated against cells bearing the sensitizing surface antigens kill only the homologous targets. Bystander cells which do not express the immunizing antigens are not killed, even when intimately mixed with appropriate target cells.[5-7] In addition to the lack of bystander killing, the CTL itself is not killed during the lytic process and can recycle to kill other antigen-bearing target cells.[8-10]

These experimental observations demonstrate two important characteristics of CTL-mediated cytolysis. First, killing is unidirectional; only appropriate target cells are killed, CTL and bystander cells are not. Second, a simple, nonspecific, soluble mediator cannot be involved in the lytic process.[11] If a nonspecific mediator exists, then a process of highly focused factor must be hypothesized to explain the lack of bystander killing.[12] A possible explanation for sparing of the effector cell (at whose surface, of course, the factor would be most highly concentrated) during target cell lysis would be that CTLs are immune to their own killing factor. This is clearly not the case; cytotoxic T cells are fully susceptible to killing by other CTL populations.[7,12-16]

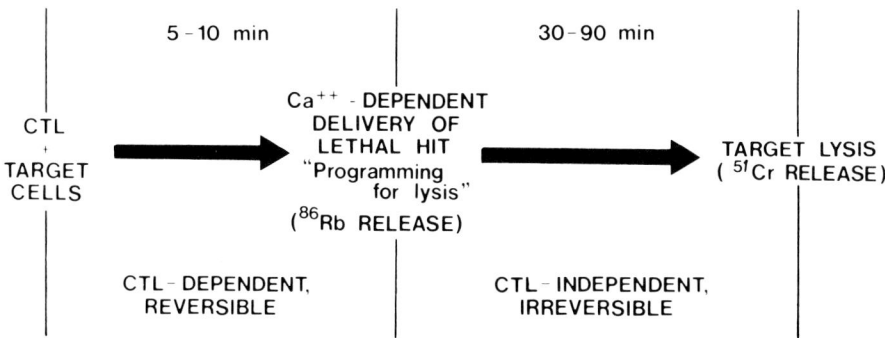

FIGURE 1. Schematic representation of the two stages of CTL-mediated cytolysis.

B. Effector Cell-Dependent and Independent Phases of CTLMC

CTLMC may be divided into two distinct phases (Figure 1). The first phase requires the physical presence of the CTL. It begins with CTL-target cell binding, and culminates in delivery of the lethal hit.[17,18] Delivery of the lethal hit is strictly Ca^{++}-dependent and programs the target cell to die.[11,19,20] Once the target cell has been programmed to die, the CTL is no longer required in order for lysis to occur.[20] Thus, the second phase of CTLMC is killer cell-independent and terminates in target cell lysis.

CTL can be removed during the killing process by EDTA, which breaks up conjugates and prevents new conjugate formation[21-25] by heating, which inactivates the CTL,[17,26] or by direct killing of the CTL with anti-Thy-1 antibody plus complement.[23,27] While these treatments abrogate CTLMC if performed prior to delivery of the lethal hit, they have no effect on target cell lysis if performed after the target is programmed to die.

In the first, relatively short (5 to 10 min) phase of CTLMC, programming for lysis occurs. This corresponds in time with the biochemical parameter of ^{86}Rb release. Release of this potassium analog has been taken to imply either that a small membrane lesion has been induced[28-31] or that a calcium flux has occurred.[32] The delivery of the lethal hit follows first order kinetics and is independent of the number of CTL bound to the target cell.[33] By definition, all of the required CTL-derived lytic signals or mediators are passed to the target cell during the first phase of CTLMC. In addition, CTL-mediated cytolysis is independent of protein and RNA synthesis,[34,35] and therefore, any CTL-derived factors must be preformed.[20]

The second phase of CTLMC, lysis of the target cell as measured by ^{51}Cr release, follows a protracted course after delivery of the lethal hit. In contrast to delivery of the lethal hit, this phase, although it does not require CTLs, may be shortened somewhat if the CTL remains bound to the target cell[1,36] or if more than one CTL interacts with the target.[33,37] There is, however, a minimum lag time before lysis occurs (approximately 30 min after programming) which appears to be truly CTL-independent.[33]

These experiments point out at least two more characteristics of CTLMC which must be incorporated into models. First, programming for lysis is strictly dependent upon direct interaction between the CTL and its target cell. However, once programming has occurred, the target cell lyses independent of the physical presence of the CTL. Second, there is a significant lag period between delivery of lethal hit and actual lysis of the target cell, which may be shortened but not eliminated by the presence of the CTL. This last point indicates that the CTL-dependent lethal hit is not lytic but rather induces changes in the target which eventually lead to lysis. Programming for lysis, while not immediately lethal, is nonetheless irreversible.[20]

C. Differences between CTL- and Complement-Mediated Cytolysis: Colloid Osmotic Lysis

Cytolysis mediated by antibody and complement has often been used as a model for

CTLMC. Indeed more than one model has been put forward which suggest that the CTL like complement produces primary membrane damage which is followed by colloid osmotic lysis.[30,38-40] In the case of antibody and complement, colloid osmotic lysis is said to occur when the permeability barrier provided by the plasma membrane becomes compromised so that equilibration of ions (e.g., K^+) takes place between the cell and the medium. The macromolecules inside the cell now exert an unbalanced osmotic pressure across the membrane, leading to a rapid influx of water and release of cytoplasmic contents following membrane rupture.

There has been much debate upon whether colloid osmotic lysis *per se* occurs during CTLMC. While the potassium analog ^{86}Rb is released very early during CTLMC, there does not appear to be a sequential release of cytoplasmic contents according to molecular weight.[41,42] ^{51}Cr-associated material is released at the same time as phosphoryl choline, phosphorylated 3-0-methyl-glucose (a nonmetabolized glucose analog), sucrose, proteins (greater than 25,000 MW) and RNA. These results suggest that cell lysis is an explosive event with cell contents being suddenly released rather than slowly leaking out.[43]

Colloid osmotic lysis is still being used as a model for CTLMC, although it seems most likely that simple colloid osmotic lysis does not account for the death of target cells following interaction with CTL. There is, however, no evidence to rule out that primary damage to the target cell plasma membrane contributes to CTLMC, and much to support such a view.

Several other dissimilarities exist between CTLMC and complement-mediated lysis, some of which focus on internal changes in the target cell which precede ^{51}Cr release:

1. In contrast to CTLMC which is not inhibited by EDTA once lethal hit has been delivered, the lytic phase of complement-mediated lysis can be blocked by EDTA even after release of ^{86}Rb.[24,44]
2. Complement-mediated lysis induces calcium-dependent serotonin release from mast cells, whereas CTL-mediated killing of the same cells does not induce degranulation.[45,46] This is strong evidence that the two mechanisms are fundamentally different.
3. Zeiosis, which is thought to be indicative of cytoskeleton breakdown, occurs during CTLMC but is not observed during antibody and complement-mediated killing of the same target cell.[43]
4. Cells undergoing complement-mediated lysis have the morphology of necrosis, whereas cells killed by CTL have the morphology of apoptosis.[47]
5. The morphological appearance of the nucleus remains unchanged during complement-mediated lysis.[47] Changes in nuclear structure are evident during CTLMC.[48]
6. Very little DNA is released from cells lysed with antibody and complement even after all of the cytoplasmic contents have been released.[50,51] In CTLMC, the slow release of DNA was used to argue in favor of colloid osmotic lysis, based on its large size. The important point which may have been missed was that a massive proportion of target cell DNA is released during CTLMC,[28,29] and its size is much smaller than intact chromatin.[2,3,49]

D. Changes in Nuclear Structure

One of the earliest morphological changes in targets of CTL is widespread condensation of nuclear chromatin, the hallmark of apoptosis.[52] Apoptosis is the term which denotes the morphology of "programmed" cell death and is used to differentiate certain forms of cell death from accidental death or necrosis.[47,52,53]

Apoptosis and necrosis can be differentiated on the basis of both induction and morphology. It can be generalized that necrosis is induced in circumstances of wide departure from physiological conditions including: hypoxia;[54] inhibition of oxidative phosphorylation, glycolysis or Krebs cycle enzymes;[55-57] hyperthermia;[58] and following damage induced by antibody and complement.[47,59,60] The dominant event in necrosis appears to be loss of control of cell volume. Intracellular organelles, in particular mitochondria, as well as the cell itself are observed to swell. This culminates in the rupture of plasma and internal membranes and leakage of cellular contents.[47]

Apoptosis, in contrast to necrosis, occurs in normal tissue turnover,[61-63] embryogenesis,[64,65] metamorphosis,[66,67] hormone-induced tissue atrophy,[62,63,68,69] upon removal of growth factors from dependent cells,[70,71] and following low doses of X-irradiation.[72] The morphological characteristics of apoptosis are progressive contraction of cellular volume and extensive chromatin condensation with preservation of the integrity of cytoplasmic organelles. Eventually the cell lyses, and membrane-bound cellular contents are released.

In addition to the morphological characteristics associated with apoptosis, Wyllie has shown that fragmentation of the nuclear chromatin into oligonucleosomes correlates with chromatin condensation in thymocytes treated with glucocorticoids.[68]

CTL-mediated cytolysis, in contrast to complement-mediated lysis, has the morphology of apoptosis.[2,49,53,73-79] Killing is associated with chromatin condensation in the target cell nucleus. Russell et al.[2,49,80,81] have shown that nuclear damage occurs during CTLMC. Nuclear damage was detected by the appearance of detergent-soluble DNA, and it was suggested that breakdown of the target cell nuclear membrane breakdown occurs during CTLMC. Detergent soluble DNA was not observed during complement-mediated cytolysis, once again indicating significant differences between the two types of death.[80,81]

Work in our laboratory has confirmed Wyllie's observations that DNA fragmentation is an early event during glucocorticoid-induced killing of thymocytes,[69] and we have extended these studies to demonstrate that DNA fragmentation is prominent after low-dose irradiation of lymphocytes[82] and removal of IL-2 from dependent T cells.[4] In order to clarify the role of nuclear changes during CTLMC, we decided to examine the changes in nuclear chromatin in the targets of CTL.

III. DNA FRAGMENTATION INDUCED DURING CTLMC

A. DNA Fragmentation Assay

Assays of CTL-mediated cytolysis have previously been described which measure release of radiolabeled DNA;[28,80,83,84] however, these assays did not establish whether the DNA released during target cell lysis was fragmented. Wyllie[68] had described a chemical method for determination of fragmented DNA during glucocorticoid-induced thymocyte death. This assay was not suited for use in CTL studies. A new isotopic assay was devised, based on Wyllie's technique, to determine the proportion of target cell DNA fragmented during CTL-mediated cytolysis.

In this assay, target cells are labelled in their DNA with ^{125}IUdR and/or in their cytoplasm with ^{51}Cr, mixed with CTL, and placed in microfuge tubes. The cells are subjected to very slow speed centrifugation to establish cell-to-cell contact[18] and are placed at 37°C. At the end of the incubation period, intact cells and large cell debris are separated from the culture medium by centrifugation (200 × g; 10 min). The medium contains fragmented but not intact DNA[3] and ^{51}Cr-associated material which has been released from lysed target cells.[6,34] Release of ^{51}Cr from target cells is commonly used as a measure of target cell lysis.

Since the cells which contain fragmented DNA may not yet have undergone lysis during the incubation period, it is necessary to do one more procedure in order to calculate the total fragmented DNA induced in the target cells during CTL-mediated cytolysis. Therefore, the pelleted cells are lysed by addition of hypotonic buffer, and the lysates subjected to high speed centrifugation (13,000 × g; 10 min). The 13,000 × g supernatant contains only fragmented DNA, whereas the 13,000 × g pellet contains predominantly intact DNA. The percent fragmented DNA is calculated as the proportion of the total radioactivity (incubation

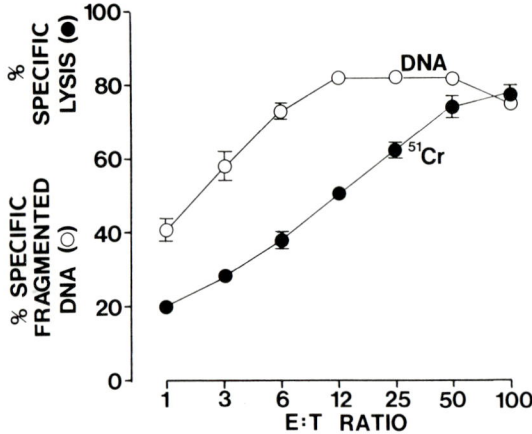

FIGURE 2.. Dose-response curve of induction of DNA fragmentation during CTL-mediated cytolysis. P815 cells labelled with ^{125}IUdR and ^{51}Cr were incubated with CBA/J anti-BALB/cJ MLR blasts at various E:T ratios. Specific DNA fragmentation (○) and ^{51}Cr release (●) were determined after 4 hr incubation.

medium + 13,000 × g supernatant and pellet) present in the incubation medium and 13,000 × g supernatant. Thus, percent released DNA and fragmented DNA are calculated from the following formulae:

$$\% \text{ released DNA} = \frac{^{125}\text{I in incubation medium}}{\text{total }^{125}\text{I}} \times 100$$

$$\% \text{ fragmented DNA} = \frac{^{125}\text{I in (inc. med. + 13,000 × g supernatant)}}{\text{total }^{125}\text{I}} \times 100$$

Target cells incubated in the absence of CTL release very small amounts of ^{125}I-labeled material and are found to contain up to 20% ^{125}IUdR-associated material which does not sediment upon centrifugation of cell lysates. In order to correct for spontaneous release and apparent fragmentation of DNA from control samples, the following formula is used:

$$\% \text{ specific released or fragmented DNA} = \frac{e - s}{m - s} \times 100$$

where e = the experimental value for percent fragmented DNA, s = the spontaneous value for percent fragmented DNA, and m = the maximum value for percent fragmented DNA. In contrast to maximum ^{51}Cr release, which is quantitated by lysing the cells by freeze/thawing or with hypotonic buffer, the maximum value for fragmented DNA cannot be readily determined. However, based upon experimental observations and theoretical considerations, the maximum value for DNA fragmentation can be set at 90%.

B. Induction of DNA Fragmentation in Target Cells by CTL

To investigate the changes in target cell DNA during CTL-mediated cytolysis, DNA fragmentation and ^{51}Cr release were determined during 4 hr dose-response experiments employing various effector to target (E:T) ratios. With increasing numbers of CTL added to a constant number of ^{125}IUdR and ^{51}Cr labeled target cells, there is a concomitant increase in both the percent specific fragmented DNA and in the percent specific ^{51}Cr released from the targets (Figure 2). Similar results have been obtained with a variety of target cells and

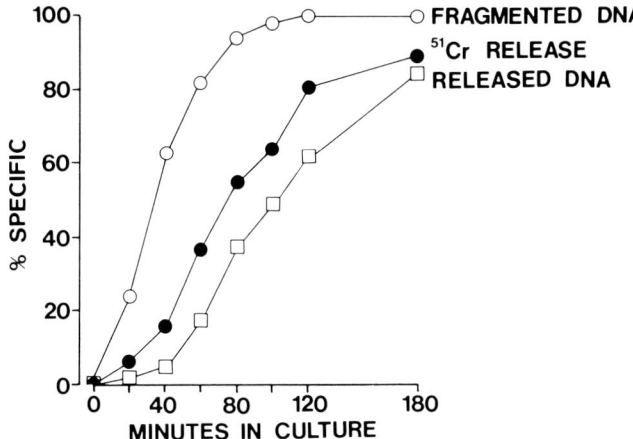

FIGURE 3. Time course of induction of DNA fragmentation during CTL-mediated cytolysis. P815 cells labeled with ^{125}IUdR and ^{51}Cr were incubated with CBA/J anti-BALB/cJ cytotoxic T lymphocytes. Specific fragmented DNA (○), released DNA (□), and ^{51}Cr release (●) were determined at various times after initiation of culture.

CTLs.[3,4] In all instances, the induction of DNA fragmentation, as well as ^{51}Cr release, requires that the CTLs be specific for the target cells used. No DNA fragmentation is observed in bystander cells or in the CTLs themselves during the lytic process.

Cleavage of target cell DNA is induced only by CTL of appropriate specificity, and is not seen when targets are killed by heating, freeze/thawing, interruption of energy production, or lysing with antibody and complement.[3] Thus, DNA fragmentation is the consequence of a specific effector-target cell interaction and not merely a result of cell death.

1. DNA Fragmentation is an Early Event in CTL-Mediated Cytolysis

In order to better understand the induction of DNA fragmentation during CTLMC, time course experiments were performed at constant E:T ratios. DNA fragmentation is always found to be an early event in CTLMC, preceding ^{51}Cr release by 30 to 120 min (Figure 3). The timing of the initiation of DNA fragmentation in target cells, often within minutes of establishment of cell-to-cell contact, suggests that DNA fragmentation is induced very soon after delivery of the lethal hit.

Release of fragmented DNA into the incubation medium was found to parallel ^{51}Cr release. It is apparent from the time course studies that DNA fragmentation, once initiated, always goes rapidly to completion in the target cell, and it is suggested that no lysed target cells contain unfragmented DNA.

2. DNA Fragmentation is Characterized by Production of Oligonucleosomes

After interaction with CTL, DNA in the target cells is fragmented, as evidenced by its failure to sediment upon centrifugation. The size distribution of the DNA fragments isolated from ^{125}IUdR-labeled target cells following interaction with CTL was examined by agarose gel electrophoresis (Figure 4). Only intact DNA is observed when target cells are incubated alone (lane 2), whereas a decreased amount of intact chromatin is seen when CTL are added (lane 4). The fragmented DNA isolated from target cells following interaction with CTL (lane 4) migrates as discrete bands which, by comparison to DNA markers, are multiples of an approximately 200-base pair subunit.[3] Release of DNA fragments into the incubation medium occurs during CTLMC, and this DNA also consists of oligonucleosome-sized subunits (lane 3).

These findings suggest that DNA fragmentation results from activation of an endonuclease

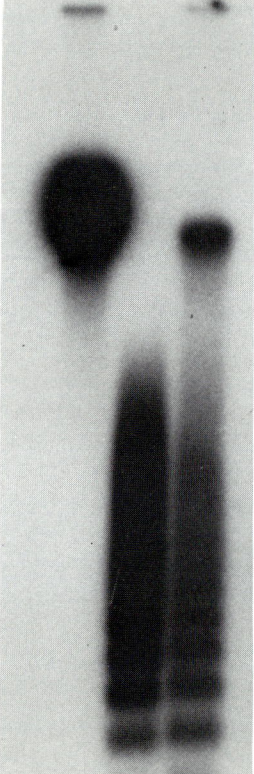

FIGURE 4. Electrophoresis of DNA isolated from incubation medium (lanes 1,3) or from ^{125}IUdR-labeled P815 cells (lanes 2,4) after 90 min incubation alone or with CTL. Electrophoresis in 0.75% agarose was for 2 hr at 85 V. DNA was visualized by autoradiography.

in the target cell nucleus which cleaves DNA in the linker region between nucleosomes. These results are in agreement with those of Russell et al.,[2,49] who have found that a "nuclear lesion" involving degradation of target cell DNA occurs during CTLMC. DNA fragmentation does not appear to go beyond production of nucleosome-sized fragments, indicating that the endonuclease activated during CTLMC is restricted in its activity by chromatin superstructure. The electrophoretic pattern of target cell DNA fragments following interaction with CTL is identical to that found by Hewish and Burgoyne[85] in isolated liver, thymus, and spleen nuclei after activation of the endogenous, Ca^{++} and Mg^{++}-dependent endonuclease and by Wyllie[68] in thymocytes being killed by glucocorticoids. In addition, we have found this pattern after low dose-irradiation of lymphocytes and following removal of growth factor from IL-2-dependent T cells.[4,69]

Table 1
REQUIREMENTS FOR RELEASE OF DNA FRAGMENTS FROM INTACT CELLS OR ISOLATED NUCLEI FOLLOWING VARIOUS EXPERIMENTAL TREATMENTS

			Release of DNA from:			
			Intact cells[a]		Isolated nuclei[b]	
Buffer	Mg^{++}	Triton	Alone	+ CTL	Alone	+ Nuclease
1. Isotonic	+	−	No	No	No	No
2. Isotonic	+	+	No	Yes	No	No
3. Hypotonic	−	−	No	Yes	No	Yes
4. Hypotonic	−	+	No	Yes	ND	ND
5. Isotonic	−	−	ND	ND	No	Yes
6. Hypotonic	+	−	ND	ND	No	No
7. Isotonic + trypsin	+	−	ND	ND	No	Yes

Note: ND, not determined.

[a] P815 cells labeled with ^{125}IUdR were incubated in tissue culture medium alone or with CBA anti-BALB/c CTL. After 30 min, Trition X-100 (final conc. 0.5%) was added to some of the cultures, or the cells were harvested by centrifugtaion and resuspended in hypotonic buffer (10 mM Tris, 1 mM EDTA, pH 7.4) with (line 4) or without (line 3) Triton X-100. The cells from each condition were then centrifuged (200 × g; 10 min), and the radioactivity present in the supernatants was measured. Release of fragmented DNA from target cells incubated for 30 min in the presence or absence of CTL was negligible (line 1).

[b] Nuclei isolated from ^{125}IUdR-labeled P815 cells were incubated in isotonic buffer (150 mM NaCl, 10 mM Tris, 10 mM MgCl$_2$, 5 mM CaCl$_2$, pH 7.4) with or without murine spleen endonuclease.[4] After 90 min, Triton X-100 (line 2) or trypsin (line 7) was added to some of the cultures, or the nuclei were harvested by centrifugation and resuspended: in isotonic buffer containing MgCl$_2$ (150 mM NaCl, 10 mM Tris, 10 mM MgCl$_2$; line 1); in isotonic buffer lacking MgCl$_2$ (150 mM NaCl, 10 mM Tris; line 5); in hypotonic buffer containing MgCl$_2$ (10 mM Tris, 10 mM MgCl$_2$; line 6); or in hypotonic buffer lacking MgCl$_2$ (10 mM Tris, 1 mM EDTA; line 3). After vortexing, the nuclei were centrifuged (200 × g; 10 min) and the radioactivity present in the supernatants was measured. Release of fragmented DNA from nuclei incubated in the presence or absence of endonuclease and harvested in isotonic buffer containing MgCl$_2$ was negligible (line 1).

3. Breakdown of DNA-Nucleoprotein Interactions in Target Cells is an Early Event in CTLMC

CTL induce other nuclear damage besides DNA fragmentation. When target cells containing fragmented DNA are lysed by addition of Triton X-100, the fragmented DNA does not co-sediment with the nuclear fractions.[2,4,49,80,81] This means that the DNA fragments are already in the cytoplasm or are still in the nucleus but are readily released from it by the detergent. This is a very different result from that obtained when DNA in isolated normal nuclei is cleaved into oligonucleosome-sized fragments with endogenous or added endonuclease:[4,86,87] almost all of the fragmented DNA under these circumstances remains associated with the nuclei, even when treated with Triton X-100 (Table 1). To release fragmented DNA from these nuclei requires treatment with trypsin or removal of magnesium. These treatments disrupt the DNA-nucleoprotein interactions which are responsible for the overall structure of chromatin;[87-90] even extensively fragmented DNA is not released from nuclei unless there is a breakdown in the nucleoprotein backbone that stabilizes chromatin superstructure.[87]

The appearance of detergent-soluble DNA after exposure to CTL indicates that normal DNA-nucleoprotein interactions have been disrupted; that is, breakdown of overall nuclear structure occurs in addition to (not as a consequence of) DNA fragmentation during CTL-mediated cytolysis. The rapid onset of DNA fragmentation[3] and the fact that all the DNA

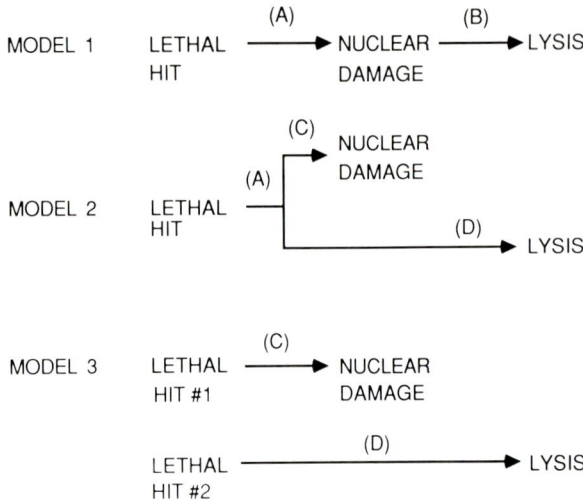

FIGURE 5. Schematic representation of models which can be used to investigate the relationship between induction of DNA fragmentation and ^{51}Cr release during CTL-mediated cytolysis. Letters represent possible sites of action of inhibitors.

fragments are detergent-soluble[4] have not yet allowed us to ascertain which biochemical change is induced first by CTL. These results confirm those obtained by Russell et al.[2,49] although he explained detergent-soluble DNA as resulting from nuclear membrane breakdown rather than disruption of DNA-nucleoprotein interactions.

IV. THE RELATIONSHIP BETWEEN DNA FRAGMENTATION AND TARGET CELL LYSIS

A. Testable Models

The results presented so far have shown that changes in nuclear structure precede target cell death by a significant amount of time. The key question is: What is the relationship between nuclear damage and lysis of the target cell? In this section we will discuss the results of studies performed to investigate this relationship, first by examining simple models. Figure 5 shows the three models which can be drawn to relate DNA fragmentation and ^{51}Cr release to one another and to the lethal hit.

In model 1, the binding of the CTL and target cell leads to delivery of a single lethal hit which induces target cell nuclear damage. DNA fragmentation leads directly to and is the cause of lysis. In model 1 some inhibitors might block DNA fragmentation and therefore lysis (A) while others would block only lysis (B). This model predicts that lysis could not take place in the absence of prior DNA fragmentation; thus, if conditions could be found in which lysis occurred while the nucleus remained intact, this model will be disproved.

In model 2 a single lethal hit triggers both nuclear damage and lysis, although the pathways to these events are separate. In model 3 the lethal hit for each event is also separate. Models 2 and 3 can only be differentiated by studies on the mechanism of lethal hit. For practical purposes only model 2 will be considered. In this model a single lethal hit event induces both DNA fragmentation and ^{51}Cr release; but lysis is not directly dependent upon DNA fragmentation. DNA fragmentation could merely be an early marker of lethal hit delivery, or might synergize with the lytic process to hasten or ensure cell death. This question will be discussed further.

The use of inhibitors might help determine whether model 1 or model 2 is more likely to be correct. Inhibitors of lethal hit delivery would block both DNA fragmentation and ^{51}Cr

Table 2
REQUIREMENT FOR EXTRACELLULAR CALCIUM IN THE INDUCTION OF DNA FRAGMENTATION DURING CYTOTOXIC T LYMPHOCYTE-MEDIATED CYTOLYSIS

Buffer	Mg^{++} (mM)	Ca^{++} (mM)	Ions added	% Specific fragmented DNA	% Specific ^{51}Cr release
TCM[a]	—	—	—	95	89
CMF[b]	—	—	—	2	13
	5	—	—	0	6
	—	2	—	62	65
	5	2	—	87	85
	5	—	5 mM Sr^{++}	65	82

[a] TCM = RPMI 1640 tissue culture medium supplemented with 50 μM 2-mercaptoethanol and 5% fetal calf serum. RPMI 1640 contains 2 mM Mg^{++} and 2 mM Ca^{++}.

[b] CMF = calcium- and magnesium-free medium (135 mM NaCl, 5 mM KCl, 4 mM glucose, phenol red, 25 mM Hepes, pH 7.4) supplemented with 50 μM 2-mercaptoethanol and 5% fetal calf serum which had been dialyzed exhaustively against 150 mM NaCl. P815 target cells labeled with $^{125}IUdR$ and ^{51}Cr were incubated wtih CBA anti-BALB CTL. CTL and target cells were washed extensively in CMF prior to addition to culture tubes. DNA fragmentation and ^{51}Cr release were determined after 4 hr incubation at 37°C.

release, while other inhibitors could, as in model 1, block only ^{51}Cr release (D). Unlike model 1, however, in model 2 it is possible for an inhibitor to exist which can block DNA fragmentation (C) without blocking ^{51}Cr release.

B. The Induction of DNA Fragmentation and Target Cell Lysis Require Extracellular Calcium

When CTL and target cells were incubated in calcium- and magnesium-free medium, DNA fragmentation and ^{51}Cr release were not observed until calcium and magnesium were added back (Table 2). Since the lethal hit event in CTL-mediated cytolysis is strictly calcium-dependent,[11,20] this result indicates that nuclear changes and plasma membrane damage are, as all models assume, post-lethal hit events.

C. Only Target Cells Which have Already Been Induced to Fragment Their DNA Lyse During the Killer Cell-Independent Phase of CTLMC

In order to study the timing of post-lethal hit events more precisely, CTL pretreated with anti-Thy-1 antibody were incubated with target cells (Figure 6). At various times after initiation of culture, the CTL were rapidly killed by addition of complement and the targets incubated for a total of 4 hr before determination of DNA fragmentation and lysis (dotted lines). This treatment, as reported in the literature,[20] stopped further delivery of the lethal hit signal, but did not effect killer cell-independent lysis. At the time of addition of complement, DNA fragmentation and ^{51}Cr release were determined in parallel cultures (solid lines). Comparing the two curves generated by this protocol showed that removal of CTLs prevented further DNA fragmentation, while ^{51}Cr release eventually caught up to the level of DNA fragmentation; that is, only those target cells which had fragmented their DNA went on to lyse in the absence of CTLs. Since the numbers do not allow the alternative explanation — that separate but equal numbers of targets are either fragmenting their DNA or lysing, but not both — this observation suggests that DNA fragmentation and ^{51}Cr release are induced in the same cell as a result of the same lethal hit event. While these experiments

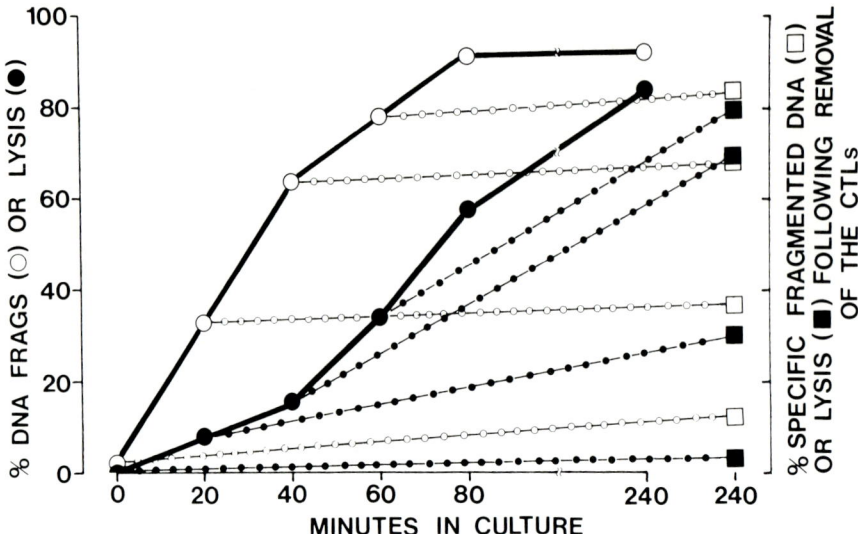

FIGURE 6. Effect of addition of complement to conjugates of target cells and anti-Thy-1 pre-treated cytotoxic T lymphocytes on DNA fragmentation and ^{51}Cr release. C57B1/6 anti-BALB/c CTL were treated with monoclonal anti-Thy-1 antibody for 30 min at 4°C prior to incubation with P815 target cells. At various times after initiation of culture DNA fragmentation (○) and ^{51}Cr release (●) were determined in some cultures (solid lines), while guinea pig complement was added to parallel samples. DNA fragmentation (□) and ^{51}Cr release (■) were determined in cultures to which complement was added after a total of 4 hr incubation (dotted lines).

were very helpful in establishing a single lethal hit event, and thus making model 3 unlikely, they do not yet allow us to differentiate between models 1 and 2 in Figure 5.

D. The Effect of Various Inhibitors on DNA Fragmentation and ^{51}Cr Release During CTLMC

Several other experimental treatments and inhibitors were tested in order to further characterize the linkage between DNA fragmentation and target cell lysis. The results of these studies are summarized in Figure 7, and are similar to what has been reported in the literature.[43,46] The majority of the inhibitors of CTL-mediated cytolysis (EDTA, EGTA, TLCK, TPCK, zinc[3] and cold) apparently block delivery of the lethal hit, as they abrogated both DNA fragmentation and ^{51}Cr release (data not shown).

In addition to blocking delivery of the lethal hit, cold temperatures appeared to block ^{51}Cr release independent of lethal hit delivery. In these experiments cultures of CTL and target cells were transferred to the cold at various times after delivery of the lethal hit had occurred, as determined by induction of DNA fragmentation. At every time-point, transfer to cold temperatures blocked further DNA fragmentation and prevented lysis of target cells which had already fragmented their DNA. These results are in agreement with those in the literature concerning the inhibition of post-lethal hit target cell lysis by cold temperature,[27,29] but still do not help us choose model 1 or model 2.

One inhibitor, manganese, prevented target cell lysis without blocking the induction of DNA fragmentation.[4] Manganese appears to block an as-yet-undetermined event. This could be at step (B) in model 1 or step (D) in model 2. Manganese shows that lysis is not an inevitable rapid response to DNA fragmentation in target cells.

No inhibitor was found which blocked DNA fragmentation without also blocking ^{51}Cr release. Since absence of evidence is not evidence of absence, the studies of inhibitors of CTL-mediated cytolysis, while interesting, do not yet allow us to choose between the models presented in Figure 7.

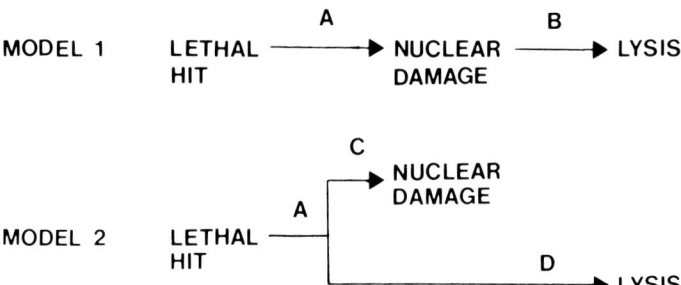

FIGURE 7. The effect of inhibitors on CTL-mediated cytolysis and their most likely site of action:

Inhibitor	Inhib. DNA fragments	Inhib. ^{51}Cr release	Most likely site of action
EDTA, EGTA	Yes	Yes	Pre-lethal hit and/or (A)
TLCK, TPCK	Yes	Yes	Pre-lethal hit and/or (A)
Zinc	Yes	Yes	Pre-lethal hit and/or (A)
Cold Temp.	Yes	Yes	All Stages of CTLMC
Manganese	No	Yes	(B) or (D)

E. Does DNA Fragmentation Inevitably Lead to Lysis?

A more direct approach was thus undertaken to answer the question: Does DNA fragmentation inevitably lead to lysis, and if so, how and with what kinetics? A cell whose DNA is extensively fragmented will be severely compromised in its ability to synthesize new proteins. Is it possible that cessation of target cell protein synthesis could account for the rapid lysis observed following interaction with CTL? When target cells were incubated with protein or RNA synthesis inhibitors, cell death did not occur for at least 24 hr.[3] Thus it is unlikely that DNA fragmentation-induced inhibition of protein synthesis is solely responsible for the rapid lysis of the target cell.

In addition to DNA fragmentation, however, the target cell nuclear structure is also damaged during CTL-mediated cytolysis. Is it possible that disruption of the DNA-nucleoprotein interactions which normally stabilize nuclei lead to cell lysis? Induction of DNA fragmentation and disruption of the stabilizing DNA-nucleoprotein interactions may allow the fragmented DNA to contribute to the overall osmotic pressure of the cell. Fragmented DNA is colloidal in nature compared to intact chromatin, and since it is rapidly solubilized, it could contribute to an osmotic influx of water into the cell, eventually leading to lysis. But as previously discussed, colloid osmotic lysis is probably not a major event in CTLMC.

In order to further investigate the idea that nuclear damage leads directly to cell death, let us compare CTL-mediated cytolysis to unrelated systems in which DNA fragmentation also precedes cell death. DNA fragmentation is an early event in glucocorticoid-induced thymocyte death and death of activated T cells following removal of IL-2. Death in these two systems also has the morphology of apoptosis,[68,70,71] and it has been suggested that both are examples of programmed cell death. Plasma membrane breakdown is observed some 4 to 6 hr after induction of DNA fragmentation.[4,61-62,68,69] The results presented in this review and those of other investigators[2,49,53,77] suggest that CTL-mediated cytolysis involves the same changes in nuclear structure (chromatin condensation and oligonucleosome production) as are observed in examples of programmed cell death. Therefore, if CTL induce the final biochemical events of programmed cell death, then lysis would be expected to begin some 4 to 6 hr after the induction of DNA fragmentation.

However, target cell lysis occurs with faster kinetics following induction of DNA fragmentation in CTL-mediated cytolysis (30 to 60 min) than in the glucocorticoid or IL-2

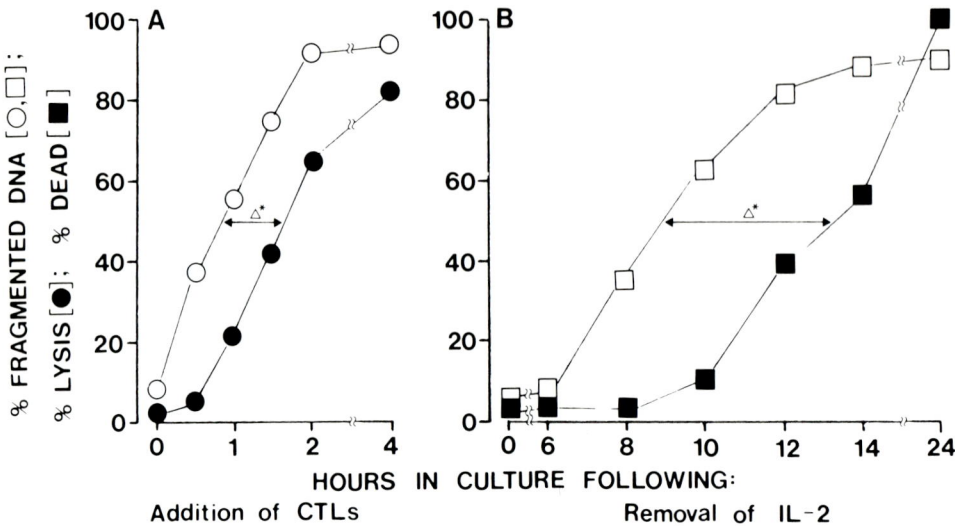

FIGURE 8. Comparison of CTL- vs. growth factor removal-mediated killing of IL-2-dependent CTLL-20 cells. (A) Time course of DNA fragmentation and ^{51}Cr release from CTLL-20 cells mediated by cytotoxic T cells. ^{125}IUdR and ^{51}Cr-labeled CTLL-20 target cells were mixed with BALB/c anti-C57B1/6 CTL. Specific DNA fragmentation (○) and ^{51}Cr release (●) were determined at various times after initiation of culture. (B) Time course of DNA fragmentation and cell death following removal of IL-2 from CTLL-20 cells. CTLL-20 cells labeled with ^{125}IUdR were incubated without IL-2. DNA fragmentation (□) and cell death (■), as measured by eosin uptake, were determined at various times after initiation of culture. DNA fragmentation and cell death in ^{125}IUdR-labeled CTLL-20 cells incubated in the presence of IL-2 were less than 10% at all time points (data not shown). *;Δ = the additional incubation times required for 50% ^{51}Cr release (●) or cell death (■) after induction of 50% fragmented DNA in CTLL-20 cells were: (A) for CTL-mediated cytolysis Δ = 45 min; and (B) for IL-2 removal-induced death Δ = 4 hr.

systems. This is a real difference in mechanism, and not just due to differences in target cell phenotype, as is readily apparent when the kinetics of lysis of the same cells (CTLL-20 cells) are compared during CTL-mediated cytolysis and following removal of IL-2 (Figure 8).

In truly programmed cell death, it is reasonable to assume that the induction of DNA fragmentation and the changes in nuclear structure observed as apoptosis, contribute directly to cell death which occurs several hours later. In CTL-mediated cytolysis, however, something beside changes in nuclear structure must occur to account for the accelerated rate of lysis. It seems probable that the CTL directly damages the target cell membrane, which either leads directly to lysis or hastens its demise. This last statement is supported by two observations in the literature:

1. Enucleated cells can serve as targets for CTL-mediated cytolysis.[91-94] Obviously, a nuclear lesion cannot play a role here.
2. The time for target cell lysis to occur, but not for delivery of the lethal hit, may be significantly shortened by increasing the number of CTLs conjugated to a single target[33,37] or by increasing the amount of time that the CTL remains conjugated to the target following lethal hit delivery.[1,36] How does the CTL, by its continued presence, shorten the time to lysis? The rapid kinetics of induction of DNA fragmentation, once lethal hit is delivered, make it unlikely that the CTL could either induce more fragmentation or more rapid fragmentation. If, however, the CTL directly induces target cell membrane damage, then the amount of time the CTL is conjugated to the target or the number of CTL conjugated to a single target could affect the time interval required for lysis to occur.

MODEL 1

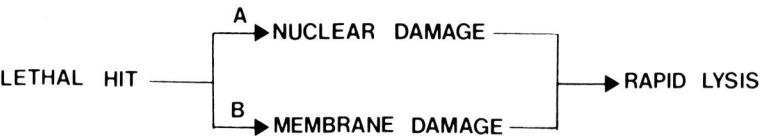

MODEL 2

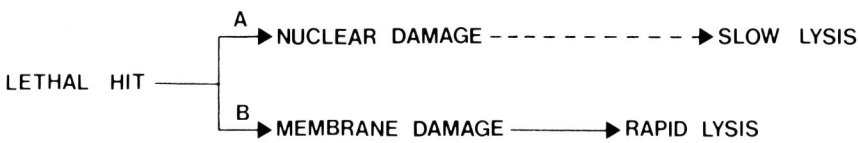

FIGURE 9. Schematic representation of models which account for rapid CTL-mediated cytolysis.

V. A MODEL OF CTLMC INVOLVING SYNERGY BETWEEN EXTERNAL AND INTERNAL DAMAGE INDUCED IN THE TARGET CELL BY CTL

In this discussion, nuclear damage has been shown to be an early event in CTL-mediated cytolysis. Target cell death, as measured by ^{51}Cr release, and changes in nuclear structure arise as a result of what is probably a single lethal hit event. As we have seen, nuclear damage alone cannot account for rapid target cell lysis. In addition, it has been suggested that the CTL can directly damage the target cell membrane. The observations which have been made during the study of CTL-mediated cytolysis suggest two closely-related models (Figure 9) whose steps are as follows:

1. The CTL and target cell bind via specific receptor-ligand interaction.
2. Following binding, a single lethal hit event occurs.
3. Two events result from the lethal hit:
   a. DNA fragmentation and breakdown of the overall nuclear structure are induced in the target.
   b. The CTL is activated such that that it inflicts direct target cell membrane damage.
4. Target cell lysis is rapid due to either synergy between nuclear changes and plasma membrane damage (model 1) or as a result of plasma membrane damage alone (model 2).

In model 1, nuclear and membrane damage synergize to produce rapid lysis. In the absence of membrane damage, lysis would occur, but with slower kinetics. What is not clear is whether lysis could occur in the absence of nuclear damage; if it did, the model predicts slower kinetics. This last point may be quite important if the membrane damage induced by the CTL is either nonlethal or reparable. Cells can repair membrane lesions, including those induced by complement.[44,95] (Volume I, Chapter 10). In CTL-mediated cytolysis, minimal target cell membrane damage might kill the target slowly unless the target cell had also undergone nuclear damage. The combination of extensive nuclear damage (increased osmotic pressure due to fragmented DNA?) and some membrane damage would cause rapid lysis of the target cell. In model 1, both nuclear and membrane damage are required for rapid lysis, although each may independently kill the target cell with somewhat slower kinetics.

In model 2, nuclear damage occurs as a result of the lethal hit, but is not at all required for rapid lysis. In this model, target cell membrane damage is not reparable but rapidly lyses the target. Due to the lethal nature of the membrane damage, model 2 requires a highly active mediator whose mechanism could account for the well-known lack of bystander killing and CTL self-destruction. In contrast, membrane damage can be sublethal in model 1 and therefore would have no demonstrable effect on the CTL itself or bystander cells.

The results which have been presented in this discussion do not allow us to choose between models 1 and 2. It is obvious that studies can be performed to see which model is correct. In model 1, blocking nuclear (A) or membrane damage (B) will abrogate rapid lysis. In model 2, blocking membrane damage (B) will prevent rapid lysis, whereas blocking nuclear damage (A) should have no effect.

The key experimental approach to deciding which model is correct would involve searching for a system in which CTLs could induce rapid lysis of target cells in the absence of nuclear changes. In brief, this could be achieved in two ways.

The first system in which the requirement for nuclear changes could be assessed is one in which either the CTL or target cell have been altered such that nuclear changes can no longer be induced during CTL-mediated cytolysis. The most obvious example is one we have already mentioned: CTL-mediated killing of enucleated cells. Nuclear changes certainly are not induced in this instance. What is not clear from the literature, however, are the kinetics of lysis of enucleated cells. In all the studies which have been reported,[91-94] fixed time point assays (4 hr) have been used, and so it is not clear whether cytoplasts are lysed as rapidly as intact target cells. Time-point studies would be crucial to determine if, in the absence of nuclear changes, lysis is still as rapid an event.

In addition to the lack of kinetic data, the relevance of CTL-mediated lysis of enucleated cells to killing of intact cells is unclear. Cytoplasts undergo a great amount of damage during the enucleation process, and therefore, the amount of membrane damage required to lyse a cytoplast may be several times less than for a normal target. This would be especially true if the membrane damage induced by the CTL was either nonlethal or reparable as suggested by model 1 in Figure 9.

Due to the problems associated with enucleated targets, a system involving true mutation of the CTL or target cell such that nuclear damage was not induced would be more appropriate to decide if nuclear changes are required for lysis. While such a mutation may be found, a much simpler test would involve finding an inhibitor which prevents nuclear damage without blocking lysis. To understand how a mutation or inhibitor would interfere with nuclear damage, the requirements which must be met in order for nuclear and/or plasma membrane damage to occur should be discussed.

VI. WHAT IS THE MECHANISM OF INDUCTION OF DNA FRAGMENTATION AND TARGET CELL LYSIS?

A. The Consequences of CTL-Target Cell Binding and Delivery of the Lethal Hit

During CTL-mediated cytolysis, the lethal hit must accomplish two things. First, it must activate the CTL so that it can cause direct damage to the target cell membrane. Activation of the CTL is probably a result of engagement of the CTL antigen receptor. Once activated, any one of several mechanisms which have been proposed to mediate external damage could be invoked. These mechanisms include direct target cell membrane damage mediated by CTL-target cell receptor-ligand interactions,[96,97] as well as secretion of toxins including lytic granules.[98,99] Any of these processes could be involved in CTL-mediated plasma membrane damage provided that they account for the unidirectional nature of the killing process. If the mediators are nonspecific, like lytic granules, then the membrane damage induced by these mediators might be minimal or even reparable to account for the lack of CTL or bystander death.

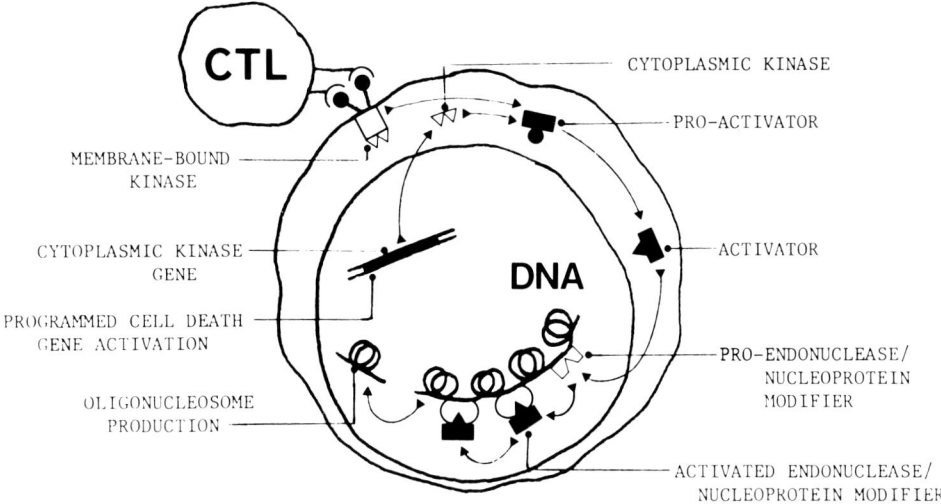

FIGURE 10. Schematic representation of a model in which the final common pathway of programmed cell death may be activated via a protein synthesis-dependent or independent mechanism.

The lethal hit must also initiate the processes which lead to induction of DNA fragmentation and breakdown of overall nuclear structure. The production of oligonucleosome-sized DNA requires an endonuclease, limited in activity by nucleosome structure, while disruption of DNA-nucleoprotein interactions most likely requires modification of nucleoproteins. Nuclear damage could be induced by one of two possible mechanisms:

1. The CTL transfers the relevant enzymes or enzyme activators to the target cell: the target cell plays a passive role.
2. The CTL signals the target cell such that an intrinsic cell death program involving nuclear damage is initiated: the target plays an active role.

B. Activation of a Cell Death Program Intrinsic to the Target Cell

While the CTL could directly transfer the nuclear-modifying enzymes to the target, there is little evidence to support such an idea.[100,101] It cannot, however, be ruled out that the lytic granules contain the endonuclease itself[102] or other factors responsible for activation of the endonuclease in target cells.[103] The similarity between the nuclear changes observed in CTL-mediated cytolysis and apoptotic death, suggest that the CTL may signal the activation of the final common biochemical pathway of programmed cell death. A schematic representation of a model involving signalling is shown in Figure 10. This model accounts for the induction of nuclear changes in programmed cell death and CTL-mediated cytolysis.

In this model, the enzymes which induce DNA fragmentation and disrupt DNA-nucleoprotein interactions are present in all cells as proenzymes. The proenzymes, when activated, encompass the final common pathway of programmed cell death. It is proposed that activation of these enzymes can occur via a protein synthesis-dependent (e.g., via programmed cell death as exemplified by glucocorticoids or IL-2 deprivation[4,69]) or independent pathway (e.g., via CTL-mediated cytolysis[3,4]). Programmed cell death induces synthesis of new proteins (perhaps a protein kinase) which leads to activation of the cell death program.

In CTL-mediated cytolysis, the CTL interacts with the target via specific target cell membrane proteins, and induces DNA fragmentation and cytolysis in a protein synthesis-independent fashion.[3] In a manner synonymous to cell activation, the CTL-target cell membrane interaction leads to activation of a pre-existing plasma membrane-associated protein kinase which in turn activates the final common pathway. Studies are now in progress to elucidate the proteins involved in the induction of nuclear damage in programmed cell death. It is hoped that once the final common pathway is understood, the results may be used to better understand the mechanism of CTL-mediated cytolysis.

C. The Lack of Double-Stranded DNA Fragmentation in Human Target Cells Supports an Intrinsic Cell Death Program

Sears and Christiaansen[104,105] have reported that while mouse and human effector cells induce oligonucleosome fragmentation of mouse target cell DNA, no fragments are observed in human targets. This appears to be the result of differences in the type and degree of fragmentation which occurs in human target cells rather than absence of nuclear damage. Gromkowski et al.[106] have reported that while mouse and human CTLs induce double-stranded breaks in mouse target cell DNA, these effector cells induce single-stranded breaks in human target DNA. Single-stranded breaks in DNA would not be observed in the quantitative assay of DNA fragmentation or in the neutral agarose gels employed by ourselves[3] and Sears and Christiaansen.

The observation of differences in DNA fragmentation patterns which are dependent on the species of the target cell and not on the species of the CTL suggest that DNA fragmentation is the result of an enzyme pathway intrinsic to the target cell which is activated by, but not transferred from, the CTL. The alternative explanation that mouse and human DNA differ dramatically in their susceptibility to a CTL-derived endonuclease is unlikely. No differences in the susceptibility of mouse or human DNA to several endonucleases including micrococcal nuclease, DNase I, or the endogenous endonuclease have been reported.[107,108] Thus, our presumption that all cells contain the proenzymes involved in the fragmentation of DNA observed in programmed cell death and CTLMC may prove to be correct. This idea requires further study.

While differences exist in the pattern of DNA fragmentation observed in human and mouse target cells, studies have not been performed to look for disruption of DNA-nucleoprotein interactions. DNA which contains predominantly single-stranded breaks would be expected to co-sediment with intact chromatin, even in the presence of detergent, and so more intricate experiments must be devised to answer this question. It is most likely that nuclear damage is induced in human target cells but that the nature of the DNA fragmentation does not allow for easy quantitation.

VII. CONCLUSIONS

Further studies must be done in order to determine whether DNA fragmentation and breakdown of nuclear structure are required for CTL-mediated cytolysis. Since DNA fragmentation is such an early and impressive event in CTL-mediated killing, one might ask why a CTL would want to induce target cell nuclear damage if membrane damage was sufficient? Fragmentation of target cell DNA may be important for several reasons including:

1. Damage to the target cell nucleus may assure killing of the target. It has been well-documented that target cells vary in their susceptibility to CTL-mediated cytolysis.[20] These differences are often reflected in the kinetics of lysis, rather than as a true resistance to killing. Recently, it has been observed that target cells vary in their susceptibility to lytic granule-induced membrane damage,[99,109-111] suggesting that target cells differ in their sensitivity to membrane damage. DNA fragmentation would increase the likelihood of killing of target cells which are somewhat resistant to CTL-mediated membrane damage. In addition, extensive DNA fragmentation condemns the target cell to eventual death even in the absence of membrane damage.

2. Damage to the target cell nucleus may contribute to rapid lysis. In addition to guaranteeing that the target cell dies, nuclear damage may also serve to kill the target cell in as short a time as possible. This would be particularly advantageous when dealing with virally infected cells. Several viruses can replicate very rapidly within cells; therefore, the kinetics of lysis of infected cells may play a very important role in the pathology of viral diseases.
3. CTL-induced DNA fragmentation may also degrade viral DNA. There is accumulating evidence that cells in vivo can be transfected directly with viral DNA.[112,113] Thus, mere lysis of a target cell containing perhaps many copies of a viral DNA genome may not assure eradication of the virus. However, activation of an endonuclease could lead to cleavage of viral DNA (and RNA?) present in the target cell and thereby prevent transfection of uninfected cells. Studies are now in progress to investigate the state of viral DNA in infected cells during CTL-mediated cytolysis.

Nature has endowed the cytotoxic T cell with an arsenal of weapons to assure killing of any virally infected or tumor cell. Future studies will continue to concentrate on these diverse mechanisms.

ADDENDUM

In Section V, it was suggested that a system involving true mutation of the CTL or target cell such that nuclear damage could not be induced would be the most appropriate way to decide if nuclear changes are required for cytolysis. Following preparation of this manuscript, David Ucker[114] apparently found such a system and has shown that a mutant clone derived from a steroid-sensitive thymoma is resistant to corticosteroids and cytotoxic T cell-mediated killing whereas the parental cells are sensitive to both. The "deathless" cell is susceptible to lysis by anti-H-2 antibodies plus complement[114] and isolated lytic granules (David Ucker, personal communication). In addition, a revertant cell has been isolated which is sensitive to both steroids and CTL. Thus it appears that the deathless condition results from a mutation which prevents activation of an intrinsic target cell suicide program. The mutant provides strong evidence that induction of target cell nuclear damage is essential for CTL-mediated killing.[115]

ACKNOWLEDGMENT

This work was supported by U.S.-NIH Grant AI-16611.

REFERENCES

1. **Sanderson, C. J.,** The mechanism of lymphocyte-mediated cytotoxicity, *Biol. Rev.*, 56, 153, 1981.
2. **Russell, J. H.,** Internal disintegration model of cytotoxic lymphocyte-induced target damage, *Immunol. Rev.*, 72, 97, 1983.
3. **Duke, R. C., Chervenak, R., and Cohen, J. J.,** Endogenous endonuclease-induced DNA fragmentation: an early event in cell-mediated cytolysis, *Proc. Natl. Acad. Sci. U.S.A.*, 80, 6361, 1983.
4. **Cohen, J. J., Duke, R. C., Chervenak, R., Sellins, K. S., and Olson, L. K.,** DNA fragmentation in targets of CTL: an example of programmed cell death in the immune system, *Adv. Exp. Med. Biol.*, 184, 439, 1985.
5. **MacDonald, H. R., Phillips, R. A., and Miller, R. G.,** Allograft immunity in the mouse. I. Quantitation and specificity of cytotoxic effector cells after *in vitro* sensitization, *J. Immunol.*, 111, 565, 1973.
6. **Cerottini, J.-C. and Brunner, K. T.,** Cell-mediated cytotoxicity, allograft rejection and tumor immunity, *Adv. Immunol.*, 18, 67, 1974.

7. **Gensheimer, G. G. and Neefe, J. R.**, Cell mediated lympholysis: a receptor associated lytic mechanism, *Cell. Immunol.*, 36, 54, 1978.
8. **Ginsburg, H., Ax, W., and Berke, G.**, Functional implications of cellular immunity. An analysis of graft reaction of cell cultures, in *Pharmacological Treatment in Organ Transplantation,* Bertelli, A. and Monaco, A. P., Eds., Excerpta Medica Foundation, Amsterdam, 1970, 85.
9. **Koren, H. S., Ax, W., and Freud-Moelbert, E.**, Morphological observations on the contact induced lysis of target cells, *Eur. J. Immunol.*, 3, 32, 1973.
10. **Zagury, D., Bernard, J., Theirness, N., Feldman, M., and Berke, G.**, Isolation and characterization of individual functionally reactive cytotoxic T lymphocytes: conjugation, killing and recycling at the single cell level, *Eur. J. Immunol.*, 5, 818, 1975.
11. **Golstein, P. and Smith, E. T.**, Mechanism of T-cell-mediated cytolysis: the lethal hit stage, *Contemp. Topics Immunobiol.*, 7, 273, 1977.
12. **Martz, E. and Benaceraff, B.**, Multiple target cell killing by the cytolytic T lymphocyte and the mechanism of cytotoxicity, *Transplantation*, 21, 5, 1976.
13. **Golstein, P.**, Sensitivity of cytotoxic T cells to T cell mediated cytotoxicity, *Nature*, 252, 81, 1974.
14. **Kuppers, R. C. and Henney, C. S.**, Evidence for direct linkage between antigen recognition and lytic expression in effector T cells, *J. Exp. Med.*, 143, 684, 1976.
15. **Kuppers, R. C. and Henney, C. S.**, Studies on the mechanism of lymphocyte mediated cytolysis. IX. Relationships between antigen recognition and lytic expression in killer T cells, *J. Immunol.*, 118, 71, 1977.
16. **Fishelson, Z. and Berke, G.**, T lymphocyte mediated cytolysis: dissociation of the binding and lytic mechanisms of the effector cell, *J. Immunol.*, 120, 1121, 1978.
17. **Wagner, H. and Rollinghoff, M.**, T cell mediated cytotoxicity: discrimination between antigen recognition, lethal hit and cytolysis phase, *Eur. J. Immunol.*, 4, 745, 1974.
18. **Martz, E.**, Early steps in specific tumor cell lysis by sensitized mouse T-lymphocytes. I. Resolution and characterization, *J. Immunol.*, 115, 261, 1975.
19. **Golstein, P. and Smith, E. T.**, The lethal hit stage of mouse T and non-T cell-mediated cytolysis: differences in cation requirements and characterization of an analytical "cation pulse" method, *Eur. J. Immunol.*, 6, 31, 1976.
20. **Martz, E.**, Mechanism of specific tumor cell lysis by alloimmune T lymphocytes: resolution and characterization of discrete steps in the cellular interaction, *Contemp. Top. Immunobiol.*, 7, 301, 1977.
21. **Mauel, J., Rudolf, H., Chapuis, B., and Brunner, K. T.**, Studies on allograft immunity in mice. II. Mechanism of target cell inactivation *in vitro* by sensitized lymphocytes, *Immunology*, 18, 517, 1970.
22. **Henney, C. S. and Bubbers, J. E.**, Studies on the mechanism of lymphocyte-mediated cytolysis. I. The role of divalent cations in cytolysis by T lymphocytes, *J. Immunol.*, 110, 63, 1973.
23. **Martz, E. and Benaceraff, B.**, An effector cell independent step in target cell lysis by sensitized mouse lymphocytes, *J. Immunol.*, 111, 1538, 1973.
24. **Martz, E.**, Inability of EDTA to prevent damage mediated by cytolytic T lymphocytes, *Cell. Immunol.*, 20, 304, 1975.
25. **MacDonald, H. R.**, Early detection of potentially lethal events in T-cell mediated cytolysis, *Eur. J. Immunol.*, 5, 251, 1975.
26. **Miller, R. G. and Dunkley, M.**, Quantitative analyses of the ^{51}Cr release cytotoxicity assay for cytotoxic lymphocytes, *Cell. Immunol.*, 14, 284, 1974.
27. **Sanderson, C. J. and Taylor, G. A.**, The kinetics of ^{51}Cr release from target cells in cell mediated cytotoxicity and the relationship to the kinetics of killing, *Cell Tiss. Kinetics*, 8, 23, 1975.
28. **Henney, C. S.**, Studies on the mechanism of lymphocyte-mediated cytolysis. II. The use of various target cell markers to study cytolytic events, *J. Immunol.*, 110, 73, 1973.
29. **Martz, E., Burakoff, S. J., and Benacerraf, B.**, Interruption of the sequential release of small and large molecules from tumor cells by low temperature during cytolysis mediated by immune T-cells or complement, *Proc. Natl. Acad. Sci. U.S.A.*, 71, 177, 1974.
30. **Ferluga, J. and Allison, A. C.**, Observations on the mechanism by which T lymphocytes exert cytotoxic effects, *Nature*, 250, 673, 1974.
31. **Martz, E.**, Early steps in specific tumor cell lysis by sensitized mouse T lymphocytes. II. Electrolyte permeability increase in the target cell membrane concomitant with programming for lysis, *J. Immunol.*, 117, 1023, 1976.
32. **Martz, E., Heagy, W., and Gromkowski, H.**, The mechanism of CTL-mediated killing: monoclonal antibody analysis of the roles of killer and target cell membrane proteins, *Immunol. Rev.*, 72, 73, 1983.
33. **Perelson, A. S., Macken, C. A., Grimm, E. A., Roos, L. S., and Bonavida, B.**, Mechanism of cell-mediated cytotoxicity at the single cell level. VIII. Kinetics of lysis of target cells bound by more than one cytotoxic T lymphocyte, *J. Immunol.*, 132, 2190, 1984.

34. **Brunner, K. T. Mauel, J., Cerottini, J.-C., and Chapuis, B.,** Quantitative assay of the lytic action of immune lymphoid cells on ^{51}Cr labelled allogeneic target cells *in vitro*; inhibition by isoantibody and by drugs, *Immunology,* 14, 181, 1968.
35. **Thorn, R. M. and Henney, C. S.,** Studies on the mechanism of lymphocyte mediated cytolysis. IV. A reappraisal of the requirement for protein synthesi during T cell mediated lysis, *J. Immunol.,* 116, 146, 1976.
36. **Macken, C. A. and Perelson, A. S.,** A multistage model for the action of cytotoxic T lymphocytes in multicellular conjugates, *J. Immunol.,* 132, 1614, 1984.
37. **Zagury, D., Bernard, J., Jeannesson, P., Thierness, N., and Cerottini, J.-C.,** Studies on the mechanism of T cell mediated lysis at the single cell level. I. Kinetic analysis of lethal hits and target cell lysis in multicellular conjugates, *J. Immunol.,* 123, 1604, 1979.
38. **Henney, C. S.,** Estimation of the sizes of a T cell lytic lesion, *Nature,* 249, 456, 1974.
39. **Mayer, M. M.,** Mechanism of cytolysis by lymphocytes: a comparison with complement, *J. Immunol.,* 119, 1195, 1977.
40. **Green, W. R. and Henney, C. S.,** The mechanism of T cell mediated cytolysis, *CRC Crit. Rev. Immunol.,* 1, 59, 1981.
41. **Sanderson, C. J.,** The mechanism of T cell mediated cytotoxicity. I. The release of different cell components, *Proc. R. Soc. London Ser. B.,* 192, 221, 1976.
42. **Martz, E.,** Sizes of isotypically labelled molecules released during lysis of tumor cells labelled with ^{51}Cr and [^{14}C]nicotinamide, *Cell Immunol.,* 26, 313, 1976.
43. **Sanderson, C. J.,** Morphological aspects of lymphocyte mediated cytotoxicity, *Adv. Exp. Med. Biol.,* 146, 3, 1982.
44. **Burakoff, S. J., Martz, E., and Benacerraf, B.,** Is the primary complement lesion insufficient for lysis? Failure of cells damaged under osmotic protection to lyse in EDTA or at low temperature after removal of osmotic protection, *Clin. Immunol. Immunopathol.,* 4, 108, 1975.
45. **Ko, L. and Lagunoff, D.,** Depletion of mast cell ATP inhibits complement-dependent cytotoxic histamine release, *Exp. Cell Res.,* 100, 313, 1976.
46. **Martz, E., Parker, W. L., Gately, M. K., and Tsoukas, C. D.,** The role of calcium in the lethal hit of T lymphocyte-mediated cytolysis, *Adv. Exp. Med. Biol.,* 146, 121, 1982.
47. **Wyllie, A. H.,** Cell death: a new classification separating apoptosis from necrosis, in *Cell Death in Biology and Pathology,* Bowen, I. D. and Lockshin, R. A., Eds., Chapman and Hall, London, 1981, 9.
48. **Goldberg, B. and Green, H.,** The cytotoxic action of immune gamma globulin and complement on Krebs ascites tumor cells. I. Ultrastructural studies, *J. Exp. Med.,* 109, 505, 1959.
49. **Russell, J. H., Masakowski, V., Rucinsky, T., and Phillips, G.,** Mechanisms of immune lysis. III. Characterization of the nature and kinetics of the cytotoxic T lymphocyte-induced nuclear lesion in the target, *J. Immunol.,* 128, 2087, 1982.
50. **Colter, J. S., Kritchevsky, D., Bird, H. H., and McCandless, R. F.,** *In vitro* studies with antisera against tumor cell protein fractions, *Cancer Res.,* 17, 272, 1957.
51. **Green, H., Fleischer, R. A., Barrow, P., and Goldberg, B.,** The cytotoxic action of immune gamma globulin and complement on Krebs ascites tumor cells. II. Chemical studies, *J. Exp. Med.,* 109, 511, 1959.
52. **Kerr, J. F. R., Wyllie, A. H., and Currie, A. R.,** Apoptosis: a basic biological phenomenon with wide-ranging implications in tissue kinetics, *Br. J. Cancer,* 26, 239, 1972.
53. **Wyllie, A. H., Kerr, J. F. R., and Currie, A. R.,** Cell death: the significance of apoptosis, *Int. Rev. Cytol.,* 68, 251, 1980.
54. **Jennings, R. B., Ganote, C. E., and Reimer, K. A.,** Ischaemic tissue injury, *Am. J. Pathol.,* 81, 179, 1975.
55. **McDowell, E. M.,** Light and electron microscopic studies of the rat kidney after administration of inhibitors of the citric acid cycle *in vivo*. I. Effects of sodium fluoroacetate on the proximal convoluted tubule, *Am. J. Pathol.,* 66, 513, 1972.
56. **McDowell, E. M.,** Light- and electron-microscope studies of the rat kidney after administration of inhibitors of the citric acid cycle *in vivo*: changes in the proximal convoluted tubule during fluorocititrate poisoning, *J. Pathol.,* 108, 303, 1972.
57. **Laiho, K. U. and Trump, B. F.,** Studies on the pathogenesis of cell injury. Effect of inhibitors of metabolism and membrane function on the mitochondria of Ehrlich ascites tumor cells, *Lab. Invest.,* 32, 163, 1975.
58. **Buckley, I. K.,** A light and electron microscopic study of thermally injured cultured cells, *Lab. Invest.,* 26, 201, 1972.
59. **Prieto, A., Kornblith, P. L., and Pollen, D. A.,** Electrical recordings from meningioma cells during cytolytic action of antibody and complement, *Science,* 157, 1185, 1967.
60. **Hawkins, H. K., Ericsson, J. L. E., Biberfeld, P., and Trump, B. F.,** Lysosome and phagosome stability in lethal cell injury, *Am. J. Pathol.,* 68, 255, 1972.

61. **Kerr, J. F. R. and Searle, J.,** Deletion of cells by apoptosis during castration-induced involution of rat prostate, *Virchows Arch. Abt. B.,* 13, 87, 1973.
62. **Wyllie, A. H., Kerr, J. F. R., Macaskill, I. A. M., and Currie, A. R.,** Adrenocortical cell deletion: the role of ACTH, *J. Pathol.,* 111, 85, 1973.
63. **Wyllie, A. H., Kerr, J. F. R., and Currie, A. R.,** Cell death in the normal neonatal rat adrenal cortex, *J. Pathol.,* 111, 255, 1973.
64. **Schweichel, J. U.,** Electron microscopical studies on the degradation of the apical ridge during the development of limbs in rat embryo, *Z. Anat. Entwicklungsges.,* 136, 192, 1972.
65. **O'Connor, T. M. and Wyttenbach, C. R.,** Cell death in the embryonic chick spinal chord, *J. Cell Biol.,* 60, 448, 1974.
66. **Kerr, J. F. R., Harmon, B., and Searle, J.,** Effect of a transient period of ischaemia on myocardial cells. II. Fine structure during the first few minutes of reflow, *Am. J. Pathol.,* 74, 399, 1974.
67. **Decker, R. S.,** Influence of thyroid hormones on neuronal death and differentiation in larval *Rana pipiens, Dev. Biol.,* 49, 101, 1976.
68. **Wyllie, A. H.,** Glucocorticoid-induced thymocyte apoptosis is associated with endogenous endonuclease activation, *Nature,* 284, 555, 1980.
69. **Cohen, J. J. and Duke, R. C.,** Glucocorticoid activation of a calcium-dependent endonuclease in thymocyte nuclei leads to cell death, *J. Immunol.,* 132, 38, 1984.
70. **Bishop, C. J., Moss, D. J., Ryan, J. M., and Burrows, S. R.,** T lymphocytes in infectious mononucleosis. II. Response *in vitro* to interleukin 2 and establishment of T cell lines, *Clin. Exp. Immunol.,* 60, 70, 1985.
71. **Moss, D. J., and Bishop, C. J., Burrows, S. R., and Ryan, J. M.,** T lymphocytes in infectious mononucleosis. I. T cell death *in vitro, Exp. Immunol.,* 60, 61, 1985.
72. **Searle, J., Lawson, T. A., Abboy, P. J., Harmon, B., and Kerr, J. F. R.,** An electron-microscope study of the mode of cell death induced by cancer-chemotherapeutic agents in populations of proliferating normal and neoplastic cells, *J. Pathol.,* 116, 129, 1975.
73. **Russell, S. W., Rosenau, W., and Lee, J. C.,** Cytolysis induced by human lymphotoxin in target cells, *J. Immunol.,* 111, 1128, 1972.
74. **Battersby, C., Egerton, W. S., Balderson, G., Kerr, J. F., and Burnett, W.,** Another look at rejection of pig liver homografts, *Surgery,* 76, 617, 1974.
75. **Slavin, R. E. and Woodruff, J. M.,** The pathology of bone marrow transplantation, *Pathol. Annu.,* 9, 291, 1974.
76. **Sanderson, C. J.,** The mechanism of T cell mediated cytotoxicity. II. Studies of cell death by time-lapse microcinematography, *Proc. R. Soc. London Ser. B.,* 192, 241, 1976.
77. **Don, M. M., Ablett, G., Bishop, C. J., Bundesen, P. G., Searle, K. J., and Kerr, J. F.,** Death of cells by apoptosis following attachment of specifically allergized lymphocytes *in vitro, Aust. Exp. Biol. Med. Sci.,* 55, 407, 1977.
78. **Matter, A.,** Microcineamtographic and electron microscopic analysis of target cell lysis induced by cytotoxic T lymphocytes, *Immunology,* 36, 179, 1979.
79. **Sanderson, C. J. and Glauert, A. M.,** The mechanism of T-cell mediated cytotoxicity. VI. T-cell projections and their role in target cell killing, *Immunology,* 36, 119, 1979.
80. **Russell, J. H., Masakowski, V. R., and Dobos, C. B.,** Mechanisms of immune lysis. I. Physiological distinction between target cell death mediated by cytotoxic T lymphocytes and antibody plus complement, *J. Immunol.,* 124, 1100, 1980.
81. **Russell, J. H. and Dobos, C. B.,** Mechanisms of immune lysis. II. CTL-induced nuclear disintegration of the target begins within minutes of cell contact, *J. Immunol.,* 125, 1256, 1980.
82. **Sellins, K. and Cohen, J. J.,** Protein synthesis-dependent induction of endogenous endonuclease in irradiated thymocytes, *Fed. Proc.,* 43, 1640, 1984.
83. **Klein, G. and Perlmann, P.,** *In vitro* cytotoxic effect of isoantibody measured as isotope release from target cell DNA, *Nature,* 199, 451, 1963.
84. **Holm, G. and Perlmann, P.,** Phytohaemagglutinin-induced cytotoxic action of unsensitized immunologically competant cells on allogeneic and xenogeneic tissue culture cells, *Nature,* 207, 818, 1965.
85. **Hewish, D. R. and Burgoyne, L. A.,** Chromatin substructure. The digestion of chromatin DNA at regularly spaced sites by a nuclear deoxyribonuclease, *Biochem. Biophys. Res. Comm.,* 52, 504, 1973.
86. **Burgoyne, L. A. and Mobbs, J.,** The reaction of the Ca-Mg endonuclease with the A-sites of rat nucleoprotein, *Nucl. Acids Res.,* 2, 1551, 1975.
87. **Burgoyne, L. A. and Hewish, D. R.,** The regular substructure of mammalian nuclei and nuclear Ca-Mg endonuclease, in *The Cell Nucleus, Vol. IV, Chromatin, Part A,* Busch, H., Ed., Academic Press, New York, 1978, 67.
88. **Simpson, R. T.,** Modification of chromatin by trypsin. The role of proteins in maintenance of deoxyribonucleic acid conformation, *Biochemistry,* 11:2003, 1972.
89. **Chattergee, S. and Walker, I. O.,** The modification of deoxyribonucleohistone by trypsin and chymotrypsin, *Eur. J. Biochem.,* 34, 519, 1973.

90. **Weintraub, H. and Van Lente, F.,** Dissection of chromatin structure with trypsin and nucleases, *Proc. Natl. Acad. Sci. U.S.A.,* 71, 4249, 1974.
91. **Berke, G. and Fishelson, Z.,** T lymphocyte mediated cytolysis: contribution of intracellular components to target cell susceptibility, *Transplant Proc.,* 9, 671, 1977.
92. **Siliciano, R. F. and Henney, C. S.,** Studies on the mechanism of lymphocyte mediated cytolysis. X. Enucleated cells as targets for cytotoxic attack, *J. Immunol.,* 121, 186, 1978.
93. **Hale, A. H. and Paulus, L. K.,** Lysis of enucleated tumor cells with allogeneic and syngeneic cytotoxic thymus-derived lymphocytes, *Eur. J. Immunol.,* 9, 640, 1979.
94. **Sanderson, C. J. and Thomas, J. A.,** The mechanism of T cell-mediated cytolysis. VII. Lysis of isolated cytoplasts and karyoplasts, *Immunology,* 37, 373, 1979.
95. **Ohanian, S. H. and Schlager, S. I.,** Humoral immune killing of nucleated cells: mechanisms of complement-mediated attack and target cell defense, *CRC Crit. Rev. Immunol.,* 1, 165, 1981.
96. **Berke, G. and Clark, W. R.,** T lymphocyte-mediated cytolysis — A comprehensive theory. I. The mechanism of CTL-mediated cytolysis, *Adv. Exp. Med. Biol.,* 146, 57, 1982.
97. **Clark, W. R. and Berke, G.,** T lymphocyte-mediated cytolysis — a comprehensive theory. II. Lytic vs. nonlytic interactions of T lymphocytes, *Adv. Exp. Med. Biol.,* 146, 69, 1982.
98. **Henkart, P. A.,** Mechanism of lymphocyte-mediated cytotoxicity, *Ann. Rev. Immunol.,* 3, 31, 1985.
99. **Podack, E. R.,** The molecular mechanism of lymphocyte-mediated tumor cell lysis, *Immunol. Today,* 6, 21, 1985.
100. **Kalina, M. and Berke, G.,** Contact regions of cytotoxic T lymphocyte target cell conjugates, *Cell. Immunol.,* 25, 41, 1976.
101. **Sanderson, C. J., Hall, P. J., and Thomas, J. A.,** The mechanism of T cell mediated cytotoxicity. IV. Studies on communicating junctions between cells in contact, *Proc. R. Soc. London Ser. B.,* 196, 73, 1977.
102. **Munger, W. E., Reynolds, C. W., and Henkart, P. A.,** DNase activity in cytoplasmic granules of cytotoxic lymphocytes, *Fed. Proc.,* 44, 1284, 1985.
103. **Konigsberg, P. J. and Podack, E. R.,** Target cell DNA fragmentation induced by cytolytic T-cell granules, *J. Leukocyte Biol.,* 38, 1091, 1985.
104. **Sears, D. W. and Christiaansen, J. E.,** Mechanism of rapid taumor lysis by human ADCC: mediation of monoclonal antibodies and fragmentation of target cell DNA, *Adv. Exp. Med. Biol.,* 184, 509, 1985.
105. **Christiaansen, J. E. and Sears, D. W.,** Lack of lymphocyte-induced DNA fragmentation in human targets during lysis represents a species-specific difference between human and murine cells, *Proc. Natl. Acad. Sci. U.S.A.,* 82, 4482, 1985.
106. **Gromkowski, S. H., Brown, T. C., Cerutti, P. A. and Cerottini, J.-C.,** DNA of human Raji target cells is damaged upon lymphocyte-mediated lysis, *J. Immunol.,* 136, 752, 1986.
107. **Burgoyne, L. A., Hewish, D. R., and Mobbs, J.,** Mammalian chromatin substructure studies with the calcium-magnesium endonuclease and two-dimensional polyacrylamide-gel electrophoresis, *Biochem. J.,* 143, 67, 1974.
108. **Noll, M.,** Subunit structure of chromatin, *Nature,* 251, 249, 1974.
109. **Henkart, P. A., Millard, P. J., Reynolds, C. W., and Henkart, M. P.,** Cytolytic activity of purified cytoplasmic granules from cytotoxic rat LGL tumors, *J. Exp. Med.,* 160, 75, 1984.
110. **Henkart, P., Henkart, M., Millard, P., Frederikse, P., Bluestone, J., Blumenthal, R., Yue, C., and Reynolds, C.,** The role of cytoplasmic granules in cytotoxicity by large granular lymphocytes and cytotoxic T lymphocytes, *Adv. Exp. Med. Biol.,* 184, 121, 1985.
111. **Podack, E. R., Konigsberg, P. J., Acha-Orbea, H., Pircher, H., and Hengartner, H.,** Cytolytic T-cell granules: biochemical properties and functional specificity, *Adv. Exp. Med. Biol.,* 184, 99, 1985.
112. **Will, H., Cattaneo, R., Koch, H.-G., Darai, G., Schaller, H., Schellekens, H., van Erd, P. M. C. A., and Deinhardt, F.,** Cloned HBV DNA causes hepatitis in chimpanzees, *Nature,* 299, 740, 1983.
113. **Dubensky, T. W., Campbell, B. C., and Villarreal, L. P.,** Direct transfection of viral or plasmid DNA into the liver or spleen of mice, *Proc. Natl. Acad. Sci. U.S.A.,* 81, 7529, 1984.
114. **Ucker, D. S.,** Cytotoxic T lymphocytes and glucocorticoids activate an endogenous suicide process in target cells, *Nature,* 327, 62, 1987.
115. **Golstein, P.,** Cytolytic T-cell melodrama, *Nature,* 327, 12, 1987.

Section II.C: Cytolytic Mechanism — Soluble Cytotoxic Factors Produced by Lymphocytes

Chapter 18

PRODUCTION AND FUNCTION OF LYMPHOTOXIN SECRETED BY CYTOLYTIC T CELLS

Donald Scott Schmid and Nancy H. Ruddle

TABLE OF CONTENTS

I.	General Overview	62
	A. Central Thesis	62
	B. Definition of Lymphotoxin (LT)	62
	1. Description and Definition	62
	2. Assay for LT	62
	3. Targets of LT Killing	62
	4. Properties of LT	63
	5. Cloning the Gene for LT	63
	C. Definition of Cytolytic T Cell Killing	63
II.	Previous Observations That Led to the Conclusion That LT Did Not Play a Role in CTL Killing	64
III.	CTLs and LT Producing Cells are Phenotypically LYT Identical and Possess the Same Antigen and MHC Activation Requirements	64
IV.	LT Can Kill Rapidly and Induce Chromium Release from Targets	65
V.	Bystander Killing Occurs in the Presence of CTLs	66
VI.	LT Producing Cells Kill Themselves	67
VII.	LT Producing Cells Contain Granules	68
VIII.	LT Induces Target Cell DNA Fragmentation	69
IX.	Conclusions	70
Note Added in Proof		72
References		72

I. GENERAL OVERVIEW

A. Central Thesis

Lymphotoxin plays an important role in cytolytic T cell killing. The extent of this role and the relationship of lymphotoxin to other recently described cytolytic mediators remains unclear. In this review we will consider arguments that alleged that soluble mediators did not play a role in cytolytic killing. Recently obtained data, much of which is summarized here, refute such contentions, and in fact provide strong evidence that such mediators are involved.

B. Definition of Lymphotoxin (LT)

1. Description and Definition

Ruddle and Waksman[1] described the production of a cytotoxic factor by rat lymphoycytes which were reexposed to specific antigen in tissue culture. The production of this factor was antigen specific, i.e., lymphocytes from rats sensitized to tuberculin produced the factor in the presence of purified protein derivative but not histoplasmin. However, the activity of the factor was not antigen specific; i.e., it killed syngenic rat embryo fibroblasts. Similar observations were made by Granger and Williams,[2] who demonstrated the presence of cytotoxic activity in the media of lymphocyte cultures activated by any one of a number of different agents, including mitogens such as phytohemagglutinin. The factor that was induced from activated T cells and killed innocent bystander cells in a species nonrestricted, antigen nonspecific manner came to be known as lymphotoxin. Ruddle and Waksman[3] and Barry and Ruddle[4] demonstrated that the factor was produced under circumstances of delayed hypersensitivity to soluble antigens, i.e., its induction was carrier specific and it was produced by T cells capable of effecting a passive transfer of a 24 hr skin test. Its production did not correlate with antibody either in terms of kinetics or conditions for elicitation of production. Lymphotoxin, along with several other lymphokines, came to be considered a positive correlate of delayed type hypersensitivity. Originally, a role for the factor in CTL killing was suggested, but over the years it was not considered very seriously as a medium of that type of killing for the reasons noted below.

2. Assay for LT

Lymphotoxin is assayed by its ability to inhibit the growth of a target cell in tissue culture. Several different targets of varying sensitivity have been used. The murine L929 cell is used most frequently to evaluate both murine and human LT. The original assay involved the addition of LT to the target and evaluation 72 hr later by counting remaining cells with a Coulter counter. Recent modifications have included the use of vital dyes, such as neutral red or crystal violet, with a spectrophotometer to quantitate cell survival. The most dramatic effects are seen three days after addition of LT to the target cell. The assay can be compressed in time by the addition of inhibitors of synthesis of DNA (mitomycin C), RNA (actinomycin D), or protein (cycloheximide). In the presence of such inhibitors, maximal killing is seen within 24 hr of addition of LT. The effect can also be enhanced by performing the assay at elevated temperatures (40° C). The experiments described in this manuscript that have been carried out in our laboratory (unless specifically noted otherwise) have not included metabolic inhibitors and have been done at 37°C. L929 survival has been evaluated 72 hr after addition of LT by counting remaining target cells.

3. Targets of LT Killing

Though the L929 cell is the most frequently employed target, several other cell lines are as sensitive, or even more sensitive to LT killing. These include rat embryo fibroblasts,[1] mouse embryo fibroblasts,[5] several lymphomas,[6,7] interleukin 2 (IL-2) maintained T cell lines,[7] lipopolysaccharide activated B cells,[7] and the mastocytoma, P815,[7] a frequent target in CTL killing. The methylcholanthrene induced sarcoma, Meth A, is also susceptible to LT induced hemorrhagic necrosis in the mouse.[8] Several targets appear to be relatively insusceptible. The basis of a cell's lack of sensitivity to LT and its relationship to CTL sensitivity remain to be determined. LT has several other activities which are probably not relevant to the topic under discussion here, its role in cytolytic T cell killing. These include stimulation of human polymorphonuclear neutrophil function noted by Shalaby et. al.,[9] and inhibition of the activity of the enzyme lipoprotein lipase, the assay for cachectin (Beutler and Ruddle, unpublished).

4. Properties of LT

The development and analysis of clonally derived cell lines such as IL-2 maintained T cell clones, T cell hybridomas, and lymphomas has allowed production of large quantities of lymphokines from the progeny of a single cell. This has provided starting material for biochemical purification of LT. The observation by Williamson and colleagues[11] that RPMI 1788, a B lymphoma, produced high titers of LT was key to the success reported elsewhere in this volume by Aggarwal and his colleagues[12,13] in characterizing the molecule. Briefly, the product of the B lymphoma is a glycosylated protein that has a M_r of 25 kDalton on SDS polyacrylamide gels.

The early descriptions of LT had suggested that there were several different classes of LT distinguishable by size and reactivity with various antibodies. The problem of heterogeneity of LT species has still not been completely resolved. However, one could now surmise that some of the earlier antigenically distinct species may have been either LT or TNF. Furthermore, Stone-Wolff et al.[10] have demonstrated that a large species of LT (68 kDalton) is resolved to smaller species (25 kDalton) on SDS polyacrylamide gels. It is quite possible that additional forms of LT will be characterized. Resolution of this problem awaits protein sequencing and gene cloning.

5. Cloning the Gene for LT

Gray and his colleagues[8] were able to use the information derived from the protein sequence of LT to prepare synthetic oligonucleotides and isolate the cDNA for LT. The genomic organization of human LT has been described in detail as well by Nedwin et al.[14] We have determined that the gene for murine LT is very similar to that of the human. This was accomplished by screening a mouse genomic library with the human LT cDNA. A murine 1.9 kilobase Bam HI fragment was isolated and sequenced and found to have a genomic organization very similar to the human counterpart. The deduced amino acid sequence of the mature protein is approximately 85% homologous to that of the human. The Bam HI fragment has been used in Northern blot analysis of RNA from a murine IL-2 maintained clone and hybridized with a 15s species of RNA, identical in size to that seen in human PHA stimulated peripheral blood cells. This RNA was used to construct a cDNA library which should prove useful in expressing the gene to compare the murine and human LT proteins.

C. Definition of Cytolytic T Cell Killing

For the purposes of discussion, cytolytic T cell killing will be defined as that effected by antigen specific cells whose activation requires the presence of that antigen presented within the context of self molecules of the major histocompatibility complex. Though the original in vitro studies of homograft immunity were carried out by counting surviving cells 72 hr after the addition of sensitized cells,[15,16] the definitive assay has been that of Brunner et al.,[17] which quantitates the rapid (4 hr) release of ^{51}Cr from target cells after the addition of sensitized T cells. CTLs also effect the release of ^{3}H-thymidine from prelabeled target cells.[18-22] This phenomenon, a manifestation of target cell DNA fragmentation, can actually be evaluated at a point earlier in time than ^{51}Cr release.

II. PREVIOUS OBSERVATIONS THAT LED TO THE CONCLUSION THAT LT DID NOT PLAY A ROLE IN CTL KILLING

Several arguments have been advanced that purport to exclude a role of LT in CTL killing. The major objections for a role of LT in the cytolytic T cell induced process included: differences in phenotypes of CTL and LT producing cells, the exquisite antigen specificity of CTLs and the lack thereof in LT killing, the fact that CTLs kill rapidly and LT kills slowly, the absence of bystander killing in CTL cultures, the unidirectional nature of CTL killing, the differences in ionic requirements between CTL and LT induced killing, the observation that granules played a role in CTL killing while they had not been demonstrated (or sought) in LT producing cells, and the demonstration of DNA fragmentation in targets of CTL killing, that again had not been demonstrated or sought in LT killing. In the remainder of the chapter we will address these arguments with recently published data obtained from our own and others' laboratories to provide a more complete picture and suggest that the bulk of the evidence indicates that LT *is* involved in CTL killing.

III. CTLS AND LT PRODUCING CELLS ARE PHENOTYPICALLY LYT IDENTICAL AND POSSESS THE SAME ANTIGEN AND MHC ACTIVATION REQUIREMENTS

The original data indicated that CTLs specific for transplantation antigens expressed the Lyt-2 differentiation antigen. Helper T cells were of the Lyt-1 phenotype. Lymphokine producing cells obtained from mice sensitized to soluble antigens, were predominately Lyt-1$^+$. It is now clear from the contributions of several workers that Lyt phenotype is more clearly a reflection of the nature of MHC restriction, than of function.[23] That is, Lyt-1$^+$ (or more accurately L3T4$^+$) cells, generally recognize antigen within the context of class II MHC molecules, and Lyt-2$^+$ cells recognize antigen within the context of class I molecules. Both can produce lymphokines.

CTL killing was antigen specific and restricted by elements coded by genes in the major histocompatability complex. The killing seen after the addition of LT to cells in tissue culture was neither antigen specific nor restricted by elements of the major histocompatibility complex. In fact it was not even species specific. Human LT killed murine cells; the reverse was also true. Thus, it was difficult to reconcile the specificity which was the hallmark of CTL killing with the apparent promiscuity of killing mediated by a soluble factor.

Several workers[24,25] have now demonstrated that L3T4$^+$, class II restricted cells can behave as cytolytic T cells. That is, if antigen is presented to such cells within the context of class II, they will effect ^{51}Cr release. Tite and Janeway[25] used L3T4$^+$ BALB/c IL2 maintained ovalbumin specific class II restricted cells and demonstrated that they killed OVA coupled A20, a B lymphoma. Ia negative variants of such lymphomas did not serve as targets. Several of these clones functioned as helper cells as well, and all produced LT. In fact the ability to produce LT was positively correlated with the ability of individual clones to effect CTL killing,[26] and the induction is just as exquisitely antigen specific and MHC restricted as that required for activation of CTLs.

The mirror image of the L3T4$^+$ CTL is the Lyt-2$^+$ LT producing cell. We have also prepared several T cell clones which are conventional CTLs. They are specific for antigen within the context of Class I MHC molecules, are Lyt-2$^+$, and kill antigen coupled targets as measured by ^{51}Cr release. These cells also make LT. We derived a number of TNP-specific, Lyt 2$^+$ cell lines in our laboratory from CBA/J mice (H-2^k) which had been sensitized to picryl chloride.[27,28] When tested in a 4 hr ^{51}Cr release assay against the appropriate syngeneic TNP-coupled target cells, most of these lines exhibited a pattern of killing characteristic of CTL. Comprehensive studies of the TNP-specific CTLs demonstrated that in every instance, cell lines and clones which are capable of killing in an antigen-specific, MHC class I-restricted fashion, also secrete LT under stimulation by antigen or mitogen.[27-30] In fact the requirements for LT production are absolutely identical to those of CTL killing. Not only are these cells restricted to class I antigens for both LT induction and CTL killing, in fact they are restricted to a particular antigen, K^k.

The observations noted above indicate that the interpretation that only Lyt-2$^+$ cells were killers and only Lyt-1$^+$ cells make lymphokines, was incorrect. There are several explanations for this misapprehension. These include the fact that targets used for CTL killing were predominately Ia$^-$ and the fact that most investigators searched for LT in culture supernatants 4 hr after CTL killing. At this time the target is absorbing most of the activity. It is more appropriate to look for LT in the supernatants at later times if the induction signal includes an LT sensitive cell. LT is produced predominately by Lyt-1$^+$ cells in the cases of sensitization with soluble antigens. It appears that such cells are preferentially stimulated by soluble proteins, probably due to the importance of macrophage (Ia$^+$) presentation. Nevertheless, even in the original experiments in which whole lymph node populations were used, a proportion of Lyt-2$^+$ cells also produced LT after ovalbumin stimulation[30] Recent work noted above with T cell clones has answered this question without a doubt and indicates that CTL activity and LT production can be carried out by the same cells under the same circumstances.

IV. LT CAN KILL RAPIDLY AND INDUCE CHROMIUM RELEASE FROM TARGETS

It was originally observed that CTLs killed rapidly and LT killed slowly. When CTL killing is measured by ^{51}Cr release from target cells, maximal killing is detected at approximately 4 hr. LT killing requires at least 24 hr, even when the time scale is compressed by the addition of metabolic inhibitors. It is difficult to evaluate ^{51}Cr release at that time because its spontaneous leakage from most targets is then quite high. The observation that the kinetics of CLT and LT killing were different was thought to be extremely important, because it was believed by some that the time course of an event indicates something about the mechanism of that event. Thus if two events have different kinetics, their mechanisms may differ.

Differences in the kinetics of LT and CTL killing could be explained if a local concentration of LT at the site of CTL apposition is very high, and/or if CTL kill by injecting a toxin. It would simply take a longer time for sufficient concentrations of LT to be reached and for the cells to take up LT in the absence of a CTL delivery system. We wished to see whether or not LT preparations from a cytotoxic T cell could cause short-term release (4 hr) of ^{51}Cr from target cells if it were first rapidly introduced into the cytoplasm. In order to approach this problem, we adopted a technique described by Okada and Rechsteiner[31] for rapidly internalizing macromolecules into the cytoplasm of fibroblasts. The basis of the technique is the incubation of target cells in a hypertonic solution (0.5 M sucrose) containing the macromolecule to be internalized, under conditions which stimulate pinocytosis (10% polyethylene glycol 1000, 37°C), and exposing the cells to a brief hypertonic shock, which has the effect of lysing the newly formed pinocytic vesicles without lysing the cells themselves.

Using this approach as indicated in Figure 1, our laboratory was able to demonstrate that LT-containing supernatant fluids of ConA-stimulated cytotoxic T cell lines could kill target cells in 4 hr, as measured by ^{51}Cr release.[29] We also tested a series of supernatant fluids taken at various points in time following ConA stimulation in both the traditional 72 hr

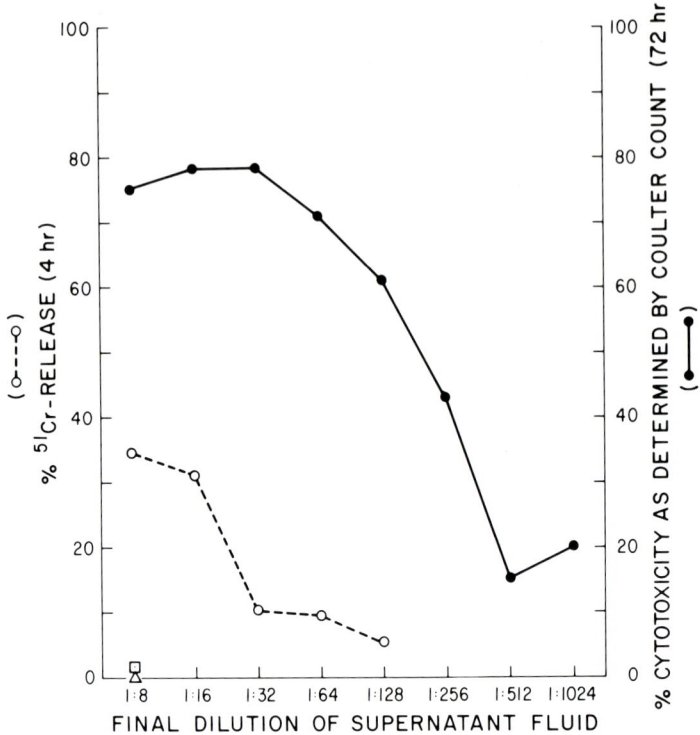

FIGURE 1. LT causes ^{51}Cr release after rapid internalization. LT was tested for activity in the standard L929 assay evaluated at 72 hr (●) and for ability to cause ^{51}Cr release from L929 4 hr after internalization using the method of Okada and Rechsteiner[31] (○). Controls include ^{51}Cr release after internalization of medium plus fetal calf serum (▫) and ^{51}Cr release after addition of LT containing supernatants that were not subjected to internalization (△). (From Schmid, D. S. et al., *Cell. Immunol.*, 93, 73, 1985.)

lymphotoxin assay and in the 4 hr rapid internalization assay. In these experiments, the ^{51}Cr pattern was similar to the cytotoxicity curve in the standard assay evaluated at 72 hr. At early time-points, little or no killing was evident in either assay, and the level of killing in both assays increased to peak with supernatant fluids recovered 48 hr post ConA stimulation. If growth medium alone was rapidly introduced into target cell cytoplasm, no appreciable ^{51}Cr release over background levels was detected in any of these experiments. Thus, it was demonstrated that LT could kill over a period of time comparable to that required by CTL if it was first forcibly internalized. This was a somewhat artificial system and might have generated subtle abnormalities in target cell physiology unaccounted for by our controls. Nevertheless, the results are consistent with the concept that LT kills just as rapidly and dramatically as CTLs if it can be rapidly introduced into the cytoplasm of target cells.

V. BYSTANDER KILLING OCCURS IN THE PRESENCE OF CTLs

Several previous observations had suggested that bystander killing did not occur in the presence of an ongoing cytolytic T cell killing reaction. If CTL killing involved a nonspecific mediator such as lymphotoxin, lysis of cells that did not express the antigen recognized by the CTLs should also take place in the same culture in which CTL killing was occurring. Thus, one should see ^{51}Cr release from "bystander cells" in such cultures. Several investigators have noted that such was not the case when the cultures were evaluated at the time (4 hr) at which peak CTL killing occurred. We have modified previous experimental con-

Table 1
BYSTANDER KILLING OF P815 CELLS OCCURS IN CULTURES WITH PC1 KILLING OF L929 CELLS

	% Specific release from ^{51}Cr P815 in reactions with	
Effector: target	PC1 59:TNP-L929	PC1 59:L929
1:1	64	12
0.5:1	54	7

Note: PC1 59 cells (TNP-specific, H-2K^k restricted) were added to TNP-L929 cells at the indicated ratios. This results in as much as 60% specific ^{51}Cr release from TNP-L929 targets at 4 hr, and less than 10% ^{51}Cr release from the nonspecific target, L929, at that time. In the experiment described above, PC1 59 cells were added to TNP-L929 or L929 in the presence of ^{51}Cr labeled P815 bystander cells. Isotope release was measured 24 hr later.

ditions by extending their duration and have demonstrated that bystander kill does occur both in the case of Class II[26] and Class I restricted CTLs.[32] Table 1 includes data generated in the course of an experiment in which bystander killing was demonstrated. The TNP-specific H2K^k restricted CTLs killed TNP-L929 and also destroyed bystander P815 cells, as demonstrated by ^{51}Cr release. The killing of P815 is somewhat delayed in time behind the 4 hr peak ^{51}Cr release from comparable cultures of effector cells and prelabeled specific targets. That is, more time, on the order of an additional 6 to 12 hr, is needed to readily demonstrate high levels of nonspecific killing in the course of an ongoing specific cytotoxic reaction. This is consistent with the concept that specific targets are killed rapidly because of high local concentrations of toxic factors. Once the specific target receptors (extra- or intracellular) are occupied by LT, additional LT diffuses to adjacent cells. We have previously demonstrated that the ability of a T cell to cause bystander kill is positively correlated with its ability to produce LT under comparable circumstances.[26] Furthermore, the ability of a cell to serve as an effective target in bystander kill is proportional its LT sensitivity.[7,26] There are several possible explanations for the relative dearth of previously described examples of bystander kill. They concern the brevity of most experiments and in some cases the use of LT insensitive targets as bystanders.

VI. LT PRODUCING CELLS KILL THEMSELVES

When CTLs kill targets, they themselves are not usually killed in the 4 hr course of the experiment, and the concept arose that CTL killing is unidirectional. One would expect such death to occur if a soluble mediator were involved, because that substance would kill by diffusion back to the CTL or it might even kill those cells manufacturing it before release. Heretofore, there was not a great deal of evidence that cells stimulated to secrete LT were killed in the course of antigen activation. In fact, one could study proliferation of such cells which also were producing LT. The concept evolved that CTLs and LT producing cells were immune to the killing process. We have now shown that this is not the case.[7,28] If very few target cells are used to present antigen, and large amounts of LT are produced, the producing cells are killed. Thus we have determined that the best way to maintain a T cell clone that can be induced by antigen to produce LT is to use fairly high numbers of

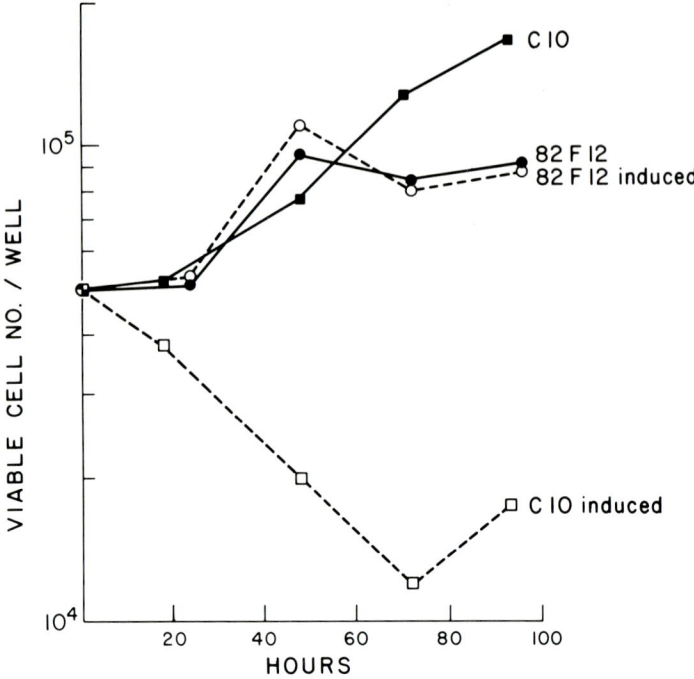

FIGURE 2. ConA induction results in suicide if a clone makes LT. T cell clones C10 and 82F12 were grown in the presence of 8 U IL2/mℓ and were induced (– –) or not (—) with 5 μg/mℓ ConA. Under these conditions, C10 makes 512 U/mℓ interferon and 16 U/mℓ LT and dies. 82F12 makes 512 U/mℓ interferon and no LT and survives. Experiment carried out by Drs. B. Conta and N. Ruddle.

antigen presenting cells, rather low amounts of antigen, infrequent antigen stimulation, and relatively low cell density. It is not known whether the cytotoxic effect of cultures grown under conditions of high amounts of antigen and low amounts of feeders is due to destruction from within, or to an autodestruction by LT after release. A dramatic example of autodestruction of LT producing cells is seen in Figure 2. In this case C10, a cloned T cell line, is agglutinated by ConA and induced to make LT and IFN. 82F12 also is agglutinated and induced to make IFN by ConA, but it does not make LT. The inability to make LT is reflected in the continued growth of 82F12 in the presence of activation. Clone C10 dies in identical circumstances because it makes LT. These conclusions are buttressed by the fact that 82F12 survives under conditions of antigen stimulation, which are lethal to cells of clone C10.

Autodestruction of CTLs was probably previously not commonly seen because their antigen was an integral part of their target. It is likely that most of the LT induced in such circumstances is delivered to the target, and does not act back on the T cells in the course of the experiment. The conclusion of the observations reported here and in previous publications[7,28] is that LT producing cells can be killed by the LT that they produce.

VII. LT PRODUCING CELLS CONTAIN GRANULES

Dennert and Podack have described the existence of granules in CTLs.[33] Such granules are likely to be involved with the killing mechanism.[34] A number of proteins have been isolated from these granules.[34] Recently Podack has demonstrated that isolated cytolytic granules kill L929 cells and induce target cell DNA fragmentation, properties shared with

Table 2
KINETICS OF GRANULE FORMATION AND LT PRODUCTION IN 21C11 HELPER T CELL CLONE FOLLOWING CON A STIMULATION

Time (hr)	Granule formation	Lt U/mℓ
0	Faint, but clearly visible thin corona of granules present in most cases. Represents baseline level of granule production.	0
4	Thin, dully staining corona. No intense staining.	388
8	Corona thickened. Staining more intense.	1098
12	Thickness of granule corona is on average twice that seen with 4 hr cells. Bright staining.	1522
18	Cells already in decline. Intact cells stain no more brightly than at 8 hr.	2702
24	Cells quite sickly. Some intact, but they do not stain brightly.	8192

Note: T cell clone 21C11 cells were grown in the presence of IL-2. Cells were stimulated with 5μg/mℓ Conconavalin A, and culture supernatants were harvested for LT by assaying killing of L929 cells. Cells were stained for granules at the indicated times according to the method of Podack and Konigsberg, with a polyclonal rabbit anti-granule antibody (1:100 dilution) for 20 min and a fluoresceinated goat anti-rabbit immunoglobulin (1:10 dilution) for 10 min.

From Ruddle, N., McGrath, K., James, T., and Schmid, D. S., in UCLA Symposium New Series, Bonavida, B. and Collier, R. J., Eds., 45, 379, 1986. With permission.

LT, suggesting that LT may be one of the 7 proteins associated with such structures.[35] Self-assembling tubules are formed from one of the proteins, perforin. The granules have been found fairly consistently in activated CTL and NK clones,[33-37] though they had not previously been observed in cells that would be expected to make LT; however a systematic search had not taken place. We hypothesized that the differences in the kinetics of killing by LT and CTL could reflect differences in the mode of toxin delivery. For example, secreted LT may depend largely on target cell pinocytosis for entry into the cell, whereas the LT delivered by cytolytic cells may be prepackaged into cytolyic granules. We have now found granules to be invariably present in our mitogen-activated LT-secreting helper cell clones (Table 2). Individual clones can vary considerably. One ovalbumin-specific helper clone, 153-E11, attained peak granule formation only 4 to 6 hr following mitogen stimulation.

The postulated presence of LT in these granules, coupled with the formation of pore-like complexes by other components in the granules[34] has led us to propose that the granules provide killer cells with a mechanism for rapidly introducing LT into the target cell. In addition, the experiments cited here provide compelling evidence for a role of LT in killing mediated by cytotoxic T cells and T helper cells with cytotoxic activity. TNF may be involved in killing mediated by NK cells or macrophages but is unlikely to play a role in T cell mediated killing, as TNF secretion has not been detected from T cells.

VIII. LT INDUCES TARGET CELL DNA FRAGMENTATION

Considerable data have accumulated to suggest that CTLs induce target cell DNA degradation. Russell and co-workers[18-20] and Duke et al.[21] have shown that the release of a target cell nuclear label, [125]IUDR or ^{3}H-Tdr, occurs even before the release of cytoplasmic ^{51}Cr label in targets killed by CTLs generated in mixed leukocyte reactions. Nuclear label is also released very early from targets lethally hit by CTL when the cytoplasmic membrane is prematurely lysed under conditions which do not affect the release of nuclear labels in targets which have not been "programmed" for lysis.[18-21] This suggested an early onset compromise of nuclear membrane integrity in target cells attacked by CTL which precedes the measureable release of cytoplasmic labels. The fragmentation of target cell DNA proceeds at regular intervals along the chromatin strand, generating fragments which are approximate multiples of 200 base pairs. When electrophoresed in agarose, these fragments result in a characteristic laddered pattern.[21] These phenomena are not observed in targets which have been lysed by antibody and complement. Since target cell DNA fragmentation had not previously been sought in the case of LT killing, it was not known whether it occurred.

We began our studies by examining the ability of the TNP-specific cytotoxic T cell clones to cause fragmentation in the appropriate target cell. In all cases, TNP-specific (H-2^k) effector cells were able to fragment DNA only in H-2^k targets which had first been treated with specific hapten. We then studied the time course of fragmentation mediated by the TNP-specific effectors, finding in accordance with others[18,21] that the first fragmentation was evident at 30 min at the higher effector:target ratios, reaching peak effect by the end of 2 hr in culture. In contrast, 3 to 4 hr were required to reach peak levels of killing as measured by ^{51}Cr release at the same effector:target ratio.[22]

We also examined the ability of an ovalbumin-specific, MHC class II-restricted cell line, 5.9.24 (having the characteristic phenotype and functions of helper cells but with CTL activity[25,26] against ovalbumin-pulsed cells expressing the appropriate Ia molecules) for its ability to cause DNA fragmentation in target cells. Again, these cells were able to effect DNA fragmentation in syngeneic ovalbumin-pulsed targets, but not in unpulsed targets. The kinetics of fragmentation were virtually indistinguishable from those of the TNP-specific cytotoxic T cell lines.[22] In addition, like the TNP-specific CTL and the MLR described by Duke et al.[21] these cells caused DNA fragmentation in the characteristic laddered pattern, as indicated in Figure 3.

We next wanted to determine whether or not LT, which is produced by both the TNP-specific CTL lines and by 5.9.24 under antigen or mitogen stimulation, could cause DNA fragmentation in susceptible target cells. LT-containing supernatant fluids from either helper cell clones or CTL lines could cause fragmentation of target cell DNA in the several targets tested, although a longer time course was required (24 to 48 hr) to achieve the effect.[22] When ^{125}I UdR labeled DNA fragments from LT-treated targets were electrophoresed on agarose gels, the laddered effect was clearly evident, with the smallest fragment of around 200 base pairs more prominently represented than in the shorter (2 hr) assays. Recombinant-derived tumor necrosis factor (TNF), a soluble protein with some properties in common with LT[38] and which is 38% homologous to LT,[13,38] could also mediate target cell DNA fragmentation,[39] though less effectively than LT preparations. Recombinant-derived interferon gamma (IFNγ), another candidate molecule for mediating this activity, was unable to cause DNA fragmentation in L929 target cells.[39] Additionally, IFN-γ was unable to synergize with either LT or TNF to enhance the fragmentation of DNA in targets. No fragmentation was detectable in medium-only controls, or in target cells which had been lysed with antibody plus complement.

These experiments provide further evidence that LT is likely to be involved in the cytotoxic T cell lytic event, and that LT, CTL, and LT-secreting helper cells with cytolytic activity all mediate killing using a similar or identical process.

IX. CONCLUSIONS

In this chapter we have summarized the data that strongly implicate a role for soluble mediators in general and lymphotoxin, in particular, in CTL killing. The evidence is still largely circumstantial. There are several key experiments that remain to be done. One is the demonstration that anti-LT antibody inhibits CTL killing. Such experiments have been carried out repeatedly over the years with varying results. In several experiments, anti-LT did inhibit CLT killing,[40] in others it did not.[41] The use of recombinant derived LT and

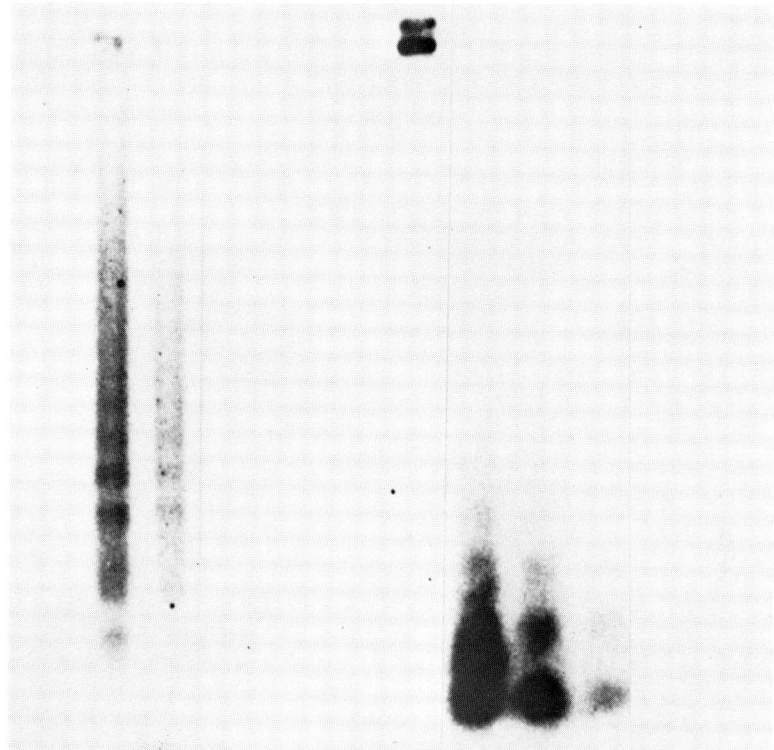

FIGURE 3. PC1 55 and LT induce fragmentation of target cell DNA. Agarose gel electrophoresis of target cell DNA fragmented by PC1 line 55 and cell-free LT-containing supernatant fluid. Target cells were labeled for 3 hr at 37°C with 50 µCi of ^{125}I UdR in 1 mℓ of RPMI 1640 medium, 5% FCS. PC1 55 with incubated for 2 hr with target cells at 37°C. LT was incubated for 24 hr with target cells at 37°C. DNA samples were prepared by extracting 2 times with phenol, and precipitated with absolute enthanol, 4×10^{-3} M MgCl$_2$, 0.12 M Na acetate. Figure shown is a composite of two experiments. (A) 2.5:1 PC1 55, BW5147-TNP target; (B) 1:1 PC1 55, BW5147-TNP target; (C) 2.5:1 PC1 55, BW5147 target; (D) 1:1 PC1 55, BW5147 target; (E and F) medium controls (2 hr) for BW5147-TNP and BW5147, respectively. (G) clone 153-E6 lymphotoxin 60 U/mℓ LT, BW5147 target; (H) 30 U/mℓ LT, BW5147 target; (I) 15 U/mℓ LT, BW5147; (J) medium control (24 hr), BW5147 target. (From Schmid, D. S. et al., *Proc. Natl. Acad. Sci. USA*, 83, 1884, 1986. With permission.)

monoclonal antibodies may resolve some of the discrepancies. However, if LT is delivered to its target by CTL in association with perforin it would be unavailable for neutralization with an antibody. Nevertheless, the bystander killing seen slightly later (vide supra) would be susceptible to inhibition with anti-LT antibody.

In this chapter we have implied that LT is delivered by the CTL to the target by means of the granule and its associated proteins. If this is the case, then what is the role of the LT receptor on target cells? It is fairly clear from experiments using ^{125}I labeled LT and TNF, that such a structure exists,[42,43] and that LT and TNF use the same receptor.[44] This suggests that the two molecules with different amino acid sequences but similar activity against a wide range of targets use the same receptor. It is also known that the presence of such a receptor is necessary but not sufficient to confer LT sensitivity to a target cell. Do cells which are LT insusceptible but susceptible to CTL lack a cell surface receptor for LT?

The different ionic requirements for LT and CTL killing have not been addressed here. It was demonstrated previously[45] that Ca^{++} was an absolute requirement for CTL killing. LT killing, on the other hand, did not require Ca^{++} and in fact was inhibited at high concentrations.[46] However, Ca^{++} probably is needed for activation of T cells to produce LT. These and other metabolic differences will have to be localized to the activation and effector steps.

The mechanisms of CTL and LT killing must be completely understood before complete understanding of their relationship is reached. DNA fragmentation is one early common event. How does this occur? It is unlikely the LT itself or any other factor delivered by the CTL is an endonuclease. The more reasonable explanation is that activation of a cellular endonuclease occurs. Does LT enter the target cell and induce a cascade of target cell events? Does the target cell play a role in its own destruction?

Are there CTLs which kill by a mechanism other than LT? Are there CTLs that are defective for LT but can still kill? In the absence of such demonstrations, and in the presence of the compelling data detailed above, we strongly suggest that the balance has shifted in favor of a role for soluble factors in CTL killing. Until one can demonstrate that LT is not required in CTL killing, we will argue that it is an important, if not the essential, component of killing.

NOTE ADDED IN PROOF

We have recently demonstrated (McGrath, K. et al., submitted) that some CTLs produce both LT and TNF. Thus, both factors probably contribute independently or in concert to CTL killing.

REFERENCES

1. **Ruddle, N. H. and Waksman, B. H.**, Cytotoxicity mediated by soluble antigen and lymphocytes in delayed hypersensitivity. III. Analysis of mechanism, *J. Exp. Med.*, 128, 1267, 1968.
2. **Granger, G. A. and Williams, T. W.**, Lymphocyte cytotoxicity in vitro: Activation and release of a cytotoxic factor, *Nature (London)*, 218, 1253, 1968.
3. **Ruddle, N. H. and Waksman, B. H.**, Cytotoxicity mediated by soluble antigen and lymphocytes in delayed hypersensitivity. II. Correlation of the in vitro response with skin reactivity, *J. Exp. Med.*, 128, 1255, 1968.
4. **Barry, W. B. and Ruddle, N. H.**, The delayed-type hypersensitivity response to (4-hydroxy-3-nitrophenyl) acetyl (NP) coupled proteins is carrier specific: In vivo and *in vitro* demonstrations, *J. Immunol.*, 131, 70, 1983.
5. **Ruddle, N. H.**, Cytotoxicity reactions mediated by antigen activated rat and mouse lymphocytes, in *Mechanisms of Cell-Mediated Immunity*, McCluskey, R. T. and Cohen, S., Eds., J. Wiley & Sons, 401, 1974.
6. **Smith, M. E., Laudico, R., and Papermaster, B. W.**, A rapid quantitative assay for lymphotoxin, *J. Immunol. Meth.*, 14, 243, 1977.
7. **Powell, M. B., Conta, B. S., Horowitz, M., and Ruddle, N. H.**, The differential inhibitory effect of lymphotoxin and immune interferon on normal and malignant lymphoid cells, *Lymphokine Res.*, 4, 13, 1985.
8. **Gray, P. W., Aggarwal, B. B., Benton, C. V., Bringman, T. S., Henzel, W. S., Jarrett, J. A., Leung, D. W., Moffat, B., Ng, P., Sverdsky, L. P., Palladino, M. A., and Nedwin, G. E.**, Cloning and expression of the cDNA for human lymphotoxin: A lymphokine with tumor necrosis activity, *Nature (London)*, 312, 721, 1984.
9. **Shalaby, M. R., Aggarwal, B. B., Rinderknecht, E., Svedersky, L. P., Finkle, B. S., and Palladino, M. A.**, Activation of human polymorphonuclear neutrophil functions by interferon-γ and tumor necrosis factors, *J. Immunol.*, 135, 2069, 1985.
10. **Stone-Wolff, D. S., Yip, Y. K., Chroboczek Kelker, H., Le, J., Henriksen-Destafano, D., Rubin, B. Y., Rinderknecht, E., Aggarwal, B. B., and Wilcek, J.**, Interrelationships for human interferon-gamma with lymphotoxin and monocyte cytotoxin, *J. Exp. Med.*, 159, 828, 1984.

11. **Williamson, B. D., Carswell, E. A., Rubin, B. Y., Prendergast, J. S., and Old, L. J.**, Human tumor necrosis factor produced by human B-cell lines: Synergistic cytotoxic interaction with human interferon, *Proc. Natl. Acad. Sci. U.S.A.*, 80, 5397, 1983.
12. **Aggarwal, B. B., Moffat, B., and Harkins, R. N.**, Human lymphotoxin production by a lymphoblastoid cell line, purification, and initial characterization, *J. Biol. Chem.*, 259,686, 1984.
13. **Aggarwal, B. B., Henzel, W. J., Moffat, B., Kohr, W. J., and Harkins, R. N.**, Primary structure of human lymphotoxin derived from 1788 lymphoblastoid cell line, *J. Biol. Chem.*, 260, 2334, 1985.
14. **Nedwin, G., Naylor, S. L., Sakaguchi, A. Y., Smith, D., Nedwin, J. J., Pennica, D., Goeddel, D. V., and Gray, P. W.**, Human lymphotoxin and tumor necrosis factor genes: structure, homology and chromosome localization, *Nucleic Acids Res.*, 13, 6361, 1985.
15. **Rosenau, W. and Moon, H.**, Lysis of homologous cells by sensitized lymphocytes in tissue culture, *J. Natl. Canc. Inst.*, 27, 471, 1961.
16. **Wilson, D. B.**, Quantitative studies on the behavior of sensitized lymphocytes in vitro. I. Relationship of the degree of destruction of homologous target cells to the number of lymphocytes and the time of contact in culture and consideration of the effects of isoimmune sera, *J. Exp. Med.*, 122, 143, 1965.
17. **Brunner, K. T., Manuel, J., Cerrottini, J. C., and Chapuis, B.**, Quantitative assay of the lytic action of immune lympoid cells on 51 Cr-labeled allogenic target cells *in vitro*: inhibition by isoantibody and by drugs, *Immunology*, 14, 181, 1968.
18. **Russell, J. H., Masakowski, V. R., and Dobos, C. B.**, Mechanisms of immune lysis. I. Physiological distinction between target cell death by cytotoxic T lymphocytes and antibody plus complement, *J. Immunol.*, 124, 1100, 1980.
19. **Russell, J.H. and Dobos, C. B.**, Mechanisms of immune lysis. II. CTL-induced nuclear disintegration of the target begins with minutes of cell contact, *J. Immunol.*, 125, 1256, 1980.
20. **Russell, J. H., Masakowski, V. R., Rucinsky, T., and Phillips, G.**, Mechanisms of immune lysis III. Characterization of the nature and kinetics of the cytolytic T lymphocyte-induced nuclear lesion in the target, *J. Immunol.*, 128, 2028, 1982.
21. **Duke, R. C., Chervenak, R., and Cohen, J. J.**, Endogenous endonuclease-induced DNA fragmentation: An early event in cell-mediated cytolysis, *Proc. Natl. Acad. Sci. U.S.A.*, 80, 6361, 1983.
22. **Schmid, D. S., Tite, J. P., and Ruddle, N. H.**, DNA fragmentation: Manifestation of target cell destruction mediated by cytotoxic T cell lines, lymphotoxin-secreting helper T-cell clones and cell-free lymphotoxin-containing supernatant, *Proc. Natl. Acad. Sci. U.S.A.*, 83, 1881, 1986.
23. **Swain, S. L.**, T cell subsets and the recognition of MHC class, *Immunol. Rev.*, 74, 129, 1983.
24. **Swain, S. L., Dennert, G., Wormsley, S., and Dutton, R. W.**, The Lyt phenotype of long term allospecific T cell lines. Both helper and killer activities are mediated by Ly-1 cells, *Eur. J. Immunol.*, 11, 175, 1981.
25. **Tite, J. P. and Janeway, C. A.**, Cloned helper T cells can kill B-lymphoma cells in the presence of specific antigen: Ia-restriction and cognate vs. non-cognate interactions in cytolysis, *J. Immunol.*, 14, 878, 1984.
26. **Tite, J. P., Powell, M. B., and Ruddle, N. H.**, Protein-antigen specific Ia-restricted cytolytic T cells: Analysis of frequency target cell susceptibility, and mechanism of cytolysis, *J. Immunol.*, 135, 25, 1985.
27. **Conta, B. S., Powell, M. B., and Ruddle, N. H.**, Production of lymphotoxin, IFN-γ and IFN-α,β by murine T cell lines and clones, *J. Immunol.*, 130, 2231, 1983.
28. **Conta, B. S., Powell, M. B., and Ruddle, N. H.**, Activation of Lyt-1$^+$ and Lyt-2$^+$ T cell cloned lines: Stimulation of proliferation, lymphokine production, and self-destruction, *J. Immunol.*, 134, 2185, 1985.
29. **Schmid, D. S., Powell, M. B., Mahoney, K. A., and Ruddle, N. H.**, A comparison of lysis mediated by Lyt-2$^+$ TNP-specific cytotoxic T lymphocyte (CTL) lines with that mediated by rapidly internalized lymphotoxin-containing supernatant fluids: Evidence for a role of soluble mediators in CTL-mediated killing, *Cell. Immunol.*, 93, 68, 1985.
30. **Eardley, D. D., Shen, F. W., Gershon, R. K., and Ruddle, N. H.**, Lymphotoxin production by subsets of T cells, *J. Immunol.*, 124, 1199, 1980.
31. **Okada, C. Y. and Rechsteiner, M.**, Introduction of macromolecules into cultured mammalian cells by osmotic lysis of pinocytic vesicles, *Cell*, 29, 33, 1982.
32. **Ruddle, N. H. and Homer, R.**, The role of lymphotoxin in inflammation, *Prog. Allergy*, 40, in press, 1987.
33. **Dennert, G. and Podack, E. R.**, Cytolysis by H-2 specific T killer cells: Assembly of tubular complexes on target membranes, *J. Exp. Med.*, 157, 1483, 1983.
34. **Podack, E. R. and Konigsberg, P. J.**, Cytolytic T cell granules: Isolation, structural, biochemical and functional characterization, *J. Exp. Med.*, 160, 695, 1984.
35. **Podack, E.**, Personal communication, 1985.
36. **Henkart, P. A., Millard, P. J., Reynolds, C. W., and Henkart, M. P.**, Cytolytic activity of purified cytoplasmic granules from cytotoxic rat large granular lymphocyte tumors, *J. Exp. Med.*, 160, 75, 1984.

37. **Blumenthal, R., Millard, P. J., Henkart, M. P., Reynolds, C. W., and Henkart, P. A.,** Liposomes as targets for granule cytolysin from cytotoxic large granular lymphocyte tumors, *Proc. Natl. Acad. Sci. U.S.A.,* 81, 5551, 1984.
38. **Aggarwahl, B. B., Kahr, W. J., Hass, P. E., Moffat, B., Spencer, S. A., Henzel, W. J., Bringman, T. S., Nedwin, G. E., Goeddel, P. V., and Harkins, R. N.,** Human tumor necrosis factor. Production purification, and characterization, *J. Biol. Chem.,* 260, 2345, 1985.
39. **Schmid, D. S., Hornung, R., McGrath, K. M., Paul, R., and Ruddle, N. H.,** Target cell DNA fragmentation is mediated by the cytokines lymphotoxin and tumor necrosis factor, *Lymphokine Res.,* 6, 1987.
40. **Walker, S. M. and Lucas, Z. J.,** Role of soluble cytotoxins in cell-mediated immunity, *Transplant. Proc.,* 5, 137, 1973.
41. **Gately, M. K., Mayer, M. M., and Henney, C. S.,** Effects of anti-lymphotoxin on cell-mediated cytotoxicity, *Cell. Immunol.,* 27, 82, 1976.
42. **Kull, F. J., Jacobs, S., and Cuatrecasas, P.** Cellular receptor for ^{125}I labeled tumor necrosis factor: Specific binding, affinity labeling and relationship to sensitivity, *Proc. Natl. Acad. Sci. U.S.A.,* 82, 5756, 1985.
43. **Tsujimoto, M., Yip, Y. K., and Vilcek, J.,** Tumor necrosis factor: Specific binding and internalization in sensitive and resistant cells, *Proc. Natl. Acad. Sci. U.S.A.,* 7626, 1985.
44. **Aggarwal, B. B., Eessalu, T. E., and Hass, P. E.,** Characterization of receptors for human tumor necrosis factor and their regulation by γ-interferon, *Nature,* 318, 665, 1985.
45. **Plaut, M., Bubbers, J. E., and Henney, C. S.,** Studies on the mechanism of lymphocyte-mediated cytolysis. VII. Two stages in the cell-mediated lytic cycle with distinct cation requirements, *J. Immunol.,* 116, 150, 1976.
46. **Okamoto, M. and Mayer, M. M.,** Studies on the mechanism of action of guinea pig lymphotoxin. II. Increase of calcium uptake rate in LT-damaged target cells, *J. Immunol.,* 120, 279, 1978.

Chapter 19

TUMOR NECROSIS FACTOR/CACHECTIN

Frederick C. Kull, Jr.

TABLE OF CONTENTS

I.	Introduction	76
II.	Historical Considerations	76
III.	Physical Properties	77
	A. Gene and Message Structure	77
	B. Primary and Secondary Structure	77
	C. Tertiary Properties	78
IV.	Biologic Activities	78
	A. Acute Phase Response Protein	78
	1. Induction of TNF	78
	2. Shock	79
	B. Tumor Necrosis	80
	C. In Vitro Properties	80
	1. Toxicity and Proliferation	82
	2. Adipocyte Differentiation/Metabolism	82
	3. Activation and Maturation Functions	83
V.	Mechanism of Action	83
	A. Cellular Receptor	83
Addendum		86
References		86

I. INTRODUCTION

Numerous discoveries revolutionized tumor necrosis factor/cachectin research in 1985. These discoveries include its isolation, amino acid sequencing, the cloning of the gene, the expression of its product (and the more widespread availability of it in purified form), the identification of it as cachectin, the identification of its cellular receptor, and other properties relating to its mechanism of action. These discoveries have dramatically enhanced our understanding of the phenomena of the necrosis which can be induced in solid tumors by endotoxin. Additionally, these discoveries have provided superb opportunities for enriching our understanding of infectious/inflammatory processes.

This review will condense these discoveries and relate them to historical developments. (Some early aspects of TNF research have been reviewed previously.[1]) Many of the biological properties summarized here are shared by lymphotoxin, which is a structurally and functionally related hormone (see preceding and following chapters). I will refer to tumor necrosis factor/ cachectin as TNF for the sake of brevity, although both names are appropriate.

II. HISTORICAL CONSIDERATIONS

Clinicians marvel at the miraculous regression which infrequently arises in cancer patients who acquire a bacterial infection. Such observations led William Coley, a turn-of-the-century physician, to treat cancer patients with infectious bacteria and bacterial extracts. His results were remarkable.[2] They encouraged the informative studies by Shear[3] in the 1940s and others, which showed that bacterial endotoxins caused necrosis and regression in experimental rodent tumors.

In contrast to the bacterial toxins, Valey Menkin, a contemporary of Shear's, introduced the notion of an endogenous tissue necrotizing factor. Menkin was the pioneer of modern lymphokine research. He extracted proteinaceous mixtures from chemically induced sites of inflammation, and he observed that the extracts were necrotizing to both normal and malignant tissue. He ascribed the activity to a factor which he called "necrosin."[4] He also characterized a "leucotaxin," an endogenous chemotactic factor. The popularity of Menkin's work may have been undermined by the revelations that endotoxin caused similar effects. Endotoxin is a ubiquitous contaminant of biologic materials.[5] We now know that endotoxin elicits the production of TNF and other acute phase reactants. We also recognize the minute concentrations of these factors in biologic fluids, and we appreciate their extraordinary potency.

TNF, an endogenous, alledged tumor-specific necrotizing factor, was described in 1976 in the serum of hypersensitive mice undergoing endotoxin-induced shock.[6] Hypersensitive shock sera was a common and enriched source of interferon and colony stimulating activities. The mice were made hypersensitive to endotoxin by pretreating them with bacillus Calmette-Guerin, which induced granulocyte/macrophage proliferation. (The TNF discovery has been reviewed elsewhere.[7]) The originators described two distinct properties in the hypersensitive shock sera: (1) the capacity to passively induce the necrosis of solid intradermal tumor implants in vivo, and (2) toxicity to cultured tumor cell lines. The originators correctly attributed these properties to the same molecular entity. Furthermore, they speculated that macrophages were the cellular source.

Most of the subsequent TNF research focused on its cytotoxic activity. Cytotoxicity was easily and accurately measured, while the in vivo necrosis was relatively cumbersome to study.[8] Matthews[9] and Mannel et al.[10] gathered evidence that macrophages and cell lines of myeloid lineage were cellular sources of TNF. A substantial purification was achieved from rabbit hypersensitive shock serum.[11] It has been purified to homogeneity from a similar source.[12] It was also isolated from the supernatants of a murine macrophage-like cell line[13]

Table 1
HETEROGENEITY CARBOXYL TO THE CYSTEINES

Human:	cys_{69}	pro	—	ser	thr	his	val_{74}
Rabbit:	cys_{67}	—	arg	ser	—	tyr	val_{71}
Mouse:	cys_{69}	pro	asp	—	—	tyr	val_{73}
Human:	cys_{101}	gln	arg	glu	pro_{105}
Rabbit:	cys_{99}	his	arg	glu	pro_{102}
Mouse:	cys_{100}	pro	lys	asp	pro_{104}

Note: Gaps (—) are introduced to align the sequences. References are noted in the text.

and a human promyelocytic leukemia.[14] Within months of one another, several groups announced purifications of TNF, its gene cloning, and the expression of cDNAs for human TNF.[15-18]

III. PHYSICAL PROPERTIES

A. Gene and Message Structure

The genes encoding human TNF and lymphotoxin (a structurally and functionally related hormone, see the relevant chapters) are located as single copy genes on chromosome 6 in a closely-linked portion near the HLA genes.[19] The significance of these juxtapositions is not yet appreciated. Both genes consist of approximately 3000 base pairs and they contain 3 introns. The third and the fourth exons contain the bulk of the coding sequence for the mature proteins, and the two genes are 56% homologous in these regions. The other regions are not appreciably homologous, except for the putative control and processing signal regions. The mRNA of TNF is ~1600 bases. It encodes for an unusually long leader sequence of 76 amino acids and a mature protein of 157 amino acids (M_r 17,000). The significance of the long leader sequence is not yet appreciated. The mRNA of interleukin-1, an acute phase response monokine, also codes for a long leader peptide.[20] (See addendum.)

B. Primary and Secondary Structure

The amino acid sequences of human, rabbit, and mouse TNFs have been deduced from their respective cDNAs. Much of the sequence of human TNF has been confirmed by amino acid sequencing.[14] Comparison of the cDNAs of mouse,[18,21] rabbit,[22] and human[15-17] TNF reveal ~80% overall amino acid homology. Comparison of the species' sequences shows that amino acid differences occur sporadically, except for two variant regions. One occurs at the amino terminus. In fact, this region may not be required for activity, since an active, truncated form of lymphotoxin lacks the homologous region.[23] All the TNFs contain two cysteine residues, which almost certainly form a disulfide bond. Murine TNF migrates in denaturing detergent polyacrylamide gels with the predicted 17,000 M_r upon reduction. However, it migrates as a more condensed 15,000 M_r protein without reduction. Sulfhydryl reducing agents inactivate TNF.[8] Additional evidence is reported based on the sequencing of tryptic peptides.[14] Thus, the cysteines create a loop within the middle third of the primary structure (for example, human TNF cys_{69} and cys_{101}). The second variant region of the TNFs occurs in those amino acids carboxyl to the cysteines (Table 1).

Human and rabbit TNF do not contain glycosylation sites. Mouse TNF contains a glycosylation site at asn_7, but it is not yet reported whether mouse TNF is glycosylated naturally.

The TNFs contain ~30% homology with human lymphotoxin, which is larger (M_r 25,000) and glycosylated.[23] The homology is substantial in portions of the molecule (see related chapter). For example, lymphotoxin lacks cysteine and the disulfide loop, but it is homologous in 5 of 8 positions with the carboxyl portion of the TNF loop (human TNF val_{91}-lys_{98}).

Secondary structural analyses of the TNFs and lymphotoxin generate algorithms of considerable similarity. They predict relatively small areas of ordered structure. Analysis of the relative hydrophilicity/phobicity of the primary structure yields a mixture consistent with those of globular proteins. These exercises and the relatively high percentages of leucine, glycine, and proline residues suggest a molecule with intriguing tertiary structure.

C. Tertiary Properties

Purified natural mouse TNF migrates in native polyacrylamide gel electrophoresis (Laemmli system, no detergent or reducing agent) anodal to albumin.[13] (The isoelectric point of murine TNF is 4.5.) The activity is pH labile and stable at pH 7 to 8.5. The activity is heat labile (70°, 15 min). The native molecular size requires some explanation. Radio-iodinated active TNF percolates through HPLC-gel filtration with an apparent M_r of 40,000 when it is applied at a "physiologic" concentration (1 nM). (Purified, active human TNF,[14] active recombinant human TNF,[17] and purified rabbit TNF[12] are also reported to be dimeric.) Gel filtration of more concentrated solutions of murine TNF yields apparent M_rs of 70,000 and 50,000 (Figure 1). Additional size heterogeneity is observed in crude sources,[8,24] which can be seen in Figure 1. These studies, chemical cross-linking studies,[68] and our experience recovering activity from denaturing gels suggest that in renaturing conditions, the purified monomer aggregates into active dimers, trimers and/or tetramers.

IV. BIOLOGIC ACTIVITIES

A. Acute Phase Response Protein

1. Induction of TNF

Cell lines of myeloid lineage shed TNF into the culture medium.[9,10,14,24] (The activity derived from human B lymphoblastoid cells termed "human TNF" has the molecular characteristics of lymphotoxin.[25]) The activity was dependent upon treatment with endotoxin. In our experience with murine macrophage-like lines, the concentrations of endotoxin which solicited production ranged from nanograms to micrograms per milliliter. The higher concentrations were toxic to the cells. Different sources of endotoxin varied in their potency.[24] TNF production was inhibited by cycloheximide (an inhibitor of protein synthesis). Its synthesis was monitored by biosynthetic radiolabeling techniques and immunoreactivity (unpublished work). The results indicated that TNF was synthesized following endotoxin treatment. It was not synthesized constitutively, stored, and then secreted. Production peaked by 6 hr. TNF was but a minor fraction of the total protein shed by macrophage-like cell lines in response to endotoxin.[13,14]

TNF was produced by peripheral blood monocytes.[9,26] The production of TNF and lymphotoxin by peripheral blood mononuclear cells (lymphocytes and monocytes) in culture has been studied in some detail.[26] Endotoxin was not the only agent capable of soliciting production. Induction was accomplished by endotoxin, lectins, or interleukin-2. The amount of TNF was increased about 10-fold by the addition of phorbol myristate acetate. It was also enhanced by addition of thymosin alpha-1, gamma interferon, or combinations of these reagents. Gamma interferon alone did not induce TNF. TNF was produced during the first 2 days of culture, whereupon lymphotoxin became the predominant cytotoxin shed by the mixed populations. Nonadherent cells (lymphocytes) were reported to produce TNF; however, there may have been contaminating monocytes or NK cells in the preparation. A soluble cytotoxic activity derived from NK cells has been attributed to TNF.[27] (See the relevant chapter herein. The lineage of NK cells is disputed.) TNF and lymphotoxin have

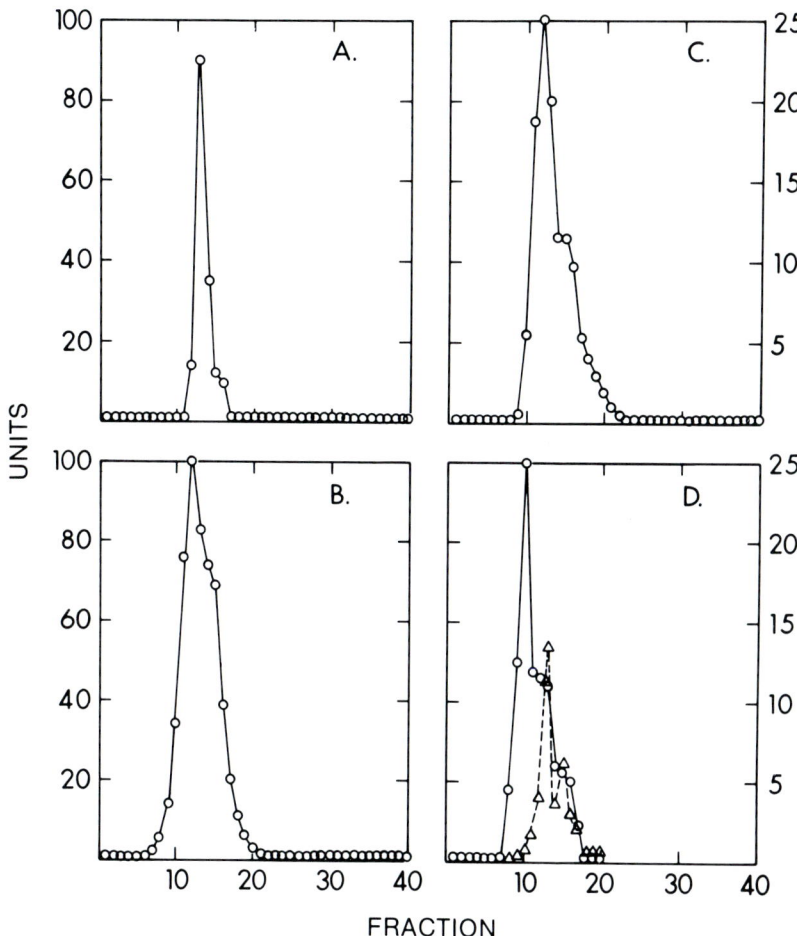

FIGURE 1. HPLC-gel filtration of murine TNF. Samples were dialized and run in 100 mM Na$_2$SO$_4$, 50 mM Tris-HC1, pH 7.4. 20 µℓ volumes were applied to a TSK-250 column (Bio-Rad). The flow rate was 1 mℓ/min, and 0.2 mℓ fractions were collected. They were measured for cytotoxicity on L-M cells as described.[13] The ordinate shows the units recovered. Recoveries were approximately 50%. (A) purified TNF; (B) crude J774.1 100 × concentrated supernatant; (C) crude RAW 264.7 75× concentrated supernatant; (D) mouse hypersensitive shock sera. The dashed line shows the activity partially purified from the same sera. Fractions correspond to the following M$_r$s as determined from calibrated standards: 10, 110,000; 12, 70,000; 16, 45,000.

been detected during the production of gamma interferon by mixed populations of leukocytes.[28]

In vivo, rodent serum TNF levels peaked in 2 hr following endotoxin administration.[29,30] For example, nanomolar concentrations were detected in the blood of normal rabbits. The TNF was rapidly cleared from the circulation. Liver, kidneys, skin, and gastrointestinal tract took up most of the TNF, and it was rapidly degraded in the tissues.[30] Considerable variation occurred in the amounts of TNF which were produced by the different strains of rodents.[29] Also, TNF levels were higher when the animals had been rendered hypersensitive by prior treatment with an adjuvant. Some of the strain variability may have been related to a given strain's response to a particular type of endotoxin. Lipid A was the required component of the endotoxin.[31]

2. Shock

While small quantities of murine TNF induced the necrosis of intradermal tumors (see below), 1 μg was lethal when it was injected i.v. into the tumor-bearing mice. Histopathologic evaluation of the tissues indicated that the mice died of acute respiratory distress. The symptoms were similar to endotoxin shock: ruffling, diarrhea, and accumulation of neutrophils and fluid in the lungs. The TNF preparation was highly purified and it contained less than 1% by weight endotoxin (F. Kull and G. Szczech, unpublished results). Similar observations on the lethality of TNF to tumor-bearing mice have been made with recombinant material.[7,74]

Anti-TNF antiserum ameliorated the lethal effects of endotoxin-induced shock when the antibodies were administered i.v. prior to the endotoxin.[32]

One concludes from these studies that TNF is an acute phase response protein, and that it conveys some of the activities seen in endotoxin shock. (Endotoxin, notably the lipid A component, activates the complement and coagulation cascades. Its properties are the focus of intense study.[33]) The acute phase response constitutes those physical and biochemical changes which occur in vivo in response to infectious/inflammatory stimuli. It is reviewed elsewhere with respect to interleukin-1 (IL-1).[34] While TNF and IL-1 are distinct molecules, many features of their production and biologic activities are similar. Both are made by myeloid cells in response to endotoxin and/or lectin-like stimuli. Both solicit neutrophilia in vivo. Other similar in vitro properties are noted below.

B. Tumor Necrosis

Intradermal tumor necrosis is perhaps the most dramatic and vivid property of TNF (Figure 2). Mice bearing solid tumor implants are injected i.v. with test material. The tumor turns blue within hours, and by 24 hr, the core contains an area of necrosis which may nearly cover the diameter of the tumor. The extent of necrosis is quantitively related to the amount of test material. Necrosis is accompanied by symptoms of shock. If the tumor is immunogenic, the necrosis may be followed by regression and cure.[35] In our hands, approximately one third of the mice who reject a methylcholanthrene-induced fibrosarcoma are cured following necrosis. Our results are similar to those originally reported for crude TNF.[6] TNF has necrosed syngeneic and xenogenic tumor transplants (human tumors in nude mice).[36] It was most effective when introduced intratumorally.

Endotoxin elicits a similar effect,[35] which may be mediated through endogenous production of TNF. The amount of TNF required to produce the effect is approximately 0.01% by weight the amount of endotoxin required to produce an equivalent response (unpublished results).

The intradermal tumor may represent a specialized case of effectiveness. Tumor-bearing mice are more sensitive to endotoxin.[37] Implantation of the tumor may serve to prime mice like an adjuvant, or it may prime them in the sense of the initial phase of the Schwartzman reaction.[38] It is tempting to speculate that one or more of the fulminant aspects of shock necrose the tumors. Algire hypothesized hypotension.[39] The skin, and especially the burdened vasculature of a growing tumor,[40] may be unusually sensitive to disseminated intravascular coagulation. Many processes may be involved. Complement[41] and alpha adrenergic requirements[42] have been implicated. Finally, we should consider a direct effect of TNF on the tumor cells. Recent results provide some clues as to how the hormone might exert its in vivo properties.

C. In Vitro Properties

Cytotoxicity is but one of several properties which have been observed in culture (Table 2). The pleiotropic nature of these responses is surprising because of their variety and opposite appearances. The variety is simplistically explained. TNF appears to be a general catabolic hormone. It may induce metabolic changes which are toxic, growth promoting, or overlooked, and some of the changes (such as endothelial cell modulation and bone resorbtion) appear to be common among distinct molecular entities (TNF, IL-1, and interferon).

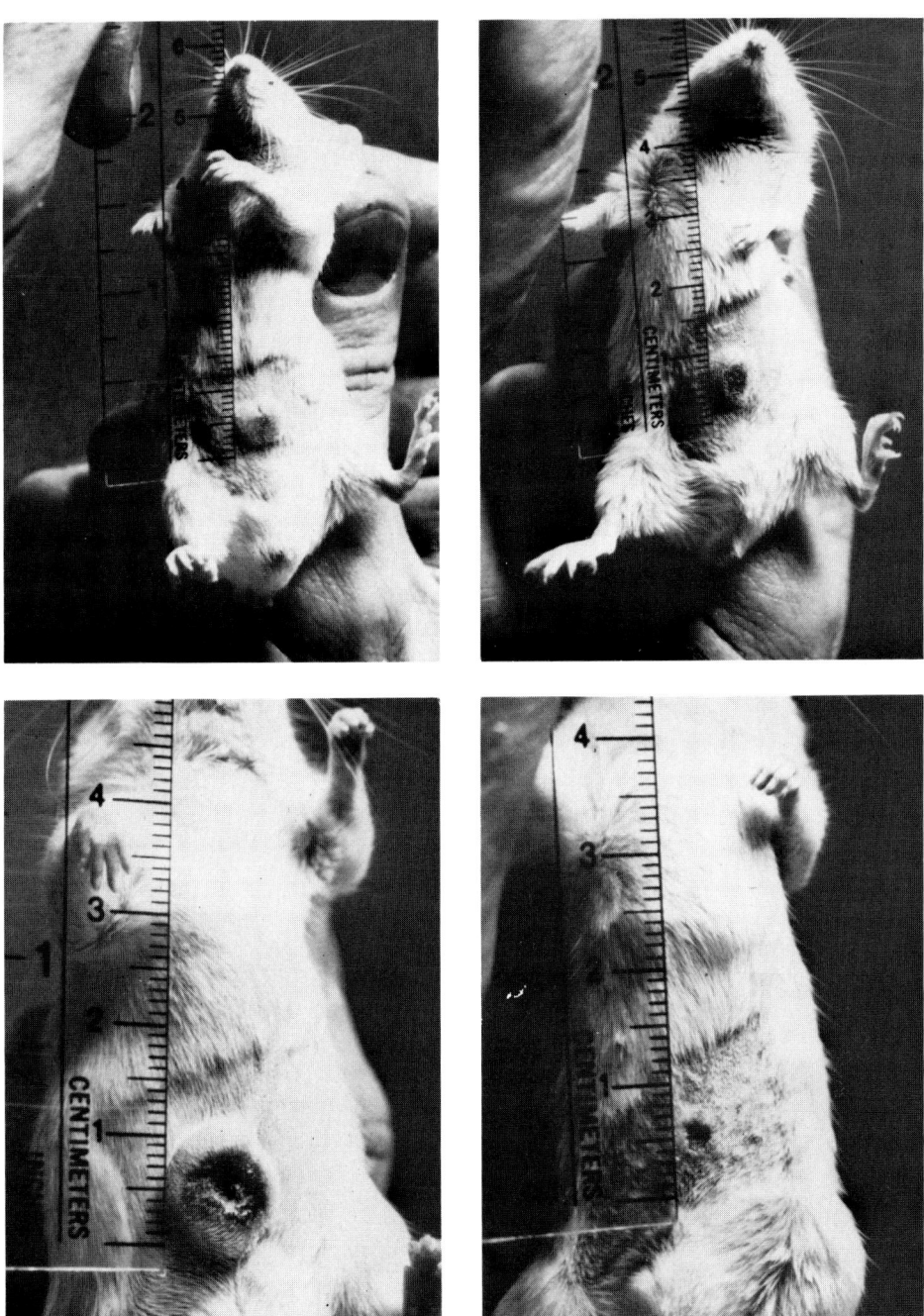

FIGURE 2. Intradermal tumor necrosis. BALB/c mice were implanted with a methylcholanthrene-induced fibrosarcoma. Eight days later they were injected i.v. with 100 ng highly purified murine TNF (right photos) or saline (left photos). Top photos show the appearance 1 day later, and bottom photos show the appearance 7 days later.

Table 2
SUMMARY OF IN VITRO PROPERTIES

Property	Target cell	Ref.
Phagocytosis and ADCC	Neutrophils	65
Adherence to endothelia	Neutrophils	66
Antigen modulation	Endothelium	67
Bone resorption	Bone fragments	63
Differentiation	Adipocytes	57,58
Proliferation	Diploid fibroblasts	45
Death	Tumorigenic fibroblasts	49

1. Toxicity and Proliferation

Cell death requires hours to days of exposure. Toxicity surveys of established cell lines concluded that many (but not all) tumor lines were sensitive, that the species of origin was irrelevant, and that normal cells were insensitive.[43,44] Claims of tumor specificity may have been premature because the "normal" lines were under-represented. In fact, diploid bovine endothelial lines and contact-inhibited murine fibroblasts were sensitive to killing by purified natural murine TNF.[13] The growth rates of some normal human lines was enhanced by recombinant human TNF.[45] The ability to stimulate fibroblast growth has been reported for partially purified IL-1 (reviewed in Reference 34). In view of the possibility of TNF contamination, these latter studies should be repeated with recombinant IL-1. The toxicity of TNF and lymphotoxin to tumor cell lines has been enhanced or manifest by combination with interferon.[25,46,47]

The L-M line, a murine tumorigenic fibroblast, is very sensitive to killing by murine TNF. L-M cells are killed during prolonged incubation (24 hr) by concentrations of TNF in the range of 0.1 to 10 pM.[13] They can be grown in the absence of any proteinaceous additives (Higuchi's medium),[48] and they are killed by TNF as readily as L-M grown in the presence of serum (unpublished observation).

A variety of altered growth conditions and metabolic inhibitors were employed to examine the mechanism of TNF-induced killing.[49] Lysosomotropic amines (which impede lysosomal functions such as degradation and receptor recycling), oxidative metabolic poisons, and reduced temperature (34°) inhibited killing. Increased temperature (40°) and inhibitors of protein and RNA synthesis enhanced killing. (Actinomycin D has been incorporated in routine assays for lymphotoxin and TNF.[23,50]) Thus, L-M cells actively participated in their own demise, and internalization of TNF may have been required for toxicity. (Radioiodinated TNF was internalized and degraded by target cells.[52]) Calcium-free medium had no appreciable effect.

The latter result contrasts with a number of lytic toxins, such as phalloidin, which require extracellular calcium to drive the lytic process.[51] This distinction may provide a clue as to the mechanism. Lytic toxins disrupt the integrity of the membrane, whereas toxins like diptheria and ricin require internalization. The work on cachexia provides additional refreshing insights into the metabolic processes which may underlie sensitivity.

2. Adipocyte Differentiation/Metabolism

Beutler et al.[55] were struck by the general dissipation (cachexia) which accompanied an experimental trypanosomal infection. The condition is commonly associated with infectious diseases and terminal cancer. It is accompanied by a tissue depletion of the enzyme lipoprotein lipase (LPL), which clears lipid from the circulation and supplies it for uptake by cells. These investigators sought a macrophage factor which depleted LPL in differentiated 3T3-L1 cells.

The 3T3-L1 line is a murine preadipocyte which can be induced to form mature adipocytes.[53] Over a period of days, the maturing cells accumulate lipid in vesicles, and they express marked metabolic changes, such as expression of LPL[54,55] and increased numbers of insulin receptors.[56]

They uncovered a factor from a murine macrophage-like cell line which they named cachectin. Cachectin completely suppressed the LPL activity of mature cells within 6 hr.[54] Additionally, it prevented preadipocyte differentiation.[57] The effects appeared to be mediated at the transcription level.

Cachectin is similar if not identical to murine TNF. The amino terminal sequence of cachectin is virtually identical to published murine TNF sequences, its physical properties are similar to TNF, and it has the cytotoxic property attributed to TNF.[58] In confirmation, murine TNF has properties attributed to cachectin (Figure 3). (See addendum.)

In addition to their immune/inflammatory functions, macrophages play a prominent part in lipid metabolism. Apolipoprotein E is a major secretory product, and macrophages provide a lipid sink via the salvage low-density lipoprotein receptor.[60] "Activated" macrophages secrete a host of factors along with TNF.[61] TNF may be a part of their endocrine-like functions. Beutler et al.[58] suggest that TNF helps to mobilize host energy reserves. The cachectin effort clearly identifies a catabolic hormonal role for TNF. (Interestingly, monocytes derived from human cancer patients spontaneously produced TNF.[59]) Similar suggestions are made for IL-1.[34]

Indeed, IL-1 modulated LPL activity in vitro.[62] It was effective at 10^{-15} M, whereas TNF was effective at 10^{-9} M. In contrast to TNF, IL-1 did not completely suppress LPL. TNF and lymphotoxin stimulated bone resorption in culture.[63] Likewise, IL-1 has been assessed a bone resorbing (osteoclast-activating factor) activity.[64]

In addition to the cachexic properties of TNF, we may consider the involvement of TNF in leukopenia (adherence). Leukocyte adherence accompanies all inflammatory processes. The following properties have been reported to date.

3. Activation and Maturation Functions

TNF, lymphotoxin, and gamma interferon have been shown to increase the phagocytic and antibody-dependent cellular cytotoxic capacities of human neutrophils.[65] Rapid treatment (5 min) of neutrophils enhanced their ability to bind to human umbilical vein endothelial cells.[66] The TNF appeared to induce the expression of antigens which were required for optimum adherance and for complement component C3bi receptor function. Treatment of the endothelial cells (4 hr) with TNF also increased their attractiveness to the neutrophils. TNF was seen to modulate the expression of class I major histocompatibility complex antigens on cultured endothelial cells and skin fibroblasts.[67] Expression was maximal at 4 days, and it was blocked by concomitant treatment with cycloheximide.

V. MECHANISM OF ACTION

A. Cellular Receptor

Several papers have described the binding of radio-iodinated TNF. They concluded the following:

1. Normal tissue,[55] diploid cell lines,[45,68] and tumor cell lines[52,68-70] bore a single class of specific high-affinity cell surface receptor.
2. The apparent K_Ds ranged from 3 pM[68] to 600 pM.[52]
3. The number of sites per cell was approximately 1000 to 2000.
4. The presence of receptors, while perhaps a prerequisite for sensitivity, was not sufficient to predict the cells' responsiveness.[68,52]

84 *Cytolytic Lymphocytes and Complement*

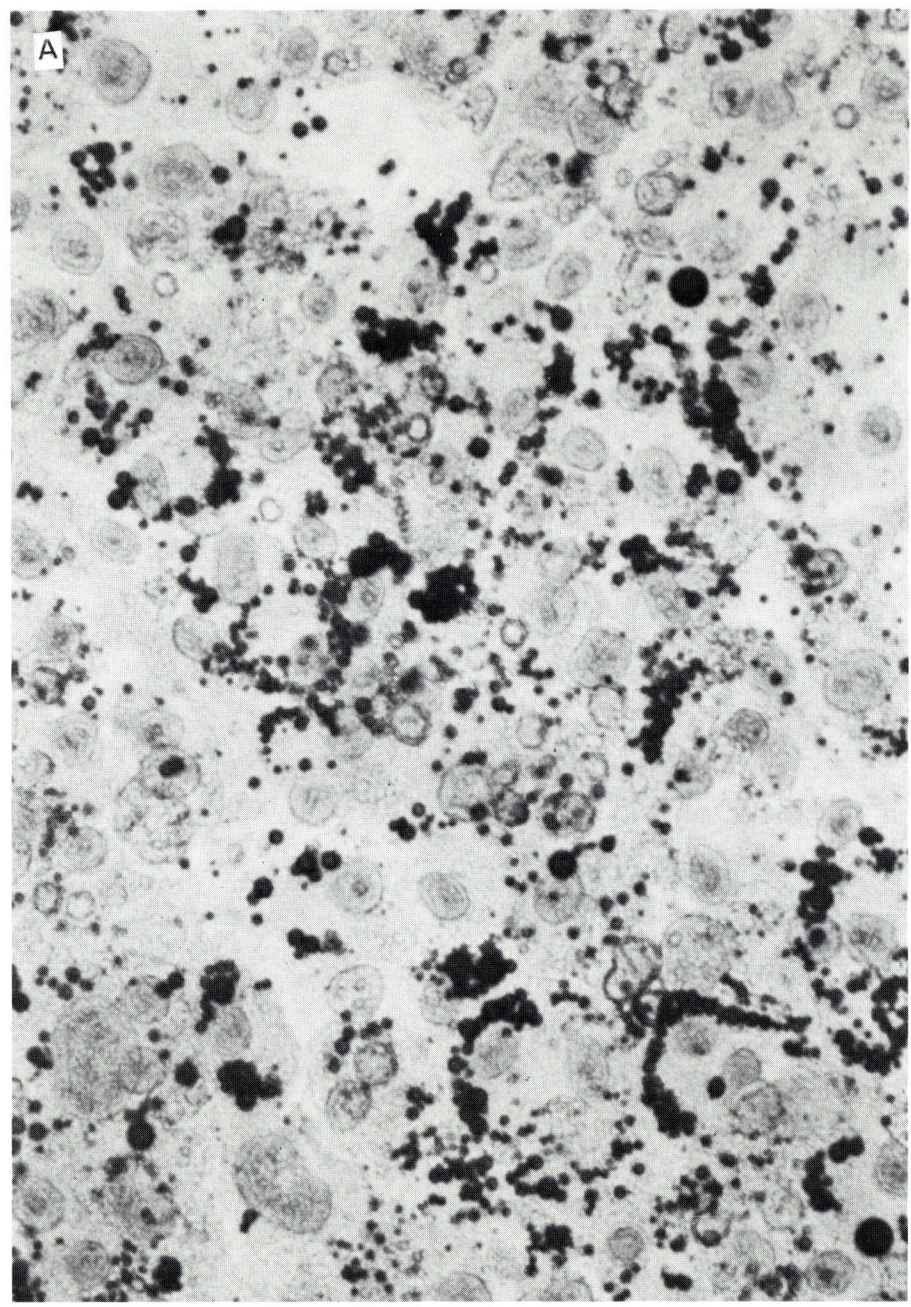

FIGURE 3. Lipid depletion in mature 3T3-L1 cells. Cells were induced to differentiate as described;[53] then fresh medium containing TNF was applied every other day. Cells were stained with oil red O, which highlighted the lipid vesicles (dark circles). The cells were counterstained with hematoxylin, which highlighted the nuclei (large faint circles). (A) control; (B) 30 pM TNF after 1 week. Magnification was 200 ×. Note the relative depletion in the lipid vesicles. Concomitant treatment with actinomycin D was toxic within 1 day, and prolonged incubations with high concentrations of TNF alone (1 n*M*) were toxic.

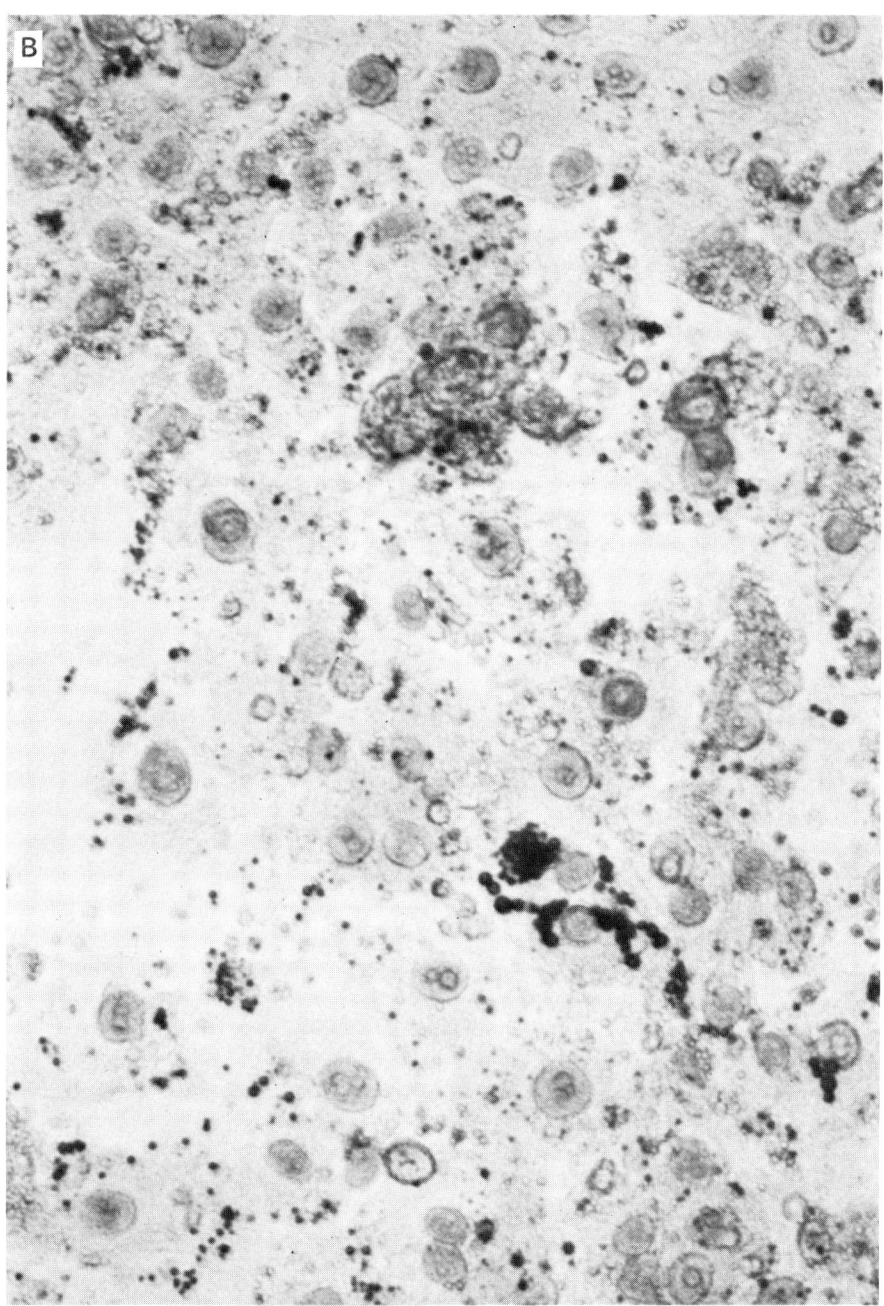

FIGURE 3B.

Cells which demonstrated a response to TNF were found to possess receptors, and no responsive cells were found which lacked receptors. Lymphotoxin and TNF competed with one another for occupancy of the same receptor, but gamma interferon did not compete.[70] Radio-iodinated murine TNF was chemically cross-linked to its putative receptor.[68] The receptor was identified as an approximately 80,000 M_r polypeptide.

Two additional considerations suggest that the binding sites were, in part, required for biologic activity. First, the affinities were in the range of the concentrations required for biologic activity. The affinities were comparable to other lymphokine ligands (such as gamma interferon and interleukin-2), and they were greater than those reported for the growth factors insulin and epidermal growth factor. Secondly, treatment of target cells with gamma interferon doubled the number of TNF receptors.[70] Interferon was reported to enhance sensitivity to TNF and lymphotoxin.[46,47]

We had speculated that internalization may be required for cytotoxicity, based on metabolic inhibitor studies.[49] Radio-iodinated TNF was internalized and degraded in both sensitive (to cytotoxicity) and resistant cells.[52] Thus, TNF may have behaved like other polypeptide hormones (for example, epidermal growth factor and insulin, which are internalized via coated pits). In like manner, we may expect both immediate and long-term effects.

ADDENDUM

Quite expectedly, many fine studies have been published since the original writing. While the majority amplify the observations noted above, a few selected works address questions raised herein.

The enigmatic long leader sequence of TNF may be a presequence used for intracellular sorting. Indeed, the complete TNF gene product (26,000 Dalton) appears to be a transmembrane protein. It was immunoprecipitated from membrane solubilizates (M. Kriegler, submitted). Also, paraformaldehyde-fixed macrophages were toxic to target cells, and toxicity was quenched by anti-TNF antisera.[71,72] Such results suggest that cell-associated (pre)TNF may have properties beyond those of the mature secreted form. Several mediators may be involved in macrophage-mediated cytotoxicity depending on the sensitivity of target cells.[73]

Shock and cachexia have been amply demonstrated. The LD_{50} of intravenously-administered human recombinant TNF in rats was estimated to be 700 μg/kg.[74] The pathophysiological and histological findings mimicked endotoxin shock. Nude mice that bore a tumor that produced 1 to 10 ng TNF/mℓ sera were found to lose weight and die more quickly than mice bearing control tumors.[75]

Despite dramatic experimental revelations, Phase I cancer trials of TNF in humans have yet to suggest an indication. Perhaps humans are less sensitive than rodents. Perhaps the role of host defense cooperation ("priming") is not sufficiently understood to predict its manipulation by TNF. At least in rodents, TNF could replace endotoxin in the eliciting phase but not in the priming phase of the Shwartzman reaction.[76]

Other reviews/compilations are suggested.[77-80]

REFERENCES

1. **Ruff, M. R. and Gifford, G. E.**, Tumor necrosis factor, in *Lymphokines*, Vol. 2, Pick, E., Ed., Academic Press, New York, 1981, 235.
2. **Nauts, H. C., Swift, W. E., and Coley, B. C.**, The treatment of malignant tumors by bacterial toxins as developed by the late William B. Coley, M. D., reviewed in the light of modern research, *Cancer Res.*, 6, 205, 1946.
3. **Shear, M. J.**, Chemical treatment of tumors; reactions of mice with primary subcutaneous tumors to injection of hemorrhage-producing bacterial polysaccharide, *J. Natl. Cancer Inst.*, 4, 461, 1944.
4. **Menkin, M.**, *Biochemical Mechanisms in Inflammation*, 3rd ed., Charles C Thomas, Springfield, Ill., 1956, 195.
5. **Atkins, E.**, Pathogenesis of fever, *Physiol. Rev.*, 40, 560, 1960.
6. **Carswell, E. A., Old, L. J., Kassel, R. L., Green, S., Fiore, N., and Williamson, B.**, An endotoxin-induced serum factor that causes necrosis of tumors, *Proc. Nat. Acad. Sci. USA*, 72, 3666, 1975.

7. **Old, L. J.,** Perspective Tumor necrosis factor (TNF), *Science,* 230, 630, 1985.
8. **Kull, F. C., Jr., and Cuatrecasas, P.,** Preliminary characterization of the tumor cell cytotoxin in tumor necrosis serum, *J. Immunol.,* 126, 1279, 1981.
9. **Matthews, N.,** Tumor-necrosis factor from the rabbit. II. Production by monocytes, *Br. J. Cancer,* 38, 310, 1978.
10. **Mannel, D. N., Moore, R. N., and Mergenhagen, S. E.,** Macrophages as a source of tumoricidal activity (tumor-necrotizing factor), *Infect. Immunol.,* 30, 523, 1980.
11. **Ruff, M. R. and Gifford, G. E.,** Purification and physico-chemical characterization of rabbit tumor necrosis factor, *J. Immunol.,* 125, 1671, 1980.
12. **Haranaka, K., Satomi, N., Sakurai, and Nariuchi, H.,** Purification and partial amino acid sequence of rabbit tumor necrosis factor, *Int. J. Cancer,* 36, 395, 1985.
13. **Kull, F. C., Jr., and Cuatrecasas, P.,** Necrosin: purification and properties of a cytotoxin derived from a murine macrophage-like cell line, *Proc. Nat. Acad. Sci. USA,* 81, 7932, 1984.
14. **Aggarwal, B. B., Kohr, W. J., Hass, P. E., Moffat, B., Spencer, S. A., Henzel, W. J., Bringman, T. S., Nedwin, G. E., Goeddel, D. V., and Harkins, R. N.,** Human tumor necrosis factor: production, purification, and characterization, *J. Biol. Chem.,* 260, 2345, 1985.
15. **Pennica, D., Nedwin, G. E., Hayflick, J. S., Seeburg, P. H., Derynk, R., Palladino, M. A., Kohr, W. J., Aggarwal, B. B., and Goeddel, D.,** Human tumor necrosis factor: precursor structure, expression and homology to lymphotoxin, *Nature (London),* 312, 724, 1984.
16. **Wang, A. M., Creasey, A. A., Ladner, M. B., Lin, L. S., Strickler, J., Van Arsdell, J. N., Yamamoto, R., and Mark, D. F.,** Molecular cloning of the complementary DNA for human tumor necrosis factor, *Science,* 228, 149, 1985.
17. **Shirai, T., Yamaguchi, H., Ito, H., Todd, C. W., and Wallace, B.,** Cloning and expression in *Esherichia coli* of the gene for human tumor necrosis factor, *Nature (London),* 313, 803, 1985.
18. **Fransen, F., Muller, R., Marmenout, A., Tavernier, J., Van der Heyden, J., Kawashima, E., Chollet, A., Tizard, R., Van Heuverswyn, H., Van Vliet, A., Ruysschaert, M., and Fliers, W.,** Molecular cloning of mouse tumor necrosis factor cDNA and its eukaryotic expression, *Nucleic Acids Res.,* 13, 4417, 1985.
19. **Nedwin, G. E., Naylor, S. L., Sakaguchi, A. Y., Smith, D., Jarrett-Nedwin, J., Pennica, D., Goeddel, D. V., and Gray, P. W.,** Human lymphotoxin and tumor necrosis factor genes: structure, homology and chromosomal localization, *Nucleic Acids Res.,* 13, 6361, 1985.
20. **March, C. J., Mosley, B., Larsen, A., Cerretti, D. P., Braedt, G., Price, V., Gillis, S., Henney, C. S., Kroneim, S. R., Grabstein, K., Conlon, P. J., Hopp, T. P., and Cosman, D.,** Cloning, sequence and expression of two distinct human interleukin-1 complementary DNAs, *Nature (London),* 315, 641, 1985.
21. **Pennica, D., Hayflick, J. S., Bringman, T. S., Palladino, M. A., and Goeddel, D. V.,** Cloning and expression *Escherichia coli* of the cDNA for murine tumor necrosis factor, *Proc. Nat. Acad. Sci. USA,* 82, 6060, 1985.
22. **Itoh, H. and Nakano, F. S.,** A novel physiologically active polypeptide, European patent application # 84105149.3.
23. **Gray, P. W., Aggarwal, B. B., Benton, C. V., Bringman, T. S., Henzel, W. J., Jarett, J. A., Leunj, D. W., Moffat, B., Ng, P., Svedersky, L. P., Palladino, M. A., and Nedwin, G. E.,** Cloning and expression of cDNA for human lymphotoxin, a lymphokine with tumor necrosis activity, *Nature (London),* 312, 721, 1984.
24. **Kull, F. C., Jr., and Cuatrecasas, P.,** Macrophage cytotoxin, in *Interleukins, Lymphokines, and Cytokines,* Cohen, S. and Oppenheim, J., Eds., Academic Press, Inc., New York, 511, 1983.
25. **Williamson, B. D., Carswell, E. A., Rubin, B. Y., Prendergast, J. S., and Old, L. J.,** Human tumor necrosis factor produced by human B-cell lines: Synergistic cytotoxic interaction with human interferon, *Proc. Nat. Acad. Sci. USA,* 80, 5397, 1983.
26. **Nedwin, G. E., Svedersky, L. P., Bringman, T. S., Palladino, M. A., and Goeddel, D. V.,** Effect of interleukin 2, interferon-gamma, and mitogens on the production of tumor necrosis factors alpha and beta, *J. Immunol.,* 135, 2492, 1985.
27. **Degliantoni, G., Murphy, M., Kobayashi, M., Francis, M. K., Perussia, B., and Trinchieri, G.,** Natural killer (NK) cell-derived hematopoietic colony-inhibiting activity and NK cytotoxic factor, *J. Exp. Med.,* 162, 1512, 1985.
28. **Kelker, H. C., Oppenheim, J. D., Stone-Wolff, D., Henrikson-DeStefano, D., Aggarwal, B. B., Stevenson, H. C., and Vilcek, J.,** Characterization of human tumor necrosis factor produced by peripheral blood monocytes and its separation from lymphotoxin, *Int. J. Cancer,* 36, 69, 1985.
29. **Haranaka, K., Satomi, N., and Sakurai, A.,** Differences in tumour necrosis factor productive ability among rodents, *Br. J. Cancer,* 50, 471, 1984.
30. **Beutler, B., Milsark, I. W., and Cerami, A.,** Cachectin/tumor necrosis factor: production, distribution and metabolic fate in vivo, *J. Immunol.,* 135, 3972, 1985.

31. **Haranaka, K., Satomi, N., Sakurai, A., and Kunii, O.,** Role of lipid A in the production of tumor necrosis factor and differences in antitumor activity between tumor necrosis factor and lipopolysaccharide, *Tohoku J. Exp. Med.,* 144, 385, 1984.
32. **Beutler, B., Milsark, I. W., and Cerami, A. C.,** Passive immunization against cachectin/tumor necrosis factor protects mice from lethal effect of endotoxin, *Science,* 229, 869, 1985.
33. **Ribi, E.,** Beneficial modification of the endotoxin molecule, *J. Biol. Response Mod.,* 3, 1, 1984.
34. **Dinarello, C. A.,** Interleukin-1, *Rev. Infect. Dis.,* 6, 51, 1984.
35. **Berendt, M. J., North, R. J., and Kirstein, D. P.,** The immunological basis of endotoxin-induced tumor regression. Requirement for T cell mediated immunity, *J. Exp. Med.,* 148, 1550, 1978.
36. **Haranaka, K., Satomi, N., and Sakuri, A.,** Antitumor activity of murine tumor necrosis factor (TNF) against transplanted murine tumors and heterotransplanted human tumors in nude mice, *Int. J. Cancer,* 34, 263, 1984.
37. **Beck, L. V., Berkowitz, D., and Seltzer, B.,** Physiological studies on tumor-inhibiting agents: effect on apparent systolic blood pressure in mice of *Serratia marcescens* tumor-necrotizing polysaccharide of Shear, *Cancer Res.,* 8, 162, 1948.
38. **Katayama, Y. and Kodama, M.,** Schwartzman model of the malignant tumor cell, *Jpn. J. Med. Sci. Biol.,* 33, 35, 1980.
39. **Algire, G. H., Legallais, F. Y., and Anderson, B. F.,** Vascular reactions of normal and malignant tissues *in vivo.* V. Role of hypotension in action of bacterial polysaccharide on tumors, *J. Natl. Cancer Inst.,* 12, 1279, 1952.
40. **Gullino, P. M.,** Influence of blood supply on thermal properties and metabolism of mammary carcinomas, *Ann. N. Y. Acad. Sci.,* 335, 1, 1980.
41. **Yamaguchi, N., Sakai, T., Yoshida, S., Katayama, Y., and Kawai, K.,** Anti-tumor activity of endotoxin depends on activation of serum complement fragments, *Gastroent. Jpn.,* 18, 436, 1983.
42. **Bloksma, N., Hofhuis, F. M., and Willers, J. M. N.,** Effect of adrenoceptor blockade on hemorrhagic necrosis of Meth A sacomata induced by endotoxin or tumor necrosis serum, *Immunopharmacology,* 4, 163, 1982.
43. **Haranaka, K. and Satomi, N.,** Cytotoxic activity of tumor necrosis factor (TNF) on human cancer cells *in vitro, Jpn. J. Exp. Med.,* 51, 191, 1981.
44. **Matthews, N.,** Production of an anti-tumour cytotoxin by human monocytes, *Immunology,* 44, 135, 1981.
45. **Sugarman, B. J., Aggarwal, B. B., Hass, P., Figari, I. S., Palladino, M. A. and Shepard, H. M.,** Recombinant human tumor necrosis factor-alpha: effects on proliferation of normal and transformed cells in vitro, *Science,* 230, 943, 1985.
46. **Stone-Wolff, D. S., Yip, Y. K., Kelker, H. C., Le, J., Henriksen-DeStefano, D., Rubin, B. Y., Rinderknecht, E., Aggarwal, B. B., and Vilcek, J.,** Interrelationships of human interferon-gamma with lymphotoxin and monocyte cytotoxin, *J. Exp. Med.,* 159, 828, 1984.
47. **Lee, S. H., Aggarwal, B. B., Rinderknecht, E., Assisi, F., and Chiu, H.,** The synergistic anti-proliferative effect of gamma-interferon and human lymphotoxin, *J. Immunol.,* 133, 1083, 1984.
48. **Higuchi, K.,** An improved chemically defined culture medium for strain L mouse cells based on growth responses to graded levels of nutrients including iron and zinc ions, *J. Cell. Physiol.,* 75, 65, 1970.
49. **Kull, F. C., Jr., and Cuatrecasas, P.,** Possible requirement of internalization in the mechanism of *in vitro* cytotoxicity in tumor necrosis serum, *Cancer Res.,* 41, 4885, 1981.
50. **Flick, D. A. and Gifford, G. E.,** Comparison of in vitro cell cytotoxic assays for tumor necrosis factor, *J. Immunol. Met.,* 68, 167, 1984.
51. **Kane, A. B., Young, E. E., Schanne, F. A. X., and Farber, J. L.,** Calcium dependence of phalloidin-induced liver cell death, *Proc. Natl. Acad. Sci. USA,* 77, 1177, 1980.
52. **Tsujimoto, M., Yip, Y. K., and Vilcek, J.,** Tumor necrosis factor: specific binding and internalization in sensitive and resistant cells, *Proc. Natl. Acad. Sci. USA,* 82, 7626, 1985.
53. **Green, H. and Kehinde, O.,** An established preadipose cell line and its differentiation in culture II. Factors affecting the adipose conversion, *Cell,* 5, 19, 1975.
54. **Kawakami, M., Pekala, P. H., Lane, M. D., and Cerami, A.,** Lipoprotein lipase supression in 3T3-L1 cells by an endotoxin-induced mediator from exudate cells, *Proc. Natl. Acad. Sci. USA,* 79, 912, 1982.
55. **Beutler, B., Mahoney, J., Le Trang, N., Pekala, P., and Cerami, A.,** Purification of cachectin, a lipoprotein lipase-suppresing hormone secreted by endotoxin-induced RAW 264.7 cells, *J. Exp. Med.,* 161, 984, 1985.
56. **Reed, B. C. and Lane, M. D.,** Insulin receptor synthesis and turnover in differentiating 3T3-L1 preadipocytes, *Proc. Natl. Acad. Sci. USA,* 77, 285, 1980.
57. **Torti, F. M., Dieckmann, B., Beutler, B., Cerami, A., and Ringold, G. M.,** A macrophage factor inhibits adipocyte gene expression: an *in vitro* model of cachexia, *Science,* 229, 867, 1985.
58. **Beutler, B., Greenwald, D., Hulmes, J. D., Chany, M., Pan, Y.-C. E., Mathison, J., Ulevitch, R., and Cerami, A.,** Identity of tumor necrosis factor and the macrophage secreted factor cachectin, *Nature (London),* 316, 552, 1985.

59. **Aderka, D., Fisher, S., Levo, Y., Holtmann, H., Hahn, T., and Wallach, D.**, Cachectin/tumour necrosis factor production by cancer patients, *Lancet*, 1190, Nov. 23, 1985.
60. **Brown, M. S. and Goldstein, J. L.**, Lipoprotein metabolism in the macrophage: implication for cholesterol deposition in atherosclerosis, *Ann. Rev. Biochem.*, 52, 233, 1983.
61. **Adams, D. O. and Hamilton, T. A.**, The cell biology of macrophage activation, *Ann. Rev. Immunol.*, 2, 283, 1984.
62. **Beutler, B. A. and Cerami, A.**, Recombinant interleukin 1 suppresses lipoprotein lipase activity in 3T3-L1 cells, *J. Immunol.*, 135, 3969, 1985.
63. **Bertolini, D. R., Nedwin, G. E., Bringman, T. S., Smith, D. D., and Mundy, G. R.**, Stimulation of bone resorption and inhibition of bone formation in vitro by human tumor necrosis factors, *Nature (London)*, 319, 516, 1986.
64. **Dewhirst, F. E., Stashenko, P. P., Mole, J. E., and Tsurumachi, T.**, Purification and partial sequence of human osteoclast-activating factor: identity with interleukin 1 beta, *J. Immunol.*, 135, 2562, 1986.
65. **Shalby, M. R., Aggarwal, B. B., Rinderknecht, E., Svedersky, L. P., Finkle, B. S., and Palladino, M. A.**, Activation of human polymorphonuclear neutrophil functions by interferon-gamma and tumor necrosis factors, *J. Immunol.*, 135, 2069, 1985.
66. **Gamble, J. R., Harlan, J. M., Klebanoff, S. J., and Vadas, M. A.**, Stimulation of the adherence of neutrophils to umbilical vein endothelium by human recombinant tumor necrosis factor, *Proc. Natl. Acad. Sci. USA*, 82, 8667, 1985.
67. **Collins, T., Lapierre, L. A., Fiers, W., Strominger, J. L., and Pober, J. S.**, Recombinant human tumor necrosis factor increases mRNA levels and surface expression of HLA-A,B antigens in vascular endothelial cells and dermal fibroblasts *in vitro*, *Proc. Natl. Acad. Sci. USA*, 83, 446, 1986.
68. **Kull, F. C., Jr., Jacobs, S., and Cuatrecasas, P.**, Cellular receptor for ^{125}I-labeled tumor necrosis factor: specific binding, affinity labeling, and relationship to sensitivity, *Proc. Natl. Acad. Sci. USA*, 82, 5756, 1985.
69. **Baglioni, C., McCandless, S., Tavernier, J., and Fiers, W.**, Binding of human tumor necrosis factor to high affinity receptors on HeLa and lymphoblastoid cells sensitive to growth inhibition, *J. Biol. Chem.*, 260, 13395, 1985.
70. **Aggarwal, B. B., Eessalu, T. E., and Hass, P. E.**, Characterization of receptors for human tumour necrosis factor and their regulation by gamma-interferon, *Nature (London)*, 318, 665, 1985.
71. **Decker, T., Lohmann-Matthes, M., and Gifford, G. E.**, Cell-associated tumor necrosis factor (TNF) as a killing mechanism of activated macrophages, *J. Immunol.*, 138, 957, 1987.
72. **Espevik, T. and Nissen-Meyer, J.**, Tumour necrosis factor-like activity on paraformaldehyde-fixed monocyte monolayers, *Immunology*, 61, 443, 1987.
73. **Klostergaard, J., Leroux, M. E., Ezell, S. M., and Kull, F. C, Jr.**, Tumoricidal effector mechanisms of murine *Bacillus Calmette-Guerin*-activated macrophages: mediation of cytolysis, mitochondrial respiration inhibition, and release of intracellular iron by distinct mechanisms, *Cancer Res.*, 47, 2014, 1987.
74. **Tracey, K. J., Beutler, B., Lowry, S. F., Merryweather, J., Wolpe, S., Milsark, I. W., Hariri, R. J., Fahey, T. J., Zentella, A., Albert, J. D., Shires, G. T., and Cerami, A.**, Shock and tissue injury induced by recombinant human cachectin, *Science*, 234, 470, 1986.
75. **Oliff, A., Defeo-Jones, D., Boyer, M., Martinez, D., Kiefer, D., Vuocolo, G., Wolfe, A., and Socher, S. H.**, Tumors secreting human TNF/cachectin induce cachexia in mice, *Cell*, 50, 555, 1987.
76. **Rothstein, J. L. and Schreiber, H.**, Synergy between tumor necrosis factor and bacterial products causes hemorrhagic necrosis and lethal shock, *Immunobiology*, 175, 31, 1987.
77. **Beutler, B. and Cerami, A.**, Cachectin and tumour necrosis factor as two sides of the same biological coin, *Nature (London)*, 320, 584, 1986.
78. **Gemsa, D., Ed.**, Abstracts, International Conference on Tumor Necrosis Factor and Related Cytotoxins, *Immunobiology*, 175, 1, 1987.
79. **Beutler, B. and Cerami, A.**, Cachectin: more than a tumor necrosis factor, *N. Engl. J. Med.*, 316, 379, 1987.
80. **Le, J. and Vilcek, J.**, Tumor necrosis factor and interleukin-1: cytokines with multiple overlapping biological functions, *Lab. Invest.*, 56, 234, 1987.

LIBRARY
UNIVERSITY OF TEXAS
SOUTHWESTERN MEDICAL SCHOOL
DALLAS, TEXAS

Chapter 20

NATURAL KILLER CYTOTOXIC FACTOR (NKCF) AS MEDIATOR IN THE LYTIC PATHWAY OF NK CELL MEDIATED CYTOTOXICITY*

Benjamin Bonavida and Susan C. Wright

TABLE OF CONTENTS

I.	Introduction	92
II.	Methods	92
	A. Production of NKCF	92
	1. Stimulation with Target Cells	93
	2. Stimulation with Mitogens	93
	3. Enhanced Production of NKCF	94
	B. Assay of NKCF activity	94
	1. Trypan Blue Exclusion	94
	2. The Microcytotoxicty ^{51}Cr Release Assay	94
III.	Model for the Mechanism of NK CMC Involving NKCF as Mediators	95
IV.	Experimental Evidence Supporting the Proposed Model of the Mechanism of NK-CMC	95
	A. Recognition and Binding of the NK Effector Cells to Target Cells	95
	B. Activation of the NKCF Release Mechanism	95
	C. Mechanism of Release of NKCF	96
	1. Involvement of Proteases	96
	2. Kinetics of Secretion of NKCF	96
	3. Biochemical Pathways of Activation of NKCF	97
	4. Interaction of NKCF with Binding Sites on NK Target Cells	97
V.	Mechanism of Action of NKCF	98
	A. Kinetic of Lysis	98
	B. Kinetic of NKCF Binding to Target Cells	98
	C. Lysis of NK-Resistant Target Cells by Fusion with Liposomes Containing NK-Sensitive Membranes	98
	D. Lysis of NK-Resistant Target Cells by NKCF Containing Liposomes	98
	E. Pore Formation	99
VI.	Biochemical Characterization of NKCF	99
VII.	Relationship Between NKCF and Other Cytotoxins	99
VIII.	Diagnostic and Clinical Implications	100
	A. Diagnostic implications	100
	1. Defective NK Effector Function	100
	2. Resistance of Target Cell Lysis by NK Cells	101
	B. Therapeutic Implications	102
References		102

---

* This review was made possible by grant support CA-35791 and CA-37199 awarded by the National Cancer Institute.

I. INTRODUCTION

It is becoming increasingly clear that several immune effector systems participate in the host defense against invading microorganisms and against spontaneous neoplasia. One effective effector system is mediated by cytotoxic cells having the ability to interact with and destroy unwanted cells such as infected cells, foreign cells, and sometimes cancerous tissue. Several cytotoxic effector systems have been described and characterized and include the cytotoxic T cells, natural killer (NK) cells, macrophages, neutrophils, platelets, etc. Based on reported data, these various cytotoxic cells exert their lytic activity presumably by different processes. However, the exact mechanisms by which they mediate target cell lysis is not known and has been an area of intense investigation in recent years. One of the difficulties encountered in such studies has been the requirement of cell-cell contact for lysis to take place, and because of this dependency, several limitations have been imposed on the system for study. Not until recently has it been possible to advance in this area of investigation because of the discovery of various soluble cytotoxic mediators that appear to participate in the lytic reaction.

Our studies have focused on the mechanism of NK-mediated cytotoxic reaction, and in particular our description and characterization of soluble natural killer cytotoxic factors (NKCF) secreted by the NK cells that lyse only NK sensitive target cells and appear to be the soluble mediators in the NK-CMC reaction.

Our initial studies were influenced by the stimulus secretion model proposed for the NK lytic mechanism.[1] This model proposes that after the effector cell binds to the target, it releases cytotoxic molecules which then lyse the target cells. This minimal model for cytotoxicity was supported by various lines of evidence when applied to assays containing NK effector and NK target cells. However, there was no evidence or attempt to demonstrate the existence of such postulated cytotoxic molecules.

Our studies were also influenced by the numerous reports characterizing various cytotoxic molecules derived from different cell types (but not NK cells) such as the lymphotoxin family of molecules, macrophage cytotoxins, and tumor necrosis factors.[2-6] Our laboratory undertook a systematic examination in search of cytotoxic mediators secreted by the NK effector cells which played a role in the NK-CMC reaction. It was essential that such molecules were also compatible with the known characteristics of the NK-CMC system.

Our initial studies identified cytotoxic mediators, termed NKCF, that were selectively specific for NK sensitive target cells.[7-9] The specificity of the NKCF prompted us to pursue several studies in an effort to establish or rule out the role of NKCF as meditors in the NK-CMC system. Our studies to date indicate that NKCF are intimately involved in the lytic mechanism of NK-CMC.[10]

In this review, we will present evidence that we have accumulated in the NKCF system. Based on these studies, we have proposed a model for the mechanism of NK-CMC in which NKCF participate in the lytic process[11] (Figure 1).

For simplicity and coherence, the presentation here is not chronological, but rather we present various lines of evidence that support each component of the proposed model. Also, we discuss briefly the mechanism of killing by NKCF and potential diagnostic and therapeutic implications of the NKCF system.

II. METHODS

A. Production of NKCF

Production of NKCF has been accomplished by both human peripheral blood and by rodent spleen cells (mouse and rat). Stimulation of NKCF can be achieved either by stimulation of NK cells with target cells or by mitogens.[7-9,12]

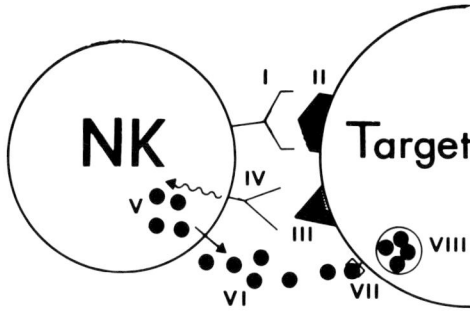

FIGURE 1. Model proposed for mechanism of NK CMC: (I) NK recognition structure; (II) NK target structure(s); (III) stimulating target cell structure; (IV) "receptor" for activation of NK effector; (V) secretory apparatus; (VI) release of NLCF; (VII) NKCF binding site; (VIII) NKCF processing; (IX) target cell death.

1. Stimulation with Target Cells

Effector cells obtained from mice or rat spleen cells are depleted of plastic-adherent cells by incubating in tissue culture flasks in RPMI 1640 with 10% FCS for 1 hr at 37°C. Human peripheral blood lymphocytes obtained from normal individuals are prepared by Ficoll-Hypaque density gradient centrifugation, followed by removal of adherent cells as described for spleen cells. Subsequent steps for the production of NKCF are identical for all 3 species. Cells are cultured in the absence of FCS in RPMI-1640 supplemented with 1% L-glutamine, 1% sodium pyruvate, 1% nonessential amino acids, and 1% penicillin-streptomycin. Effector cells are mixed with the stimulator cells to obtain a 25:1 effector to stimulator ratio. The final density of the effector cells in all cultures is 5×10^6 cells/mℓ. Cultures are started in a total of 1 to 3 mℓ in 17 × 100 mm tissue culture tubes (Falcon #2057). For larger production, tissue culture flasks are used. After 24 hr incubation at 37°C in 5% CO_2 and 95% air, the cell free supernatants are harvested and stored at either 4°C or −20°C until assaying for NKCF activity. Very often, dialysis of NKCF prior to the assay removed an inhibitor and the dialysed supernatant showed enhanced NKCF cytotoxic activity.

All cell lines used for stimulation of NKCF by NK cells are propagated in suspension in RPMI 1640 supplemented with 1% L-glutamine, 1% sodium pyruvate, 1% nonessential amino acids, and 10% FCS. All adherent cell lines are cultured in Dulbecco's modified Eagle's medium, supplemented with 10% FCS. All cell lines used are mycoplasma free and routinely tested for mycoplasma by the technique developed by Chen[13] and confirmed by a second test based on adenosine phosphorylase-mediated nucleoside toxicity.[14]

2. Stimulation with Mitogens

Lectins (Con A) is added to NK effector cells culture at 2.5 μg/mℓ and cultures incubated at various times. Significant cytotoxic activity is obtained in supernatants after 2 to 4 hr of culture.

Important considerations for the production of NKCF — Since our initial discovery and description of the NKCF system, our experience has resulted in the accumulation of several pertinent observations. A certain degree of variability from experiment to experiment is observed in the generation of NKCF in the mouse, rat, and human systems. Three general categories of results have been obtained, i.e., (1) NKCF is not detected in culture supernatants. In approximately 40% of the experiments, low levels of NKCF activity (<15%) is obtained. It is not clear why this variability is seen. In the mouse system, in particular, we observe variable results depending on strains, weather conditions, and viral infection. (2) NKCF is released spontaneously in the absence of stimulation. It is possible that the effector cells have undergone an in vivo activation resulting in active secretion of NKCF. (3) High levels of NKCF are produced in response to stimulation. These levels are much higher than control unstimulated cultures.

3. Enhanced Production of NKCF

Production of NKCF can be significantly enhanced by pretreatment of effector NK cells with IFN or IL-2[15]. Short treatment (1-2 hours) or overnight treatment of the effector cells prior to stimulation is sufficient to enhance the production of NKCF.

B. Assay of NKCF Activity

The cytotoxic activity of NKCF has been assessed by two different techniques, namely, dye exclusion and radioisotope ^{51}Cr release.

1. Trypan Blue Exclusion

Ten thousand target cells in 50 µℓ of RPMI 1640 with 10% FCS are placed in each well of sterile, flat bottomed microtiter plates; 150 µℓ of each of cell free supernatant is added to each well in triplicate, then 150 µℓ PBS or RPMI is added to the control wells. After incubation for 48 to 72 hr at 37°C, 5% CO_2, samples of the target cells are removed and viability is determined by trypan blue dye exclusion. Percent cytotoxicty is calculated as follows:

$$\% \text{ cytotoxicity} = 100 \times \frac{\% \text{ viability of control} - \% \text{ viability of test}}{\% \text{ viability of control}}$$

Cytotoxicity is determined by determining the number of residual viable cells after culture.[7-8]

2. The Microcytotoxicity ^{51}Cr Release Assay

The presence of NKCF activity is determined by measuring cytotoxicity against mycoplasma free target cells. The target cells are labeled with fresh ^{51}Cr (1 mCi/mℓ) that is always used before the date of calibration. To 0.2 mℓ of ^{51}Cr is added 4×10^6 target cells in 10 mℓ of media in a 25-cm^2 tissue culture flask. The flask is incubated vertically at 37°C in 5% CO_2, 95% air for 20 to 24 hr. The target cells are then washed 3 times and suspended at a final dilution of 2×10^5 cells/mℓ in RPMI 1640 supplemented with 1% penicillin-streptomycin and 10% FCS. The assay is set up in triplicate in 96 well, U-bottomed sterile microtiter plates. Fifty microliters of target cell suspension is added to each well. Different volumes of cell free supernatants containing NKCF (100, 50, 25 µℓ) are added to each well and the final volume is adjusted to 0.2 mℓ by adding RPMI 1640 plus 1% penicillin-streptomycin. The final concentration of FCS in cell wells is 2.5%. Wells for spontaneous and total ^{51}Cr release contain target cells plus 150 µℓ medium. After 20 hr incubation at 37°C in 5% CO_2, the ^{51}Cr released into 0.1 mℓ of supernatant for each well is determined. In general, the spontaneous cytotoxicity is less than 35% of total releasable counts. The percent cytotoxicity is calculated as follows:

$$\% \text{ cytotoxicity} = 100 \times \frac{\text{test cpm} - \text{spontaneous cpm}}{\text{total releasable cpm} - \text{spontaneous cpm}}$$

Calculation of lytic activity (LU_{20}) for cultures of 10^6 cells is determined by estimating the volume of NKCF-containing supernatant required to lyse 20% of the target cells.[12]

III. MODEL FOR THE MECHANISM OF NK CMC INVOLVING NKCF AS MEDIATORS

Depicted schematically in Figure 1 is our proposed model for the mechanism of NK CMC. The first step of the lytic pathway involves the interaction of a "receptor" [I] on the NK cell which recognizes and binds to the NK target structure [II] on the cell membrane. The effector cell must then receive a signal from the target to activate the NKCF release mechanism. This is depicted as occurring through the interaction of target-cell membrane determinants [III] with corresponding "receptors" [IV] on the effector cell, and both interactions are thought to be distinct from the initial binding step. Subsequent to stimualtion of the effector cell, the secretory apparatus [V] is activated to release NKCF [VI] in close proximity to the target cell. Following release, NKCF bind to NKCF-binding sites [VII] which may then be processed (e.g., internalized) [VII], resulting ultimately in irreversible target-cell death [IX].

IV. EXPERIMENTAL EVIDENCE SUPPORTING THE PROPOSED MODEL OF THE MECHANISM OF NK-CMC

Several lines of evidence have been accumulated from our studies and those of others that support the proposed model of NK-CMC shown in Figure 1. Below, we will present briefly the experimental studies culminating in staging the various steps of the CMC reaction.

A. Recognition and Binding of the NK Effector Cells to Target Cells

The initial interaction between NK effectors and NK target cells results in the formation of conjugates which can be visualized and counted microscopically.[16,17] The formation of conjugates appears to result from the interaction of a putative recognition receptor on the NK effector with NK target-cell structures. The chemical nature of the NK recognition structure is not known; however, recent studies have ruled out a T-cell receptor-like molecule on NK cells derived from the blood. It is not clear whether other antigen-specific receptors exist on NK cells.

The NK target-cell structure is also not known. Target structures must be shared on various target cells since the NK population is not heterogeneous and one NK cell can bind to and kill various NK-sensitive target cells.[18] There have been reports characterizing target structures on NK-sensitive targets using antibodies or membrane fractions from the target that inhibit binding.[16,19] However, the universality of such structures in the recognition event by NK cells or that such structures are also involved in adhesion in addition to recognition has not been demonstrated.[20]

The ability of an NK cell to form a conjugate with a target does not necessarily lead to target-cell lysis, since conjugate formation has been observed between NK cells and a variety of NK-resistant targets.[21,18,12] This observation implies that at least some NK-resistant target cells must be lacking a property present on NK-sensitive cells that is apparently distinct from the initial recognition/binding event (i.e., in step III, VII, or VIII in Figure 1).

B. Activation of the NKCF Release Mechanism

We have provided evidence that the subpopulation enriched in NK cells is responsible for secretion of NKCF. This was shown both in the murine system and in man.[7,8] It has also been shown that human NK cells purified by selection of Fc receptors positive LGL can produce NKCF.[22]

Following the initial recognition/binding between the NK effector and the target, the target must be able to stimulate the NK cell to release NKCF. Binding alone is not sufficient to activate the NKCF release mechanism, since we have observed examples where target cells are bound but do not stimulate release of NKCF. For example, target cells pretreated with interferon are still bound by NK cells but do not stimulate release of NKCF,[23] thus accounting for their resistance to NK-CMC.[24] Therefore, we postulate that following the initial recognition/binding event, a second signal is transmitted to the NK cell through the interaction of the same set of receptors or, alternatively, through a completely different set of membrane determinants. The model depicts this interaction as occurring through the interaction of a second set of membrane determinants for the sake of clarity; however, the available data are compatible with either alternative.

It is also possible to bypass this stimulating signal through the use of mitogens to stimulate NKCF release. For example, we have observed that NK cells from AIDS patients[25] and NK cells treated with UVR[26,27] can bind NK target cells but do not subsequently induce the release of NKCF. However, in either case, these cells will secrete NKCF upon stimulation with Con A. Therefore, in addition to effector-target cell interaction, there is at least one other mechanism to induce the release of NKCF.

C. Mechanism of Release of NKCF

We have previously reported that NKCF preexist in the cell, and their release is independent of de novo protein synthesis.[15] However, interferon pretreatment of NK effector cells resulted in augmentation of NKCF production, and the enhanced production is dependent on de novo protein synthesis. This probably accounts at least in part for the interferon-induced augmentation of NK-CMC.[24] The mechanism of NKCF release was examined in various systems described below:

1. Involvement of Proteases

Numerous reports have indicated that proteases are involved in the NK lytic mechanism.[6] These studies are based on the observation that addition of certain protease inhibitors to an NK-CMC culture inhibits the cytotoxic reaction. Since these inhibitors do not affect conjugate formation, it has been suggested that they act at the postbinding or the lethal-hit stage of lysis. According to our model of NK-CMC, it appears that proteases could be involved in either the NKCF release mechanism, the activation of NKCF, or NKCF interaction with and lysis of the target cell.

To distinguish among these possibilities, we performed several experiments using protease inhibitors which have been shown to inhibit NK CMC reactions. No effect was observed when the inhibitors were added to the NKCF assay. However, pretreatment of effector cells with these inhibitors followed by washing inhibited the production of active NKCF. These results support the hypothesis that a serine-dependent protease is involved in the release and/or activation of NKCF.[30]

2. Kinetics of Secretion of NKCF

Coculture of NK cells with stimulator cells results in the release of maximal levels of NKCF activity in the culture supernatant. Maximal activity is obtained after incubation at 37°C for 18 to 24 hr.[8] If our model is correct, it is expected that sufficient amounts of NKCF should be released in a short time, i.e., 1 to 3 hr, in order to correlate with target-cell lysis in an NK CMC reaction. In an effort to answer this question, first we examined whether the effector cell could release NKCF in a short-term assay. We examined the effect of mitogens such as ConA and the effect of phorbol esters and ionophores. The results of such studies indicated that NKCF release can take place within 1 hr after stimulation with these agents.[31] Therefore, in NK CMC, the effector is capable of producing NKCF rapidly following proper stimulation. Preliminary evidence indicates that NKCF release following target cell stimulation can take place in a relatively short time under appropriate conditions (unpublished). The long time required for NKCF release may be due to the sensitivity of the assay for detection of NKCF in the supernatant or that in cell-cell contact, NKCF is delivered to the target cell via another pathway involving vesicles and cofactors.

3. Biochemical Pathways of Activation of NKCF

Recent evidence from our laboratory indicates that protein kinase C and increased cytosolic Ca^{2+} are involved in the initiation process for secretion of NKCF. We made use of TPA and Ca^{2+} ionophores A-23187 and ionomycin and demonstrated that stimulation with both TPA and ionophores together, but not separately, will induce the release of NKCF.[31] The pathway of activation is consistent with the events following effector-stimulus interaction leading to metabolism of the membrane lipid phosphatidylinositol biphosphate to inositol triphosphate and 1,2-diacyglycerol. These in turn lead to release of Ca^{2+} into the cytoplasm from the endoplasmic reticulum store, activation of protein kinase C, and protein phosphorylation. Although these studies were not done with the stimulating target, it is possible that a similar pathway is involved in the release of NKCF following interaction of NK with the target cell.

4. Interaction of NKCF with Binding Sites on NK Target Cells

Following the release of NKCF from the NK cell, these factors must interact with the target cell to lyse it. This may occur through the interaction of NKCF with specific binding sites on the target or through penetration into the target in the absence of binding sites. Various lines of evidence from our laboratory suggest that NK targets bear binding sites to which NKCF can adhere.

1. We have shown that several NK-sensitive and NK-resistant targets can adsorb NKCF from supernatants containing NKCF.[11,42] The adsorption is dependent on the temperature, time of adsorption, and number of cells used. Several target cells which are poor targets in NK CMC have also been found to adsorb NKCF poorly. Other NK-resistant targets adsorb as efficiently as NK-sensitive targets.
2. The role of NKCF binding sites in NK CMC was directly examined. We predicted that NK targets lacking NKCF binding sites would also be resistant in the NK CMC reaction. To test this hypothesis, we cultured NK-sensitive targets in media containing NKCF to select for variants resistant to NKCF. Several variant clones were selected which were resistant to lysis by NKCF and also did not adsorb NKCF.[11] These results suggested that the variants lacked NKCF binding sites or bore sites with a poor affinity for NKCF. Furthermore, such variants were found to be resistant to lysis by NK cells in a CMC reaction. This was apparently due specifically to a deficiency of NKCF binding sites, since the variants could still form conjugates and stimulate release of NKCF. These results provide additional evidence for the role of NKCF in NK CMC and the requirement for NKCF binding sites on NK-sensitive targets. Experiments were also performed to determine if variants selected for resistance ot NK CMC would also be resistant to NKCF. It was found that the NK-resistant YAC-6-28 clone derived from the susceptible parental YAC target was also resistant to NKCF. Like the NKCF-derived variant discussed above, the NK CMC variant also lacked binding sites for NKCF.[33] Therefore, there was a good correlation between the presence of NKCF binding sites on the targets and their susceptibility to lysis by NK CMC or by NKCF.
3. NKCF binding sites are papain-sensitive. We have examined the nature of the NKCF binding sites present in the NK-sensitive target cells. Following treatment with papain, the cells were insensitive to NKCF and did not adsorb NKCF, although they retained the ability to form conjugates. These results suggested that the NKCF binding sites are protein-containing structures sensitive to papain. The resistance of papain-treated NK targets to lysis by NKCF coincided with the resistance to NK CMC, again corroborating the role of NKCF binding sites in NK CMC reactions.[32]

Altogether, the above findings indicate that a target cell's sensitivity to lysis by NK cells is dependent on the presence of NKCF binding sites on the target, and that these serve as receptors for the adsorption of the soluble mediators postulated to play a role in NK CMC.

V. MECHANISM OF ACTION OF NKCF

A. Kinetic of Lysis

We have postulated all along that NKCF plays a role in the NK CMC reaction. Therefore, it is predicted that during contact of NK and target cells, fast release of NKCF and fast kinetic of lysis should take place within the 2 to 4 hr lysis assay. We have shown that, under appropriate conditions of stimulation, NK cells can produce NKCF within a short time (30 min to 1 hr[31]). Therefore, the target cell may be triggering the NKCF release mechanism within a short period in the microenvironment of the effector-target contact area. Assuming that the first prediction is verified, we are left with the second prediction, i.e. NKCF should lyse target cells rapidly. However, the overall kinetic of lysis by NKCF is 16 to 20 hr, a time kinetic not compatible with the NK CMC reaction. Several possibilities may explain the discrepancy. (1) It is possible that NKCF released in the supernatant become partially inactivated or else are too diluted to mediate rapid target cell lysis. (2) It may be that there exists a specialized NKCF delivery mechanism operating when NK effector cells are in direct contact with the target, thus facilitating target cell lysis. (3) It is possible that other cofactors play a role in NKCF mediated lysis of target cells. For instance, target cells treated with protein synthesis inhibitors are more susceptible to lysis by NKCF, and lysis can be seen in a short-term 4 to 8 hr (unpublished).

B. Kinetic of NKCF Binding to Target Cells

We have proposed that NKCF binds to target cells through NKCF binding sites, and subsequently lysis takes place. The binding of NKCF to target cells is rapid and dependent on temperature and pH. Binding was done with crude NKCF preparation and, therefore, only qualitative data were obtained.[11] Incubation of target cells with NKCF for 1 to 2 hr and wash was sufficient for lysis to take place after incubation for 18 to 20 hr. The events taking place between binding and lysis are not known.

C. Lysis of NK-Resistant Target Cells by Fusion with Liposomes Containing NK-Sensitive Membranes

We investigated whether target resistance to NK cells is a property of the membrane. We applied a recently developed technique aimed at changing the membrane structure of acceptor cells by cell-liposome fusion. Our studies demonstrate that NK resistant tumor cells acquire sensitivity to lysis by NK cells after fusion with reconstituted vesicles which contained membrane fragments derived from NK sensitive target cells. Our findings were confirmed in both the human and rodent systems.[34] These results demonstrate the feasibility of converting a resistant NK target into a sensitive target by cell liposome fusion. The susceptibility of the converted target cell to lysis by NKCF is currently being studied in our laboratory.

D. Lysis of NK-Resistant Target Cells by NKCF Containing Liposomes

NKCF-containing large unilamellar vesicles (LUV) were prepared and incubated with various NK-resistant and sensitive target cells. The treated target cells were then incubated and lysis estimated. The results show that liposome treatment renders NK-resistant cells susceptible to lysis by NKCF.[42] Variant NK targets lacking NKCF binding sites were lysed by NKCF encapsulated liposomes. These results suggest that NKCF may mediate its cytotoxic effect through internalization of NKCF into the cytosol of the target.

E. Pore Formation

We have no direct evidence that NKCF forms pores in the target cell membrane. Using time lapse cinematography, we observed that the target cells treated with NKCF undergo changes such as blebbing and zeiosis, similar to our findings with CTL-mediated lysis of target cells.[35] The exact significance of these findings is not clear.

VI. BIOCHEMICAL CHARACTERIZATION OF NKCF

We have investigated several physical and biochemical properties of crude NKCF and have achieved partial purification of these factors.[36] The activity is stable at 4° and freezing and unstable at temperatures >63°, 8 M area, or at pH 2. The factors are sensitive to trypsin and resistant to neuraminidase suggesting that NKCF are composed in part of protein. The NKCF activity is abrogated following reduction and alkylation, suggesting a role for intact disulfide bonds in cytotoxicity. Mild oxidation with sodium periodate inactivates NKCF suggesting that carbohydrate determinants are essential for cytolytic activity.

NKCF derived from human, mice and rat sources all migrate on a single broad peak of an apparent MW of 15-40,000 by HPLC gel filtration. Using different fractionation techniques, it appears that NKCF consists of more than one type of cytotoxic molecule. Further clarification and characterization of such molecules is currently under intensive investigation.

VII. RELATIONSHIP BETWEEN NKCF AND OTHER CYTOTOXINS

The relationsihp between NKCF and other cytotoxins described in cytotoxicity is not clear. Several cytotoxic factors have been reported such as the lymphotoxin (LT) family of molecules,[37] recombinant TNFα and TNFβ,[38] granule derived cytotoxin,[39] and perforin.[40,41] Since NKCF have not yet been purified to homogeneity, we have performed several functional studies aimed at correlating NKCF with some of the available toxins.

Cytolysins and perforins have been implicated as cytotoxic mediators in both NK and CTL mediated reactions. These factors have been isolated from the granules of various types of cell lines or tumors and lyse target cells by forming pores in the membrane. Their functional properties are distinct from NKCF in that (a) they lyse nonselectively all kinds of target cells; (b) lysis occurs within minutes; and (c) lysis can take place at room temperature.

The α form of LT has recently been purified and cloned and is now termed TNFβ. Comparing the target specificity of $_r$TNFβ and NKCF was found to be different. Furthermore, antibodies directed against $_r$TNFβ did not inhibit NKCF. Our studies, therefore, suggest that NKCF is different from TNFβ (manuscript in preparation). However, the relationship between NKCF and the various forms of LT described by Granger and colleagues[37] await further investigation.

Tumor necrosis factor, originally described by Carswell et al.[2] has recently been purified and cloned.[30] TNFα is primarily produced by monocytes and macrophages. Comparing $_r$TNFα (Genentec) with NKCF showed several similarities as well as differences. Overall, TNFα exhibits a similar target cell specificity as NKCF with few exceptions. Furthermore, antibodies directed against TNF mediated partial inhibition of lysis of target cells by NKCF. These results suggested that NKCF were the same or related antigenically to TNFα.

If TNFα and NKCF were related and play a role in NK-CMC, we predicted that antibodies directed against TNFα should inhibit NK-CMC and TNFα resistant variants would exhibit resistance in the NK-CMC reaction. We tested both of these predictions. Anti-TNFα antibody caused only partial inhibition of NK-CMC in a few experiments but not in others. These results suggested that TNFα may not be involved in NK CMC but did not rule out its role. It may be that TNFα delivery to the target cell is carried out in a cryptic form not accessible to the antibody neutralizing effect. We tested the second prediction by developing variants

Table 1
COMPARISON OF VARIANT TARGETS IN CYTOTOXICITY

Properties	U937	U937$_{TR}$	U937$_{NR}$
Conjugate formation	+	+	+
Stimulation of NKCF	+	+	+
Adsorption of NKCF	+		–
Cytotoxicity[a]			
NK-CMC	+	+	–
ADCC	+	+	+
LDCC	+	+	–
Macrophage + IFN	+	–	
NKCF	+	–	–
TNF	+	–	–

[a] Lysis in either a short-term (4 hr) or long-term (18 hr) ^{51}Cr assay. The U937$_{TR}$ and U937$_{NR}$ were prepared by culture in media containing TNFα or NKCF, respectively.

resistant to TNFα (U937)$_{TR}$ which were compared to NKCF resistant variants (U937)$_{NR}$. These variants were selected following culture of the sensitive target in media containing $_r$TNFα or NKCF. The variants were resistant to lysis by either TNFα or NKCF. Various characterizations were made, and the results are summarized in Table 1. One of the interesting findings is the demonstration that U937$_{TR}$ were sensitive to lysis in NK CMC, whereas the U937$_{NR}$ were resistant.

These results suggested that TNFα alone may not be involved in NK-CMC. It is possible that more than one factor may be involved, such as TNFα and NKCF. The precise relationship between NKCF and TNFα await the purification of NKCF to homogeneity and development of NKCF specific antibodies.

VIII. DIAGNOSTIC AND CLINICAL IMPLICATIONS

Several studies have shown that the NK effector system plays a major role in immune surveillance in the fight against infection and cancer. Furthermore, studies have implicated a role for NK cells in regulation of host cells, stem cell maturation, and differentiation. Consequently, maintenance of a healthy and functional NK system should reduce the risk of infection and tumor onset. Based on this premise, it becomes of paramount importance to characterize fully the NK system and the molecular mechanisms by which these effector cells mediate their lytic function, and the molecular mechanism that endows target cells to be sensitive or resistant to lysis by NK cells and their products. These mechanisms should help elucidate and diagnose cases where the NK system is defective and should also help identify means to reverse the defective stage and develop new methods for therapy.

A. Diagnostic Implications

Based on our proposed model for the mechanism of the NK-CMC reaction and the role of NKCF as a soluble cytotoxic mediator, it becomes possible to dissect the system into several steps, each of which can be identified separately from the others. Accordingly, several factors can result in a defective NK system or result in target cell resistance to NK lysis. These are listed in Table 2.

1. Defective NK Effector Function
Several factors listed in Table 2 may be identified, each of which may contribute to a

Table 2
POSSIBLE FACTORS RESULTING IN DEFECTIVE NK ACTIVITY AND IN TARGET CELL RESISTANCE

Possible factors resulting in defective NK activity
1. Reduced frequency of NK cells
2. Failure of NK precursor cells to differentiate into mature NK cells
3. Deficiency of lymphokine (IL-2, IFN) regulating NK activity
4. Defective or low affinity target recognition and adhesion receptors
5. Defective trigger for the stimulation of NKCF
6. Failure of secretory apparatus to release NKCF
7. Failure to synthesize NKCF
8. Production of inactive NKCF

Possible factors resulting in target cell resistance to NK lysis
1. Lack of NK recognition structures
2. Lack or low affinity adhesion molecules
3. Lack or low affinity trigger structure for NKCF release
4. Absence or defective NKCF binding sites
5. Failure to process bound NKCF for lysis
6. Elevated repair mechanism

defective NK system seen clinically. Techniques are available to quantitate numbers of cells by surface phenotype or by single cell analysis for conjugate formation, identification, and separation of cells at different stages of their maturation, activation of NKCF release, and quantitation of NKCF activity. The adaptation of such techniques in a clinical set-up should help identify the steps and stages of the defective effector function. The following example illustrates this point.

AIDS patients have been shown to have low or no NK activity. The mechanism of the defective activity was examined in our laboratory.[25] Several findings were made, as follows:

1. The frequency of NK cells capable of binding and forming conjugates with NK-sensitive targets was normal or slightly elevated. This suggested that NK cells are not deleted or decreased in number in AIDS patients.
2. The NK cells could not be stimulated to release NKCF following coculture with NK targets. This localized the defect at either the trigger for release or the failure to synthesize NKCF.
3. Following stimulation with Con A, the cells released NKCF, albeit at lower levels than normal, thus showing that AIDS NK cells are not completely defective in production of NKCF. They appear defective in the trigger by the stimulator cells.
4. Following treatment of cells with IL-2, the cells regain NK activity and release NKCF upon coculture and stimulation. These results suggested that the defective trigger can be modulated by IL-2 and/or that NKCF synthesis may be augmented by IL-2. Thus, it may be possible to restore NK activity by IL-2 treatment.

Clearly, defective NK activity in cancer patients, immunodeficiencies, genetic disorders, etc. have been reported and require further investigation to characterize the nature of the defect as illustrated above for AIDS patients.

2. Resistance of Target Cell Lysis by NK Cells

In several instances, tumor target cells derived from in vivo or cultured in vitro are resistant to NK target lysis. Listed in Table 2 are several factors, each of which may influence target cell sensitivity to NK or NKCF lysis. We have characterized several of these factors in well-defined systems as described above. However, if means are available to modify such tumor cells so that they can convert to sensitive targets, it may be possible to apply such means therapeutically. To our knowledge, this has not been attempted as yet in human or experimental tumor systems.

B. Therapeutic Implications

The ability to delineate the stages of the defective NK system offers opportunities to correct the defect by various modalities. For example, the use of IL-2, IFN, or biologic response modifiers should help activate the NK system in that both differentiation of pre-NK to mature NK cells and enhancement of cytotoxic activity is achieved. This has been confirmed in vivo, but such lymphokines also exert other effects which may overcome the beneficial effects. It is possible to use NKCF-like materials as therapy, and TNFα and TNFβ are currently being testing in phase I clinical trials in cancer patients.

We have also been able to convert NK resistance by liposome fusion with membranes from NK sensitive targets in vitro. It should be possible to apply this technique in vivo to modulate NK activity as well as convert resistant tumors into NK sensitive tumor cells. The combination of lymphokines with NK target membranes into liposome could have a dual effect on both the NK cell and target cell, thus optimizing the conditions for cytotoxicity. Other approaches could be devised based on the known factors listed in Table 2.

REFERENCES

1. **Roder, J. C., Karre, K., and Kiessling, R.,** Natural killer cells, *Prog. Allergy,* 28, 66, 1981.
2. **Carswell, E., Old, L., Kassel, R., Green, S., Fiore, N., and Williamson, B.,** An endotoxin-induced serum factor that causes necrosis of tumors, *Proc. Natl. Acad. Sci. USA,* 72, 3666, 1975.
3. **Devlin, J., Klostergaard, J., Orr, S. L., Yamamoto, R., Masunaka, I. K., Plunkett, J. M., and Granger, G. A.,** Lymphotoxins: After fifteen years of research in, *Lymphokines,* Vol. 9, Pick, E., Ed., Academic Press, New York, 1984, 313.
4. **Kolb, W. P. and Granger, G. A.,** Lymphocyte in vitro cytotoxicity: Characterization of human lymphotoxin, *Proc. Natl. Acad. Sci. USA,* 61, 1250, 1968.
5. **Ruddle, N. H. and Waksman, B. H.,** Cytotoxic effect of lymphocyte antigen interaction in delayed hypersensitivity, *Science,* 157, 1060, 1967.
6. **Ruff, M. and Gifford, G.,** Tumor necrosis factor, in *Lymphokines,* Vol. 2, Pick, E., Ed., Academic Press, New York, 1981, 235.
7. **Wright, S. C. and Bonavida, B.:** Selective lysis of NK sensitive target cells by a soluble mediator released from murine spleen cells and human peripheral blood lymphocytes, *J. Immunol.,* 126, 1516, 1981.
8. **Wright, S. C., Weitzen, M. L., Kahle, R., Granger, G. A., and Bonavida, B.,** Studies on the mechanism of natural killer cytotoxicity. I. Release of cytotoxic factors specific for NK sensitive target cells (NKCF) during coculture of NK effector cells with NK target cells, *J. Immunol.,* 129, 433, 1982.
9. **Wright, S. C., Weitzen, M. L., Kahle, R., Granger, G. A., and Bonavida, B.,** Studies on the mechanism of natural killer cytotoxicity. II. Coculture of human PBL with NK-sensitive or resistant cell lines stimulates release of natural killer cytotoxic factors (NKCF) selectively cytotoxic to NK-sensitive target cells, *J. Immunol.,* 130, 2479, 1983.
10. **Bonavida, B. and Wright, S.,** Natural killer cytotoxic factors (NKCF) role in cell-mediated cytotoxicity, in *Immunobiology of Natural Killer Cells,* Vol. 1, Lotzova, E., Ed., CRC Press, Boca Raton, Fla., 125, 1986.
11. **Wright, S. C., Roder, J. C., Werkmeister, J., and Bonavida, B.,** Studies on the mechanism of natural killer (NK) cell-mediated cytotoxicity. VI. The NK resistant YAC-6-28 variant binds NK cells and stimulates release of natural killer cytotoxic factors (NKCF) but is not susceptible of lysis by NKCF, submitted.
12. **Wright, S. C. and Bonavida, B.,** Studies on the mechanism of natural killer cell-mediated cytotoxicity. V. Lack of NK specificity at the level of induction of natural killer cytotoxic factors in cultures of human, murine, or rat effector cells stimulated with mycoplasma-free cell lines, *J. Immunol.,* 133, 3415, 1984.
13. **Chen, T. P.,** In situ detection of mycolasma contamination in cell cultures by fluorescent Hoechst 32258 stain, *Exp. Cell. Res.,* 104, 255, 1977.

14. **McGarrity, G. J. and Carson, D. A.,** Adenosine-phosphorylase mediated nucleoside toxicity. Application towards the detection of mycoplasmal infection in mammalian cell cultures, *Exp. Cell. Res.*, 130, 199, 1982.
15. **Wright, S. C. and Bonavida, B.,** Studies on the mechanism of natural killer (NK) cell-mediated cytotoxicity. III. Interferon-pretreatment of effector cell augments the lytic activity of natural killer cytotoxic factors (NKCF), *J. Immunol.*, 130, 2960, 1983.
16. **Roder, J. C., Rosen, A., Fenyo, E. M., and Troy, F. A.,** Target-effector interaction in the natural killer cell system: Isolation of target structures, *Proc. Natl. Acad. Sci. USA*, 76, 1405, 1979.
17. **Targan, S., Grimm, E., and Bonavida, B.,** A single cell marker or active NK cytotoxicity: Only a fraction of target binding lymphocytes on killer cells, *J. Clin. Immunol.*, 4, 165, 1980.
18. **Bradley, T. P. and Bonavida, B.,** Mechanism of cell-mediated cytotoxicity at the single cell level. IV. Natural killing and antibody dependent cellular cytotoxicity can be mediated by the same human effector cells as determined by the single cell conjugate assay, *J. Immunol.*, 129, 2260, 1982.
19. **Werkmeister, J. A., Helfand, S. A., Haliotis, T., Pross, H., and Roder, J. C.,** Specificity of natural killer (NK) cells: Nature of target cell structures, in *NK Cells and Other Natural Effector Cells*, Herberman, R. B., Ed., Academic Press, New York, 1982.
20. **Bonavida, B., Bradley, T. P., Fan, J., Hiserodt, J., Effros, R., and Wexler, H.,** Molecular interactions in T cell-mediated cytotoxicity, *Immunol. Rev.*, 72, 119, 1983.
21. **Bonavida, B., Bradley, T. P., and Grimm, E. A.,** The single cell assay in cell-medited cytotoxicity, *Immunol. Today*, 4, 196, 1983.
22. **Degliantoni, G., Murphy, M., Kobayaski, M., Francis, M. K., Perussia, B., and Trinchieri, G.,** Natural killer (NK) cell-derived hematopoietic colony-inhibiting activity and NK cytotoxic factor. Relationship with tumor necrosis factor and synergism with immune interferon, *J. Exp. Med.*, 162, 1512, 1985.
23. **Wright, S. C. and Bonavida, B.,** Studies on the mechanism of natural killer (NK) cell-mediated ytotoxicity. IV. Interferon-induced inhibition of NK target cell susceptibility is due to a defect in their ability to stimulate release of natural killer cytotoxic factors (NKCF), *J. Immunol.*, 130, 2965, 1983.
24. **Trinchieri, G., Santoli, D., Dee, R. R., and Knowles, B. B.,** Antiviral activity induced by culturing lymphocytes with tumor-derived versus transformed cells. Enhancement of human natural killer cell activity by interferon, and antagonistic inhibition of susceptibility of target cells to lysis, *J. Exp. Med.*, 147, 1314, 1978.
25. **Bonavida, B., Katz, J., and Gottlieb, M.,** Mechanism of defective NK cell activity in acquired immune deficiency syndrome (AIDS). I. Defective trigger on NK cells for NKCF production by target cells and restoration by IL-2, *J. Immunol.*, 137, 1157, 1986.
26. **Safrit, J., Wright, S. C., and Bonavida, B.,** Mechanism of defective NK activity following irradiation with ultraviolet light, submitted.
27. **Weitzen, M. L., and Bonavida, B.,** Mechanism of inhibition of human natural killer activity by ultraviolet radiation, *J. Immunol.*, 133, 3128, 1984.
28. **Goldfarb, R. H., Timonen, T. T., and Herberman, R. B.,** The role of neutral serum proteases in the mechanism of tumor cell lysis by human natural killer cells, in *NK Cells and Other Natural Effector Cells*, Herberman, R. B., Ed., Academic Press, New York, 1982, 931.
29. **Hudig, D., Redelman, D., and Minning, L.,** Evidence for proteases with specificity of cleavage at aromatic amino acids in human natural cell-mediated cytotoxicity, in *NK Cells and Other Natural Effector Cells*, Herberman, R. B., Ed., Academic Press, New York, 1982, 923.
30. **Wright, S. C. and Bonavida, B.,** Evidence for the involvement of proteolytic enzymes in the production of natural killer cytotoxic factors, in *Natural Killer Activity and Its Regulation*, Hoshino, T., et al., Eds., Excerpta Medica, Amsterdam, 1984, 145.
31. **Graves, S. C., Bramhall, J., Wright, S. C., and Bonavida, B.,** Studies on the mechanism of natural killer cell-mediated cytotoxicity. IX. Induction of release of natural killer cell cytotoxic factors (NKCF) from human peripheral blood lymphocytes by a phorbol ester and ionophores suggest a role for protein kinase C activation, *J. Immunol.*, 137, 1977, 1986.
32. **Wright, S. C., Wilbur, S. M., and Bonavida, B.,** Biochemical characterization of natural killer cytotoxic factors, in *Mechanism of Cell-Mediated Cytotoxicity*, II, Henkart, P. and Martz, E., Eds., Plenum Press, New York, 1985.
33. **Wright, S. C., Roder, J. C., Werkmeister, J., and Bonavida, B.,** Studies on the mechanism of natural killer (NK) cell-mediated cytotoxicity. VI. The NK resistant YAC-6-28 variant binds NK cells and stimulates release of natural killer cytotoxic factors (NKCF) but is not susceptible to lysis of NKCF, *Immunobiology* (in press), 1987.
34. **Roozemond, R. C., Urli, D. C., Wright, S. C., Graves, S. C., and Bonavida, B.,** Lysis of natural killer resistant tumor cells by liposome encapsulated natural killer cytotoxic factors (NKCF), submitted.
35. **Grimm, E. A., Price, A., and Bonavida, B.,** Studies on the induction and expression of T-cell meditaed immunity. VIII. Effector-target junctions and target cell membrane disruption during cytolysis, *Cell. Immunol.*, 46, 77, 1979.

36. **Wright, S. C., Wilbur, S. M., and Bonavida, B.,** Studies on the mechanism of natural killer cell-mediated cytotoxicity. VI. Characterization of human, rat, and murine natural killer cytotoxic factors, *Nat. Immun. Cell Growth Regul.*, 4, 202, 1985.
37. **Granger, G. A., Orr, S. K., and Yamamoto, R. S.,** Lymphotoxins, macrophage cytotoxins, and tumor necrosis factors: An interrelated family of antitumor effector molecules, *J. Clin. Immunol.*, 5, 217, 1985.
38. **Gray, P., Aggarwal, B., Benton, C., Bringman, T., Henzel, W., Jarrett, J., Leung, D., Moffat, B., Ng, P., Sevedersky, L., Palladino, M., and Nedwin, G.,** Cloning and expression of the cDNA for human lymphotoxins: A lympholkine with tumor necrosis factor, *Nature*, 312, 721, 1984.
39. **Millard, P. J., Henkart, M. A., Reynolds, C. W., and Henkart, P. A.,** Purification and properties of cytoplasmic granules from cytotoxic rat LGL tumors, *J. Immunol.*, 123, 3197, 1984.
40. **Podak, E. R. and Dennert, G.,** Assembly of two types of tubules with putative cytolytic function in cloned natural killer cells, *Nature*, 302, 442, 1983.
41. **Dennert, G. and Podak, E. R.,** Cytolysis by H-2 specific T killer cells. Assembly of tubular complexes on target membranes, *J. Exp. Med.*, 157, 1483, 1983.
42. **Roozemond, R. C., Merissen, M., Urli, D. C., and Bonavida, B.,** Effect of altered membrane structure on NK cell mediated cytotoxicity, III. Decreased susceptibility to natural killer cytotoxic factor (NKCF) and suppression of NKCF release by membrane rigidification, *J. Immunol.*, 139, 1739, 1987.

Chapter 21

TUMOR NECROSIS FACTORS

Ramani A. Aiyer and Bharat B. Aggarwal

TABLE OF CONTENTS

I.	Introduction	106
II.	Bioassays	106
III.	Nomenclature	108
IV.	Sources	109
V.	Purification	110
VI.	Physicochemical Characterization	111
VII.	Gene Structure	114
VIII.	Biological Properties	114
	A. Antitumor Effects	114
	B. Proliferation of Normal Cells	116
	C. Cachectin/TNF-α	117
	D. Antipathogenic and Antiviral Effects	117
	E. Activation of Polymorphonuclear Neutrophils (PMN)	117
	F. Effects on Endothelial Cells	118
	G. Hematopoietic Cell Differentiation	118
	H. Bone Resorption	118
	I. Miscellaneous Effects	119
	J. Relationship of TNFs to Other Cytokines	119
	K. TNF Receptors	120
IX.	Mechanism of TNF Action	122
	A. In Vivo Action	123
X.	Concluding Remarks	124
Acknowledgments		124
Abbreviations		125
References		126

I. INTRODUCTION*

One of the classical observations in cancer therapy was that of Professor Busch, who reported as early as 1868 two cases of sarcoma in which the tumors had shrunk markedly after a spontaneous attack of erysipelas, a skin and subcutaneous bacterial infection. Subsequently he induced erysipelas in a woman with multiple sarcomas, and this resulted in regression of large tumors at the rate of about one centimeter per day while some of the smaller tumors completely resorbed.[1] This observation of tumor regression during bacterial infections was later confirmed by several other investigators.[2-5] W. B. Coley made the most extensive use of bacteria-free filtrates for the treatment of human malignancy.[3] These preparations have been described in the literature as "Coley's Toxins". Shear and his co-workers demonstrated in 1943 that lipopolysaccharides (LPS) present in bacterial filtrates were responsible for necrosis of tumors.[6] Algire et al. postulated that necrosis of tumors in vivo was due to LPS-induced systemic hypotension leading to collapse of the tumor vasculature, hemorrhage, cell anorexia, and death.[7] This hypothesis was contradicted by O'Malley et al. who demonstrated that the endotoxin-free serum of animals injected with LPS was capable of necrotizing tumors in other animals,[3] indicating that tumor regression was not a direct effect of LPS but was mediated by another factor(s). Carswell et al. confirmed this view[9] and named this activity Tumor Necrosis Factor (TNF). Although the latter authors indicated that it was essential to prime the animals with BCG prior to LPS injection in order to elicit the production of TNF activity in the serum, Beutler et al. have recently shown that such priming is not needed.[10]

The isolation of TNF proved to be a difficult problem, since it was felt that only trace amounts were produced in the serum of LPS treated animals. Furthermore, it was also not clear whether the tumor necrosis activity was due to one or more molecules and what relationship, if any, existed between TNF and other equally less characterized TNF-like substances. Recently, using serum-free supernatants derived from continuously growing cell lines, two factors, TNF-α[11] and TNF-β (previously called lymphotoxin),[12,13] have been purified to homogeneity from monocytes and lymphocytes, respectively, and their complete primary structures were determined. Subsequently, the cDNAs of both TNF-β[14] and TNF-α[15-21] were cloned by recombinant DNA methods and expressed in *E. coli*.

Studies, in vivo and in vitro, using the pure proteins have shown that both TNF-α and TNF-β possess the unique ability to kill selectively neoplastic tissue, while sparing normal cells. The availability of highly purified preparations of TNFs, produced in large amounts by recombinant DNA methods in *E. coli*, has now made it possible to investigate their potential as therapeutic anticancer agents in human clincial trials. While the outcome of these trails is being awaited, a large number of studies from several different laboratories have documented that, in addition to their antitumor activity, these proteins mediate a diverse array of biological responses in vitro. Although their true in vivo significance is still unknown, the biologic studies strongly suggest that TNF-α and TNF-β play an important role in immunomodulatory and inflammatory responses.

II. BIOASSAYS

The initial bioassay for TNF-α involved hemorrhagic necrosis, in vivo, of a methylcholanthrene transformed sarcoma (Meth A sarcoma) in mice.[9] The name TNF is based on this assay. This assay, however, is inconvenient for screening large numbers of fractions during purification procedures. In vitro, both TNF-α and TNF-β have been found to be toxic to several tumor cells but not to normal cells (Table 1). Mouse L-929 cells have been

---

* List of abbreviations appears at end of chapter.

Table 1
EFFECTS OF TNF ON THE VIABILITY OF HUMAN AND MURINE CELLS IN VITRO

Cell type	Effect	Ref.
Mouse cells		
Normal mouse embryo fibroblasts	Null response	22
B16F10 (Melanoma)	Null response	23
CMT-93 (rectal carcinoma)	Null response	23
S49 (lymphoma)	Null response	23
Meth A (sarcoma)	Antiproliferative	23,24
L929 (fibroblast)	Antiproliferative	23,25-28
Tumor 1023 (fibrosarcoma)	Antiproliferative	25
B6M52 (sarcoma)	Antiproliferative	23
B6M55 (sarcoma)	Antiproliferative	23
CM54 (sarcoma)	Antiproliferative	23
CM516 (sarcoma)	Antiproliferative	23
WEHI-164 (sarcoma)	Antiproliferative	23
MMT (breast carcinoma)	Antiproliferative	23
SAC (maloney-transformed 3T3)	Antiproliferative	23
Erlich Ascites Tumor (EAT)	Antiproliferative	29
Friend Erythroleukemia Cells	Antiproliferative	29
Human cells		
Normal fibroblasts	Null response	22
Normal lymphocytes	Null response	30
Neuroblastoma	Null response	22
A-549 (lung carcinoma)	Null response	23,31
Calu-3 (lung carcinoma)	Null response	23
G-361 (melanoma)	Null response	23
HeLa (cervical)	Null response	23,32
HT-1080 (fibrosarcoma)	Null response	23
KB (oral epidermoid carcinoma)	Null response	23
LS174T (colon)	Null response	23
RPMI 7931 (melanoma)	Antiproliferative	22
NHIK 3025 (epithelial carcinoma)	Antiproliferative	30,33
U-205 (mesenchymal osteosarcoma)	Antiproliferative	30
K-562 (leukemia)	Antiproliferative	30,31,34
U-937 (leukemia)	Antiproliferative	34
HL-60 (leukemia)	Antiproliferative	34
Molt-4 (leukemia)	Antiproliferative	34
Normal abdominal skin fibroblasts	Antiproliferative	30
BT-20 (breast)	Antiproliferative	23,32
BT-475 (breast)	Antiproliferative	23
MCF-7 (breast)	Antiproliferative	23
ME-180 (cervical)	Antiproliferative	23,32
SK-MEL-109 (melanoma)	Antiproliferative	23
SK-OV-4 (ovarian)	Antiproliferative	23
WiDV (colon)	Antiproliferative	23
RD (Rhabdosarcoma)	Null response	23
Saos-2 (osteogenic sarcoma)	Null response	23
SK-CO-1 (colon carcinoma)	Null response	23
SK-LU-1 (lung carcinoma)	Null response	23
SK-OV-3 (ovarian carcinoma)	Null response	23,32
SK-UT-1 (uterine carcinoma)	Null response	23
T24 (bladder carcinoma)	Null response	23
WI-38 VA13 (SV40 transformed WI-38)	Null response	23
Normal mesothelial cells from pleural expression	Stimulation of proliferation	30

Table 1 (continued)
EFFECTS OF TNF ON THE VIABILITY OF HUMAN AND MURINE CELLS IN VITRO

Cell type	Effect	Ref.
CCD-18Co (normal colon)	Stim. of proliferation	23
Detroit 551 (normal fetal skin)	Stim. of proliferation	23
LL24 (normal lung)	Stim. of proliferation	23
WI-38 (normal fetal lung)	Stim. of proliferation	23
WI-1003 (normal lung)	Stim. of proliferation	23
FS-4 Fibroblasts	Stim. of proliferation	35

found to be very sensitive targets and are used routinely to assay the cytotoxic effects of TNFs.[9,36,37,169] The sensitivity of the assay can be enhanced several-fold by pre-exposing the cells to chemotherapeutic agents, including mitomycin C,[36] actinomycin D,[38,39,170] adriamycin,[170] and aclacinomycin A,[170] or by raising the temperature.[146,158,159] Various methods have been used to quantitatively monitor cytotoxicity, including cell counting, and cellular uptake of vital dyes, radiolabeled amino acids, or nucleotides. The in vitro bioassays have proved to be fairly sensitive, reproducible, quantitative and convenient for screening large numbers of fractions during purification.

III. NOMENCLATURE

In recent years, besides TNF-α and TNF-β,[12,13] several other factors cytotoxic to tumor cells have been described in the literature; this includes a series of entities that have also been called lymphotoxin,[24,39,40] holotoxin/necrosin,[28] natural killer cytotoxic factor,[41] monocyte cytotoxic factor,[42] leukoregulin,[43] and cytotoxin.[44-46] Due to lack of sufficient chemical characterization, the precise relationship of these factors to the ones described here is unclear. Two of the factors, the monocyte-derived TNF and a lymphocyte-derived LT, that have been purified to homogeneity, cloned and characterized, are the subject of this review. Both of these proteins share tumoricidal activity in the assay for necrosis of the Meth A sarcoma in vivo as well as in the in vitro L-929 cell cytotoxicity assay.[9,36,37] As will be discussed later, despite their distinct origins and distinct antigenic determinants, TNF and LT are homologous proteins that appear to bind to the same cell surface receptors and display a remarkable similarity in their various biological actions. In order to emphasize their relatedness, these factors have been recently renamed TNF-α and TNF-β, respectively.[47] The new nomenclature will, hopefully, resolve some of the confusion that currently exists in the literature on tumoricidal factors. The factors that have been described earlier as holotoxin/necrosin[28] and cytotoxin/lymphotoxin[44-46] have been shown to be the same as TNF-α, described here.[48] Interestingly, another protein, cachectin, that causes antilipolytic effects in adipocytes has also been recently shown to be identical with TNF-α.[49] On the other hand, the precise nature of the TNF isolated from a human B lymphoblastoid cell line, designated as TNF-Luk II[50,92] is not clear. The source of this factor and some of its biochemical properties strongly suggests that it may be identical with TNF-β, although without primary structural information or unequivocal antibody neutralization data, its relationship will remain uncertain. The relationship between TNFs and various forms of LT described by Granger and his co-workers[24,40] is also unclear. However, these investigators reported recently that the cytotoxic activity of these factors could be completely neutralized by antibodies to TNF-α and TNF-β.[171,172]

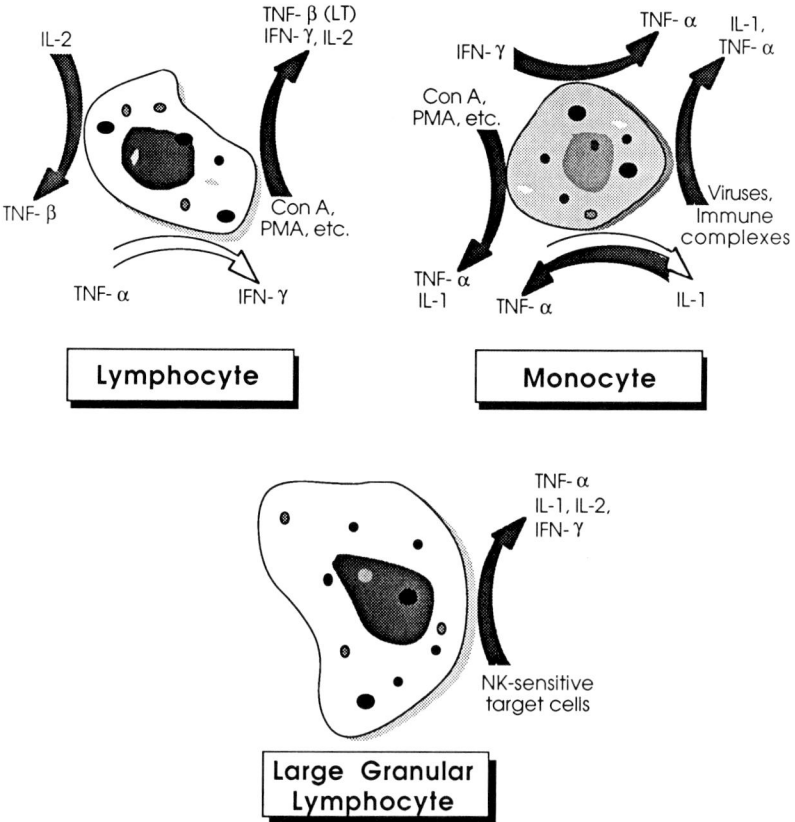

FIGURE 1. Production of TNF-α and TNF-β by cells of the immune system.

IV. SOURCES

Since massive tumor macrophage hyperplasia was observed in animals injected with LPS, Carswell et al. proposed initially that macrophages were the probable source of TNF-α.[9] This hypothesis was supported by subsequent observations of other workers that mouse peritoneal macrophages could be activated by a variety of stimuli to become toxic to tumor cells but not normal cells.[51] Recent studies using anti-TNF-α antibodies[52,53] and tumor cell variants selected for resistance to killing by TNF-α or activated macrophages[52] strongly indicate that TNF-α is the major tumoricidal factor secreted by activated macrophages. Furthermore, since TNF could not be induced by endotoxin in athymic nude mice, it appears that T-lymphocytes are also essential for TNF production.[54] Lymphocytes may be involved in TNF production in two ways: (1) lymphocytes themselves secrete a factor toxic to tumor cells called TNF-β[12,13,24,39,47] and (2) T cells secrete the lymphokines, IL-2 and IFN-γ, which potentiate the production of both TNF-α and TNF-β in vitro[55-57] (Figure 1).

The relationship between TNF-α and TNF-β was not clear until recently, when it was found that the two proteins, although biologically similar, were biochemically and antigenically distinct entities. Separation of human peripheral blood leukocytes (PBL) into monocytes (adherent cells) and lymphocytes (nonadherent cells) by elutriation techniques showed that TNF-α originated from the former and TNF-β from the latter.[58] The production of TNF-α, however, is not restricted to monocytes. A recent study has found that NK cell-sensitive tumor target cells can induce large granular lymphocytes to produce TNF-α.[59]

Due to the limited supply of PBLs in blood, several continuously growing monocytic and lymphocytic cell lines were screened. It was found that the human cell lines HL-60 (myeloid) and RPMI 1788 (lymphoid) were excellent sources for TNF-α and TNF-β, respectively.[11-15] Whereas a variety of agents could stimulate these cell lines, phorbol esters were found to be optimal for the induction of these proteins.

Several other agents have also been reported to cause induction of TNFs in vitro[48,60] and in vivo.[61,62] They include Sendai virus,[48] muramyl dipeptide derivatives,[60] immune complexes using SRBC,[61] and OK-432, a cell wall preparation from *Streptococcus pyogenes*,[62] the common cause of erysipelas (see "Introduction").

V. PURIFICATION

Early purification attempts involved the use of sera from LPS-treated mice[63-65] and rabbits[66,67] or supernatants of in vitro activated peripheral blood monocytes[68] as sources for TNF-like activity, and the supernatants from mitogen-stimulated lymphocytes[69-77] as sources for lymphocyte cytotoxin(s). None of these sources yielded sufficient purified material. As mentioned earlier, human TNF-α and TNF-β were recently purified to homogeneity from several hundred liters of serum-free conditioned media obtained from the human monocytic cell line HL-60[11] and the human lymphoblastoid cell line RPMI-1788, respectively.[12,13] Subsequently, two different groups reported the purification of rabbit TNF-α from serum of rabbits primed first with bacterial and then induced with LPS.[77-80] There are also two reports on the purification of mouse TNF-like activity from a macrophage cell line[28] and from mouse serum,[81] but no amino acid sequence data was provided, so homology with the human TNF-α could not be unequivocally established.

The schemes most frequently employed for the purification of these cytotoxic factors have involved gel filtration, ion-exchange, and lectin affinity chromatography.[63-75] These conventional procedures were inadequate to handle trace amounts of proteins present in large volumes of cell supernatants. A criterion that has played a major role in the purification of these proteins is their hydrophobic nature. Since TNF-α and TNF-β bind to glass, these cytokines could be conveniently adsorbed onto controlled pore glass beads (CPG) from several hundred liters of cell supernatants. After batch adsorption the glass beads were packed in a column and the active fraction eluted with ethylene glycol. This method provided several advantages, including rapid concentration of the activity, the ability to handle large volumes of cell supernatants, stability of the activity in the elution buffers, removal of nonhydrophobic contaminants, and the suitability of the effluents for the next step of purification. This method also avoided dialysis which could be time consuming and may destabilize the biological activity.

Ion exchange chromatography has been used routinely for the purification of these cytotoxic factors.[63-75] This step was convenient after CPG chromatography due to the low ionic strength of the eluate. Both TNF-α and -β bind to DEAE and can be eluted with 0.1-0.2 M NaCl. Another step that has been routinely employed in the purification of these cytokines is lectin affinity chromatography, particularly using Concanavalin A-Sepharose.[63,73-76] It has been found that human TNF-β,[12] but not human TNF-α,[11] binds to lectins, indicating that the former is a glycoprotein. Furthermore, among lectins, lentil lectin was found to be a far better adsorbant than Con A. The binding of the protein to lentil lectin can be reversed by α-methyl mannoside. Lectin affinity chromatography has yielded 80-3100 fold purification of TNF-β, depending on the specific activity of the starting material.[12,82] Gel filtration has also been used for purification of the cytotoxic factors.[63-75] However, this step has proven to be an inefficient purification step due to its limited capacity, poor resolution, and the oligomeric nature of these cytotoxic proteins.

High resolution ion exchange chromatography, chromatofocusing, and reverse phase high performance liquid chromatography (HPLC) are some of the more recent techniques for

Table 2
MOLECULAR CHARACTERISTICS OF TNF-α AND TNF-β

Properties	TNF-α Natural	TNF-α Recombinant	TNF-β (LT) Natural	TNF-β (LT) Recombinant
Source	Monocytes (HL-60)	E. coli	Lymphocytes (RPMI-1788)	E. coli
Protein				
Molecular weight (SDS PAGE)	17,000	17,000	20,000 / 25,000	16,000 / 18,000
Amino acid length	157	157	148 (20 kD) / 171 (25 kD)	148 (16 kD) / 171 (18 kD)
Glycoprotein	No	No	Yes	No
Disulfide bridges	One	One	None	None
Sensitivity to trypsin, chymotrypsin, and V8 protease	Yes	Yes	No	No
Gene				
Size	~3 kilobases	~3 kilobases	~3 kilobases	~3 kilobases
mRNA	1,672 base pairs		1,329 base pairs	
Signal sequence	76 amino acids		34 amino acids	
Number of introns	3 (607, 187, and 301 bp)		3 (287, 86, and 247 bp)	
Chromosomal location	6		6	

purification of proteins. Nearly 14,000-fold purification of TNF-α was obtained by using a combination of fast protein liquid chromatography (FPLC) with a Mono Q (anion exchange) column and reverse phase HPLC on a Synchropak RP-4 column.[11,83] One of the major disadvantages of reverse phase HPLC has been total or partial loss of biological activities of protein due to the combination of lower pH and organic solvents used for elution. However, it has provided enough material that is sufficiently pure for structural analysis. Finally, in the case of TNF-β, preparative polyacrylamide gel electrophoresis (both native and denaturing) has also played an important role in its purification.[12,13,82]

Employing the method of in vitro cytotoxicity on L-929 cells, it has been determined that both cytotoxic factors have been similar specific activities ranging from $4\text{-}10 \times 10^7$ units per mg protein.[11-13] The specific biological activity can be a useful, but not absolute, criterion for establishing the homogeneity of a given protein preparation. The uncertainty is due to the fact that the methodology for determination of the biological activity could vary a great deal from one laboratory to another. This is especially true in the case of the cytotoxic factors described here, for which different cell lines and varying end-points have been used to determine cytotoxicity.

VI. PHYSICOCHEMICAL CHARACTERIZATION

TNF-α and TNF-β differ significantly in their physical and chemical properties. TNF-α was found to have a single subunit with a molecular weight of 17,000[11] by SDS-PAGE. Under the same conditions, two different forms of TNF-β, with molecular weights 20,000 and 25,000, have been found (Table 2).[12,13] The 20 kDalton species is a proteolytic cleavage product of the 25 kDalton form.[12,13] There are no previously reported molecular weight estimates of these proteins under denaturing conditions. However, the estimate of the subunit molecular weight of natural human TNF-α has recently been confirmed by other workers.[17] The determination of the molecular weight under nondenaturing conditions has produced very different results. Purified human TNF-α has a native molecular weight of 45,000,[11] whereas TNF-β elutes at a position corresponding to a molecular weight of 60,000 to 70,000[12,13] during gel filtration. Molecular weights ranging from 10,000 to > 200,000 have

TNF-α															val	arg	ser	3
TNF-β	leu	pro	gly	val	gly	leu	thr	pro	ser	ala	ala	gln	thr	ala	arg	gln	his	pro	lys	met	20
TNF-α	ser	ser	arg	thr	pro	ser	asp	lys	pro	val	ala	his	val	val	ala	asn	pro	gln	ala	glu	23
TNF-β	his	leu	ala	his	ser	thr	leu	lys	pro	ala	ala	his	leu	ile	gly	asp	pro	ser	lys	gln	40
TNF-α	gly	gln	leu	gln	trp	leu	asn	arg	arg	ala	asn	ala	leu	leu	ala	asn	gly	val	glu	leu	43
TNF-β	asn	ser	leu	leu	trp	arg	ala	asn	thr	asp	arg	ala	phe	leu	gln	asp	gly	phe	ser	leu	60
TNF-α	arg	asp	asn	gln	leu	val	val	pro	ser	glu	gly	leu	tyr	leu	ile	tyr	ser	gln	val	leu	63
TNF-β	ser	asn	asn	ser	leu	leu	val	pro	thr	ser	gly	ile	tyr	phe	val	tyr	ser	gln	val	val	80
TNF-α	phe	lys	gly	gln	gly	cys	pro	---	---	---	---	ser	thr	his	val	leu	leu	thr	his	thr	79
TNF-β	phe	ser	gly	lys	ala	tyr	ser	pro	lys	ala	thr	ser	ser	pro	leu	tyr	leu	ala	his	glu	100
TNF-α	ile	ser	arg	ile	ala	val	ser	tyr	gln	thr	lys	val	asn	leu	leu	ser	ala	ile	lys	ser	99
TNF-β	val	gln	leu	phe	ser	ser	gln	tyr	pro	phe	his	val	pro	leu	leu	ser	ser	gln	lys	met	120
TNF-α	pro	cys	gln	arg	glu	thr	pro	glu	gly	ala	glu	ala	lys	pro	trp	tyr	glu	pro	ile	tyr	119
TNF-β	val	tyr	---	---	---	---	pro	gly	leu	gln	glu	---	---	pro	trp	leu	his	ser	met	tyr	134
TNF-α	leu	gly	gly	val	phe	gln	leu	glu	lys	gly	asp	arg	leu	ser	ala	glu	ile	asn	arg	pro	139
TNF-β	his	gly	ala	ala	phe	gln	leu	thr	gln	gly	asp	gln	leu	ser	thr	his	thr	asp	gly	ile	154
TNF-α	asp	tyr	leu	asp	phe	ala	glu	ser	gly	gln	val	tyr	phe	gly	ile	ile	ala	leu			157
TNF-β	pro	his	leu	val	leu	ser	pro	ser	thr	---	val	phe	phe	gly	ala	phe	ala	leu			171

FIGURE 2. Amino acid sequence of human TNF-α and TNF-β.

been reported for cytotoxic factors derived from the sera of mice and rabbits and from the supernatants of lymphocytes and monocytes.[63,75] The precise reason for such a tremendous variation is not clear. Several possibilities exist, including the existence of cytotoxic substances other than TNF-α or TNF-β, aggregation of the cytotoxic proteins with themselves or with other proteins, proteolytic cleavage of the intact molecules as is the case with TNF-β (20 vs 25 kDalton),[12,13] and differences in the degree of glycosylation.

The isoelectric points (pI) of these cytotoxic factors have been reported to be in the range of 4.5 to 6.5. TNF-β has a pI of 5.8, and 5.3 is the pI determined for TNF-α. The variations in the pI of a given protein can be caused by factors similar to those that affect its apparent molecular weight (mentioned in the previous paragraph), as well as deamidation of protein during purification.

The complete primary structure of the two proteins derived from human lymphocytes and monocytes has been elucidated[11,13] and confirmed by cDNA cloning and expression in *E. coli*[14,15] (Figure 2). The amino acid compositions derived from the structures are shown in Table 3. TNF-α is 157 amino acids long,[11,15] and sequences of 171 and 148 amino acids, respectively, have been found for the 25 and 20 kDalton species of TNF-β.[13,14] Comparison of the amino acid sequences of the two proteins revealed that they are 36% identical and 51% homologous to each other. Both TNF-α and TNF-β contain two tryptophans at approximately similar locations in the sequence, and contain equal numbers of tyrosine residues (Table 3). TNF-β has a high content of histidine and phenylalanine residues and no cysteine, whereas TNF-α has a low content of histidine and phenylalanine, two cysteines, and no methionine residues.

Recently, other investigators have also reported the amino acid sequence of human TNF-α either determined from the protein[16,17,21] or predicted from the nucleotide sequence[16,17,20,21] (see below). Some variations in the protein sequences at the amino terminal end have been observed which are shown in Figure 3. The N-terminal protein sequence of the natural human TNF-α purified from HL-60 cells obtained by Wang et al.,[17] has two discrepancies with the sequence reported earlier[11] and that predicted from the cloned cDNA sequence.[15,17] Two out of the three serines in positions 3 to 5 of the mature protein are missing, and the His-Val sequence in position 15 and 16 has been replaced by Val-Ser-Val-Ser. The reason for this

Table 3
AMINO ACID COMPOSITIONS OF TUMOR NECROSIS FACTORS FROM AMINO ACID SEQUENCE

	TNF-α	TNF-β I	TNF-β II
Asp	5	5	5
Asn	7	4	4
Thr	6	10	8
Ser	13	21	20
Glu	10	2	2
Gln	10	12	10
Pro	10	14	11
Gly	11	11	9
Ala	13	15	11
Cys	2	—	—
Val	13	10	9
Met	0	3	2
Ile	8	3	3
Leu	18	23	20
Tyr	7	7	7
Phe	4	10	10
His	3	10	8
Lys	6	6	5
Arg	9	3	2
Trp	2	2	2
Total No. residues	157	171	148
Mol			
Theoretical	17,356	18,664	15,234
(SDS-PAGE)	(17,000)	(25,000)	(20,000)
Isoelectric point:			
Theoretical	7.4	9.1	7.6
Experimental	(5.3)	(5.8)	(5.6)
Extinction coefficient 0.1% 280 nm	1.6	1.7	1.4

Note: Numbers in parentheses indicate the values obtained for recombinant molecule.

```
Predicted A.A. sequence from cDNA      V-R-S-S-S-R-T-P-S-D-K-P-V-A-H-V-V-A-N-P
(Ref. 15-17,20,21)


HL-60 derived TNF-α protein sequence   V-R-S-S-S-R-T-P-S-D-K-P-V-A-H-V-V-A-N-P
(Ref. 15)


HL-60 derived TNF-α protein sequence   V-R-S-R-T-P-S-D-K-P-V-A-V-S-V-S-V-A-N-P-N-A-E-G
(Ref. 17)


E. coli derived recombinant human      ----S-S-S-R-T-P-S-D-K-P-V-A-H-V-V-A-N-P
TNF-α protein sequence (Ref. 16,21)
```

FIGURE 3. Variation in N-terminal amino acid sequences of human TNF-α.

discrepancy is not clear. Although it has been suggested[17] that this represents the product of a second TNF-α gene, this remains unproven and is highly unlikely, since all the cDNAs for human TNF-α cloned from a number of different sources by various groups[15-17,20,21] have only the predicted sequence shown in Figure 2. Two groups[16,21] have reported the N-terminal sequence of recombinant human TNF-α expressed and purified in *E. coli* in which Val-Arg from position 1 and 2 of the natural protein sequence, respectively, are missing, even though the nucleotide codons for these amino acids are present at the corresponding positions in both the genomic[16] and cDNA[21] sequences. These investigators assumed that the N-terminal sequence of human TNF-α was Ser-Ser-Ser-Arg- . . . based on an analogy with the sequence of rabbit TNF-α purified from serum. Consequently, expression plasmids were constructed in which the nucleotides for Val-Arg were not included in the N-terminus following the initiator methionine codon. The specific activities reported for the truncated molecule expressed and purified from *E. coli* by the two groups are 1.4×10^6 units/mg[16] and 1.9×10^6 units/mg,[21] based on cytotoxic activity against L-M cells. These are about an order of magnitude lower than that obtained for the naturally derived molecule.[11]

VII. GENE STRUCTURE

Due to the limited supply of TNF-α and -β available from natural sources, it was extremely important that the genes for both the proteins be isolated, cloned, and expressed in order to make large quantities of the protein available. Therefore, oligodeoxyribonucleotide probes were syntheisized based on the amino acid sequence of both the proteins and hybridized with cDNAs prepared from the poly A rich mRNA isolated from lymphocyte and monocyte cell-lines. These results indicated that the mRNA encoding human TNF-β is approximately 1300 base pairs[14] and that of human TNF-α is about 1600 base pairs[15] in length. The primary structure predicted from the nucleotide sequence of the cDNA of both the TNFs is identical to that determined from the purified proteins themselves. The nucleotide sequence of the cDNA of TNF-α has been confirmed by several other groups.[16,17,20,21] The predicted first amino acid of the sequence of mature recombinant TNF-α has varied by two amino acid positions from one laboratory to another due to the differences in the amino terminal protein sequence obtained, as discussed in the previous section (Figure 3). There is a signal sequence of 76 and 34 amino acids before the start of the mature sequences of TNF-α and TNF-β, respectively. These are relatively long signal sequences, and their significance is currently unknown.

The genes for human lymphocyte and monocyte TNFs have also been isolated[85] (Table 2). They are both approximately three kilobases in size and contain three introns at approximately the same location. The last exons of both TNF-α and TNF-β are 80% homologous to each other. The genes for these TNFs have been localized on chromosome six within one kilobase of each other.[84,85]

VIII. BIOLOGICAL PROPERTIES

The availability of highly purified preparations of TNFs in ample quantities made by recombinant DNA technology has created interest in screening for and studying various biological activities of TNFs.

A. Antitumor Effects

One of the major biological effects of TNFs, as their names imply, is the in vivo destruction of certain tumors. In early experiments, TNF production was elicited in vivo by injecting animals first with BCG or *Corynebacterium Parvum* (CP) and then 2 weeks later with LPS. When this protocol was applied to tumor-bearing mice, they showed significant regression of their tumors as well as increased surivival times.[86-88] From a historical perspective, this is the equivalent of the use of Coley's toxins, one of the early therapeutic approaches used against human neoplasia.[3] These results were further substantiated with the use of partially purified murine TNFs against transplanted mouse tumors[27] and heterotransplanted human tumors in nude mice.[26,27] Significant anti-tumor activity was observed following intravenous or intratumor injection against several tumors transplanted in vivo, including murine Meth A sarcoma; Colon 26, colon carcinoma; sarcoma 180; Ehrlich tumor; MM46, mammary tumor; MM134, hepatoma; Lewis lung, pulmonary cancer; and B16, melanoma.[27] Similarly, human melanoma RPMI 7931 and colon carcinoma, HT-29[26] as well as malignant melanoma (SEKI, MHV-1), gastric cancer (MKN 45, KATO III), and nasopharyngeal carcinoma (KB),[27] when heterotransplanted into nude mice, could be suppressed by repeated injections of TNFs. Since homogenous pure material was not used in these experiments, it is uncertain whether these effects were entirely due to TNF-α or TNF-β, or a mixture of both, or due to other unknown agent(s). More recently,[89] purified recombinant HuTNF-α, administered daily, intratumorally in nude mice was found to cause total regression of three human tumor xenografts — breast cancers, NcMc and 1068, and bowel cancer, GFC with tumor growth totally abrogated in 75% or more of the mice. A tumor static effect was seen with the bowel cancer GF De; i.e., the size of the tumor in TNF-treated mice remained unchanged at the end of 36 days, compared to PBS-BSA-treated control mice in whom the tumor implant had grown by almost four-fold during the same period. TNF therapy was not effective in two other tumors studied, i.e., bowel cancer (GFW) and breast cancer (NCH). The same study also found that: (a) The intraperitoneal route of TNF administration was much less efficacious than the intratumoral route, even at five-fold higher doses, and (b) the combination of HuTNF-α with HuIFN-γ administered intraperitoneally was significantly more effective against the 1068 xenograft even though, by itself, HuIFN-γ alone had no significant effect on tumor growth.

Histologic examination of tumor sections following TNF administration revealed extensive necrotic areas compared to untreated controls.[26,89] In an effort to understand the mechanism of tumor necrosis and regression much attention has been focused on the in vitro ability of TNFs to directly inhibit the growth of tumor cells in culture (Table 1). The cytotoxic activity of TNFs is striking in terms of their ability to selectively kill tumor cells while sparing normal cells. The tumoricidal effect of TNF is not universal, and several tumor cell lines (e.g., T24, human bladder carcinoma) show a null response ($< 25\%$ cytostasis/cytotoxicity) in the presence of TNF.[23]

Notwithstanding the extensive ability of TNFs to specifically kill certain tumor cells in vitro, this action by itself may not completely account for the in vivo effect of rapid hemorrhagic necrosis of tumors. Whereas 1,000 U of TNF-α administered in vivo will cause complete hemorrhagic necrosis of a 10 mm-sized tumor in an animal in 24 hr, it takes 10,000 U and 72 hr to kill 5,000 ME180 cells in vitro.[90] Furthermore, for a given tumor there is no apparent correlation between its relative susceptibility to TNF killing in vitro and in vivo. For instance, the cell line L-929 that is regarded as being fairly sensitive to TNF cytotoxicity in vitro, is relatively resistant to the in vivo action of TNF,[90] whereas the reverse is the case with Meth A sarcoma.

Studies of tumor regression of Meth A sarcoma heterotransplanted into nude mice suggest the possible existence of a host-mediated factor(s) induced by TNF that contributes to the antitumor effect in addition to TNF itself.[27] This is based on the observation that when TNF was administered intravenously, Meth A sarcoma transplanted in BALB/c $nu/+$ mice was more susceptible than Meth a transplanted in nu/nu mice. On the other hand, the tumor was equally sensitive to TNF administered intratumorally in both mice. Since nu/nu mice are deficient in T cell function, a possible T cell factor in addition to TNF may be implicated in tumor killing. This observation is interesting in light of the fact that IFN-γ, a T cell

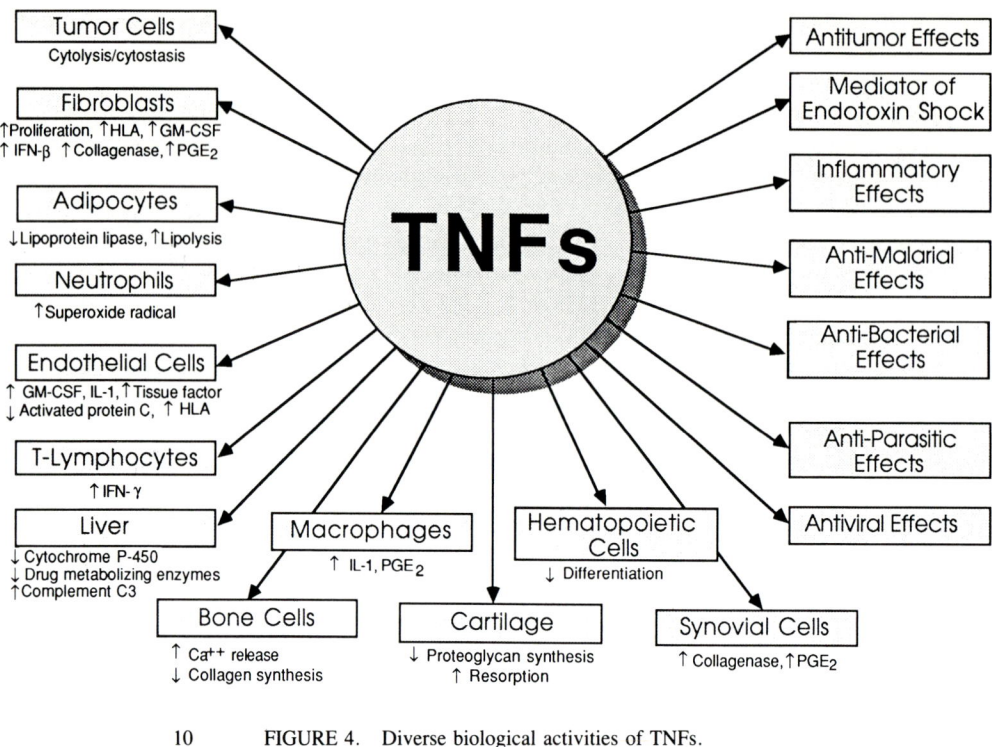

FIGURE 4. Diverse biological activities of TNFs.

lymphokine, has a pronounced synergistic effect on tumor killing by TNF in vivo,[89] and in vitro.[23,32,94,95] This confirmed previous equivocal reports in which impure preparations had been studied in vitro.[91-93] Recent studies also indicate that TNF itself can stimulate lymphocytes to secrete IFN-γ,[57] fibroblasts to secrete IFN-β_2,[96] and endothelial cells,[97] monocytes,[98] and resting macrophages[99] to secrete IL-1. Thus there may be other factors induced by TNF which are also essential for the observed antitumor activities in vivo.

Most importantly, studies with highly purified TNFs indicate that: (a) TNFs have multiple biological effects on normal cell physiology (see Figure 4), and (b) in some instances these activites resemble the actions of other cytokines, e.g., IL-1 and classical growth factors. Some of these actions are discussed below.

B. Proliferation of Normal Cells

In contrast to cytotoxic activity of TNF-α and TNF-β for a number of tumor cells, they both directly stimulate the growth of normal fibroblasts (Table 1). Growth stimulation of these cells occurred at the same low dose of TNF-α that caused inhibition of tumor cell growth,[23,35] and furthermore, the growth-stimulating activity could be inhibited by the same monoclonal anti-TNF antibody that also neutralized its tumor cell cytotoxicity. A monoclonal anti-TNF-α antibody that did not neutralize TNF-α cytotoxicity also had no effect on its growth stimulation activity of cells.[35] Insulin or insulin-like growth factors in the serum potentiated the growth stimulation produced by TNF-α, whereas EGF was shown to be ineffective.[35]

Another group of investigators found that while TNF-α by itself stimulated the growth of human diploid fibroblasts, preincubation of cells with cycloheximide (a protein synthesis inhibitor) followed by TNF-α treatment resulted in cell killing.[100] These experiments would lead one to conclude that normal cells synthesize an endogenous protein(s) that inhibits TNF-α cytotoxicity and promotes its growth factor-like activity. This kind of bi-directional regulation has also been described for TGF-β.[101]

C. Cachectin/TNF-α

Another major indication of an effect of TNF-α on normal tissue stems from studies on cachectin,[10,49,102] a macrophage secreted factor that inhibited the synthesis of enzyme lipoprotein lipase in the mouse adipocyte cell line 3T3-L1. Cachectin has been suggested to be the agent responsible for causing cachexia during certain chronic host infections and malignancies.[102,103] One of the salient features of cachexia is the loss of body weight, even with adequate food consumption. The purification of cachectin and its partial structure determination revealed that this protein was identical to TNF-α.[10,49] Subsequently it was also shown that rTNF-α exhibited cachectin-like activity in vitro.[102] Cachectin/TNF-α has been shown to suppress the expression of a number of lipogenic enzymes in adipocytes, including lipoprotein lipase, the inhibition of which prevents the uptake of free fatty acids.[102] These studies have prompted the suggestion that TNF-α is the agent responsible for cachexia during chronic host infection.[102,103] However, recent studies indicate that this activity is not unique to TNF-α, since other cytokines including IL-1,[104] IFNs,[105,106] and TNF-β[106] can also suppress lipoprotein lipase activity in 3T3-L1 adipocytes. Besides, there is no direct evidence to indicate that the administration of endotoxin-free TNF-α to an animal in a dose range responsible for tumor necrosis can induce cachexia as determined by loss of body weight.[89]

D. Antipathogenic and Antiviral Effects

Tumor necrosis serum (TNS) and partially purified preparations of TNF-α have been reported to protect animals against bacterial and parasitic infections. C3H/HeJ mice challenged with *Klebsiella pneumoniae* or *Listeria monocytogenes* showed increased survival rates following TNS injection compared to untreated controls.[107] TNF-α also appears to have a potent cytotoxic effect on the malarial parasites *Plasmodium falciparum*,[108] and *Plasmodium yoelii* and *Plasmodium berghei*.[109] Recently, recombinant TNF-α was shown to be similar to eosinophil cytotoxicity enhancing factor and it potentiated eosinophil cytotoxicity against *Schistosoma mansoni* larvae.[110]

Several investigators[96,111,112] have found that rTNF-α exhibits direct antiviral activity similar to interferons. EMCV replication in FS-4 fibroblasts was inhibited by TNF-α, and this inhibition could be completely blocked by neutralizing anti-human IFN-β antibodies.[96] However, Northern blot analysis of TNF-treated cells did not reveal mRNA for IFN-β. A new mRNA species (called IFN-β$_2$) was observed, and the antiviral activity was ascribed to it.[96] On the other hand, TNF-α protected HEP-2 cells against VSV infection,[111] and this effect was not blocked by anti-IFN antibodies.[111] Similarly, TNF-α and TNF-β were shown to directly induce resistance to infection by both RNA viruses (EMCV and VSV) and DNA viruses (Ad-2 and HSV-2) in diverse cell types.[112] Like IFNs, TNFs caused induction of mRNA for [2'-5']-oligoA synthetase mRNA. However, the antiviral effect of TNFs was not IFN-mediated since it was not abolished by anti-IFN-α, -β or -γ antibodies, there were no detectable levels of IFNs in the cell culture fluids, and no IFN mRNA was found in the cells. In addition to inducing the antiviral state, TNFs were also able to selectively kill virus-infected cells. Both the antiviral activity and virus-induced cytotoxicity of TNFs were synergistically enhanced by IFNs.[112] Furthermore, viruses as well as the polymer poly(I):poly(C) could induce the production of TNF-α in HL-60 cells and TNF-β in RPMI 1788 cells.[112]

E. Activation of Polymorphonuclear Neutrophils (PMN)

A more direct role for TNF in mediating inflammatory responses has been implicated by its effects on neutrophil functions. It has been reported[113] that pretreatment of PMN with purified TNF-α and TNF-β (free of detectable LPS contamination) induces a significant increase in their ability to phagocytose fluorescein-conjugated latex beads (1.5 micron) as well as an enhancement of PMN-mediated antibody dependent cellular cytotoxicity (ADCC) against chicken erythrocytes. More recently other investigators[114] have found significant increases in phagocytosis of unopsonized zymosan particles, degranulation, and respiratory burst activity by TNF-α treated PMN. Interestingly, these effects were inhibited by monoclonal antibodies against the C3bi receptor/adherence glycoprotein CD11.[115] TNF-α has been shown[116] to increase the expression of this protein on neutrophils resulting in their enhanced adherence to the endothelium (see below).

F. Effects on Endothelial Cells

In addition to its effects on PMN, TNF-α appears to have direct effects on endothelial cells which play a major role in inflammation and tissue injury. TNF-α induced the release of IL-1 from endothelial cells,[97] induces neutrophil adherence to endothelial cells[116,117] via the CDW18 neutrophil membrane protein complex (also called the C3bi receptor/adherence glycoprotein mentioned earlier), and increases cell surface expression of HLA-A,B antigens of the major histocompatibility complex.[118] Further evidence that the endothelium is a major site of TNF action in vivo comes from studies on effects of TNF-α on the hemostatic properties of endothelial cells[119] in culture. Incubation with rTNF-α causes the induction of two activities:[119] synthesis of tissue factor, a procoagulant cofactor protein,[120,121] and inhibition of formation of activated protein C, an anticoagulant cofactor protein.[122] Extensive changes in the morphology of human vascular endothelial cells in confluent primary culture treated with TNF-α have also been reported.[123] It is tempting to correlate these in vitro results with those observed in vivo, i.e., hemorrhagic necrosis of tumors induced by TNF-α. Two facts support the hypothesis that this may play a role in the mechanism by which TNFs cause tumor regression in vivo: (a) The administration of TNF results in hemorrhagic necrosis indicating a selective rupture of the vasculature of the tumor, and (b) similar changes in the hemostatic properties of endothelial cells in culture are also produced by IL-1;[124] and the latter has also been shown to cause hemorrhagic necrosis of tumors in vivo.[164,165]

G. Hematopoietic Cell Differentiation

A possible role for TNF-α and TNF-β in granulocyte-macrophage differentiation has been suggested from recent observations by two groups of investigators[125,127] who have found that TNF-α[125] and TNF-β[127] suppress colony formation by bone-marrow derived hematopoietic progenitor cells. Low doses (0.05 to 100 U/mℓ of rTNF-α[125] as well as TNF-(Luk II)[126] inhibited granulocyte-macrophage differentiation by both late (CFU-GM, day 7) and early (CFU-GM, day 14) precursor cells. The effect was rapid, since pulsing the bone marrow cells for only 1 hr with TNF-α was sufficient to cause suppression. Inhibition of colony formation by erythroid (BFU-E) as well as multi-potential (CFU-GEMM) progenitor cells was also observed.[125] All of these effects could be seen in nonadherent bone marrow cells substantially depleted (down to 2%) of monocytes and T lymphocytes.[125] The inhibitory effect of TNF-β on CFU-GM was observed only in the presence of IFN-γ.[127]

H. Bone Resorption

Both TNF-α and TNF-β have been shown to stimulate bone resorption and inhibit new bone formation in vitro.[128] Bone resorption activity was assayed by measuring the release of $^{45}Ca^{++}$ into the medium and was the result of osteoclast activation, since it could be inhibited by salmon calcitonin (a specific inhibitor of osteoclast activity).[129] The effect was slow (required 2 to 3 days) and needed high doses (10^{-7} M) of TNFs for optimum response. Under similar conditions, TNFs also caused a decrease in alkaline phosphatase (a marker of new bone formation) in 17/28 rat osteosarcoma cells that are phenotypically osteoblasts.[130] The authors also found that bones incubated for 48 hr with TNFs had proportionately lower levels of collagen compared to bones incubated in control medium. It was suggested[128] that TNFs may account for part or all of the activities attributed to osteoclast activating factor

(OAF), a product of activated leukocytes, and once thought to be a distinct lymphokine playing a major role in bone remodelling. Nevertheless, in view of the long time course and relatively high dose of TNFs required, one must also consider the possibility that stimulation of bone resorption may not be a primary effect of TNFs. Thus, PGE_2 has been shown to promote bone resorption,[131] as has the monokine, IL-1.[132] Furthermore, both IL-1[133] and TNF-α[134] can directly stimulate collagenase and PGE_2 production in some cell types. The effects of TNF-α, TNF-β, and IL-1 on bone resorption have been shown to be inhibited by IFN-γ,[135] whereas IFN-γ has no effect on bone resorption induced by systemic hormones such as $1,25(OH)_2$ Vitamin D_3, and parathyroid hormone.[135] Another report has recently indicated that TNF-α (and IL-1) besides stimulation of bone resorption, inhibit the synthesis of proteoglycan in cartilage,[136] as determined by incorporation of $^{35}SO_4$ into glycosaminoglycans of cartilage.

I. Miscellaneous Effects

A number of intracellular activities have been reported, some of which might provide clues to the in vivo action of TNFs. They include stimulation of IL-1 and PGE_2 production in resting macrophages,[99] induction of protein antigens of the major histocompatibility complex,[118] induction of synthesis of collagenase and PGE_2 in synovial cells and dermal fibroblasts,[134] fragmentation of target-cell DNA into discretely sized pieces,[137,138] induction of GM-CSF in normal human lung fibroblasts,[155] stimulation of complement component C3 in human hepatoma cells,[156] and depression of cytochrome P450 and drug metabolizing enzymes (ethoxycoumarin deethylase and arylhydrocarbon hydroxylase) in mouse liver.[157]

J. Relationship of TNFs to Other Cytokines

It is clear from the foregoing discussion that a simple analysis of the in vivo mechanism of action of TNFs is complicated by virtue of its various biological effects observed on different tissues in vitro. In addition, elucidation of the true physiologic role of TNFs in vivo, requires knowledge of their relationship to other monokines and lymphokines. In recent years it has become increasingly evident that cytokines acting locally, such as interleukins, interferons, etc., play an important and interdependent role in modifying biological responses. In the immune response, these mediators produce autocrine as well as paracrine effects during T and B cell activation.[139] For instance, macrophages secrete IL-1, which induces T cells to secrete IL-2, and this in turn causes secretion of IFN-γ, which can cause the production of TNF-α and TNF-β (Figure 1). Human peripheral blood mononuclear cells (PBMC) were shown to be induced by rIL-2 to secrete both TNF-β[55,56] and TNF-α,[56] and the effect of IL-2 was augmented by rIFN-γ.[55,56] In some instances IFN-γ by itself also induced TNF-α/TNF-β production.[57] TNF-α production could be seen within 3 hr after induction, reaching peak levels at 48 hr and declining thereafter; TNF-β production started at a slower rate, requiring greater than 8 hr and reached a peak in 72 hr; IFN-γ did not alter the kinetics of TNF-α/TNF-β induction by IL-2.[56] Conversely, TNF itself stimulated lymphocytes to secrete IFN-γ,[57] FS-4 fibroblasts to synthesize IFN-$β_2$,[96] and endothelial cells,[97] monocytes,[53,98] and macrophages[99] to release IL-1.

Besides regulation of TNF-α/TNF-β production by other cytokines, in order to fully comprehend the true physiological role of TNFs, one must also consider their relationship to the monokine IL-1 and the lymphokine, IFN-γ. There are many similarities between the biological action of TNFs and IL-1, and the presence of IFN-γ together with TNFs results in a markedly synergistic or antagonistic response. These actions are briefly described below.

1. Similarities Between TNFs and IL-1

TNFs share a number of biological activities with IL-1, another distinct 17,000 Dalton protein produced by monocytes, which plays a major role in mediating the immune re-

Table 4
COMPARISON OF THE BIOLOGICAL ACTIVITIES OF TNFS AND IL-1

DIFFERENCES

TNFs	IL-1
1. *Do not* stimulate proliferation of thymocytes.	1. Stimulates comitogenic proliferation of thymocytes.
2. *Do not* induce IL-2 production in lymphocytes.	2. Induces IL-2 production in lymphocytes.

SIMILARITIES

1. Endogenous pyrogenic activity, in vivo.
2. Induction of procoagulant activity in endothelial cells.
3. Stimulation of bone resprotion and cartilage resorption.
4. Stimulation of collagenase and PGE_2 production in dermal fibroblasts.
5. Suppression of lipoprotein lipase in adipocytes.
6. Stimulation of growth of normal fibroblasts.
7. Cytotoxic activity against several neoplastic cell lines.
8. Anti-tumor activity in vivo.

sponse.[140] Some common biological activities of these two monokines include: endogenous pyrogenic activity in vivo,[98] induction of procoagulant activity in endothelial cells,[119,124] stimulation of bone resorption[128,132] and cartilage resorption,[136] stimulation of collagenase and PGE_2 production in dermal fibroblasts,[133,134] suppression of lipoprotein lipase activity in adipocytes, stimulation of growth of fibroblasts,[140] while being cytocidal for several neoplastic cell lines[141,142,168] and anti-tumor activity in vivo[164,165] (Table 4).

2. Synergism Between TNFs and IFNs

Several investigators have found that the in vitro tumoricidal activity of TNFs is significantly augmented by co-incubation with IFNs.[23,32,94,95] IFN-α, -β, or-γ, while not showing any antiproliferative effects by themselves, synergistically enhanced the cytotoxicity of TNF-α/TNF-β. Synergism between IFN-γ and TNF-β has also been reported[127] for inhibition of hematopoietic cell differentiation. Furthermore, the synergistic effect of IFN-γ appears to be correlated with its ability to induce synthesis of TNF receptors in target cells.[95,144-147] It is not yet clear whether the synergism is solely explained by increased receptor number, or whether other proteins involved in the mechanism of cytotoxicity are also induced by IFN-γ. Experiments on the B16 melanoma cell line with TNF-β and IFN-γ showed some intriguing results.[94] This cell line is fairly resistant to the cytotoxic effects of both TNFs and IFNs. However a combination of the two cytokines in submaximal doses causes this tumor cell line to become a sensitive target cell for cytolysis.[94] This could be an interesting model system for studying the mechanism of synergism between TNFs and IFNs.

The synergism observed between IFN-γ and TNFs has profound implications for the mechanism by which TNFs kill tumors in vivo. It is conceivable that local production of IFN-γ or other cytokines near the tumor implant in an animal can account for the increased sensitivity of certain tumors, whereas they are relatively less sensitive to TNF killing in vitro. The synergy also opens up exciting possibilities for application in human clinical trials, where a combined lower dose of TNF and IFN-γ might provide potent antitumor activity. This has already been observed in studies with nude mice using human tumor xenografts as discussed earlier.

K. TNF Receptors

Several laboratories have used radiolabeled TNFs to demonstrate that TNFs bind to specific

Table 5
CHARACTERISTICS OF TNF RECEPTORS ON HUMAN AND MURINE CELLS

TNF type	Target cell type	Cytotoxicity (pM)	Binding kD (pM)	Binding (sites/cell)	Ref.
HuTNF-β	L-929 (murine)	70	70	3,200	143
HuTNF-α	ME-180 (human)		200	2,000	23,144
	WI-38	Resistant	220	2,200	23
	T24	Resistant	250	1,500	23
HuTNF-α	L929 (murine)	1	610	2,200	147,146
	FS-4 (human)	Resistant	320	7,500	147,146
	HeLa (human)	N.A.	160	15,000	148,147
	HT-29 (human)	N.A.	200	4,500	147
	WISH (human)	N.A.	240	6,800	147
	A673 (human)	N.A.	190	5,700	147
	RPMI-7272 (human)	Resistant	230	18,000	147
TNF[a]	HeLa52 (human)	200	200	6,000	147
	Jurkat (human)	200	250	1,100	
	Daudi (human)	Resistant	N.A.[b]		
		Resistant			
	Ht-29				95
	HeLa D98/A42				95
	SK-MEL-109				95
MuTNF-α/	L-M; (murine)	3	3	1,100	150
Necrosin	L929 (murine)	3	3	770	150
	3T3A31 (murine)	2.5	2.5	1,050	150
	CPAE (bovine)	30	3	1,500	150
MuTNF-α/	J774.1 (murine)	7,200	3	1,100	150
Necrosin		resistant			
MuTNF-α/	3T3-L1 Adipocytes	10[c]	3,000	10,000	151
Cachectin	(murine)				
MuTNF-β/	LM (murine)	100	100	200	152
LUKII[d]	HeLa (murine)	100	100	300	152
	LM (resistant)	Resistant	No[e]		

[a] Source not given.
[b] NA, data not available.
[c] The biological effect in this case was inhibition of lipoprotein lipase activity in adipocytes.
[d] This material was not homogeneous on SDS-PAGE according to the authors, hence the binding data must be interpreted with some caution.
[e] No binding observed.

cell surface receptors (Table 5). Binding is saturable, time-, temperature-, and dose-dependent with a linear Scatchard plot, indicating the presence of a single class of binding sites. The binding occurs at the physiologically relevant concentration range; the number of binding sites per cell are low (1000 to 18,000 sites/cell) and are dependent on cell type. Both TNF-α[144] and TNF-β[143] have been shown to interact with the same cell surface receptor, consistent with their similar biological actions. Receptor binding to some cell lines occurs across species; i.e., human TNFs bind to receptors on murine cells and *vice versa*.[143,146,147,150] This is consistent with the tumor cell cytotoxic effect of TNFs observed across species, and it is not too surprising in view of the high degree of sequence homology ($> 80\%$) between murine and human TNF-α.[15,18-20] The binding of TNFs to its cell surface receptors appears to be necessary, but not sufficient, for its biological activity. Thus while the human Daudi and Raji lymphoblastoid cell lines show extremely low specific binding of TNF and are also resistant to its cytotoxic effects,[148] several other TNF-resistant cell lines, including T24,[23] RPMI 7272,[146] and murine J774.1[150] possess TNF receptors comparable in affinity (Kd) and number to that observed in TNF-sensitive cells. There is also evidence indicating that binding of TNF-α to its receptor is followed by internalization and degradation of the ligand.[145,146,149] It is not known whether internalization of the TNF-receptor complex is a prerequisite for its in vitro activity. Exposure of cells to IFN-γ can up-regulate the expression of TNF-α receptors[95,144,147] with no change in the affinity of the receptor. The enhancement of receptor expression was inhibited by cycloheximide suggesting that induction of TNF-α receptors by IFN-γ occurs through the synthesis of new proteins.[144,147] A subunit molecular weight of 90,000 for the TNF-receptor complex has been determined by covalently cross-linking ^{125}I-TNF to the cell surface receptor on murine J774.1,[150] human K562,[153] and U937[153,154] cells followed by SDS-PAGE and autoradiography.

IX. MECHANISM OF TNF ACTION

As yet, not much is known regarding biochemical events that lead to each of the various effects produced by TNFs following receptor binding. One obvious question is whether all the actions of TNFs are mediated by a single receptor. The cross reactivity between TNF-α and TNF-β on binding to cell surface receptors, the linear Scatchard plots and similar Kds obtained on a wide variety of cell types, and the low doses of TNF required for biological response are all consistent with the idea of a single class of cell surface TNF binding sites. On the other hand, some of these actions, e.g., the procoagulant effects on endothelial cells, that are also mediated by IL-1, could very well be events that are secondary to the stimulation of IL-1 release by TNF.

Mechanistic studies have been most extensively carried out on the in vitro cytotoxicity of TNF to L-929 cells.[158-161] Unlike the actions of certain other cytolytic effectors (e.g., pore-forming proteins)[162,163] that act rapidly by punching holes in the plasma membrane, TNF-mediated cell killing is a slow process (24 to 72 hr)[162,163] requiring a finite, dose-dependent time-lag of 4 to 10 hr.[158,159] The lag period can be shortened by increasing the TNF dosage but to no less than 4 hr.[158,159] The lag time can also be shortened to about 4 hr by preincubation with the inhibitors of protein synthesis (cycloheximide) or RNA synthesis (Actinomycin D).[158,159] Sensitivity to TNF-mediated killing is also enhanced by raising the temperature to 39°C[158,159] and decreased by lowering the temperature to 32°C,[160] suggesting that metabolically active cells are better targets for killing by TNF. Evidence indicating that internalization of TNF may be necessary for TNF-mediated killing in vitro comes from studies that show that sensitivity is decreased by preincubation with agents that disrupt cytoskeletal elements, including colchicine, colecemid, and cytochalasin B.[160,161] Inhibitors of lysosome activity, chloroquine, methylamine, and leupeptin also lowered the sensitivity.[160,161] However, direct microinjection of TNF into target L-929 cells did not result in either disruption of internal organelles or cell death, as observed by electron microscopy.[161] The same cells, when incubated in the presence of externally added TNF, suffered extensive lysis of internal organelles, whereas the cell membrane remained relatively intact.[161] These results suggest that an orderly, time dependent, receptor-mediated sequence of events possibly followed by internalization and degradation of the TNF-receptor complex precedes the action of TNF in vitro.

The precise biochemical events that follow receptor binding have not yet been elucidated. Whether TNF action follows the cAMP/cGMP pathway or protein kinase C pathway for signal transduction is not known. Using crude preparations of TNF, induction of phospholipases and DNAse have been reported, but whether they are primary or secondary events involved in the action of TNF is not clear.

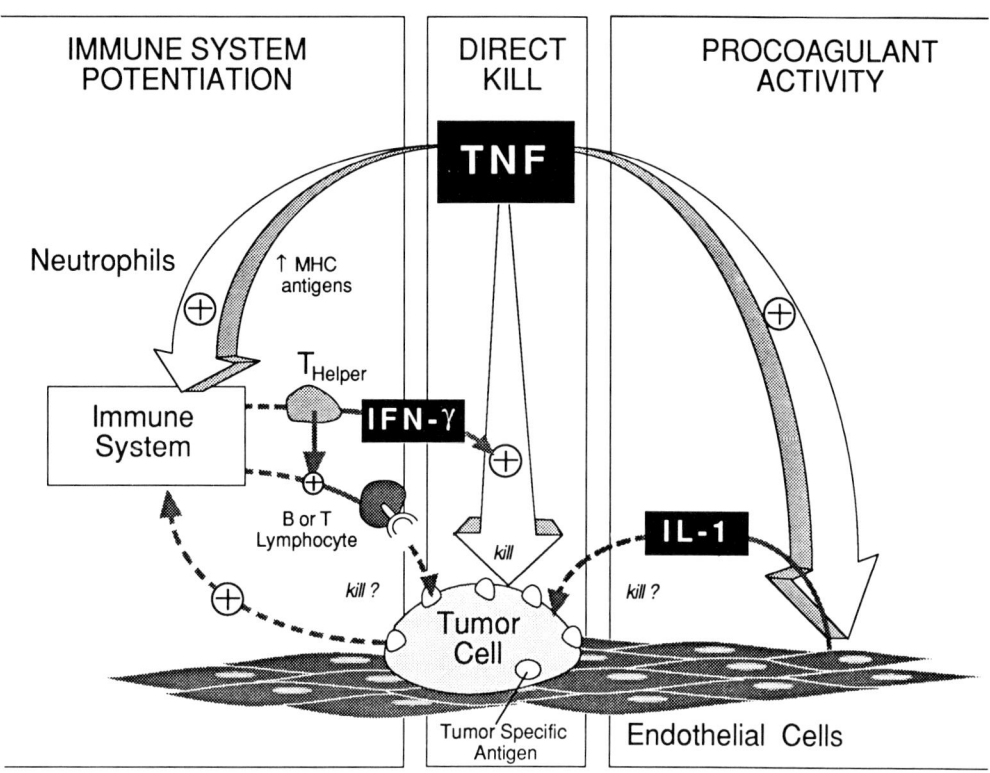

FIGURE 5.   Possible mechanism of antitumor action of TNF in vivo.

A. In Vivo Action

Perhaps the most intriguing questions on TNF action relate to the mechanism of hemorrhagic necrosis of tumors in vivo. First, there is the issue of selectivity whereby at low doses TNF lacks toxicity on normal tissue compared to the neoplastic tissue. Secondly, there is the issue of the increased susceptibility of certain tumors to TNF-mediated killing in vivo in contrast to in vitro. We propose the hypothesis that TNFs augment or potentiate the immune surveillance system of the host against a tumor implant (Figure 5). The response will be directed against tumor-specific antigens recognized as "foreign" by the host. This ensures selectivity to tumor tissue. In the absence of TNF such a response might be too weak to combat the tumor load. In the presence of TNF, the relative tumor burden is reduced probably in two ways: first, by means of its direct cytotoxic effect on the tumor cells; second, by interacting with various components of the immune system (PMNs, lymphocytes, etc.) resulting in the local production of other cytokines, particulary IFN-γ and IL-1 at the site of the tumor, and the induction of cell surface MHC antigens. This may result in augmentation of the immune response against the tumor specific antigen as well as an inflammatory response resulting in activation of PMN and the stimulation of endothelial cell procoagulant activities, producing extensive damage to the tumor vasculature and leading to hemorrhagic necrosis and eventual tumor regression. This hypothesis helps explain both the in vivo selectivity of TNF for neoplastic tissues as well as the differential susceptibility of the tumor to TNF in vivo. One of the predictions of this hypothesis is that if tumor regression is due to a TNF-dependent host-mediated immune response against a particular tumor, an animal in which the primary implant has completely regressed would be resistant to a secondary challenge with the same tumor but not to other tumors. A recent study has found this to be true in the case of BALB/c Meth A sarcoma implanted in $CB6F_1$ mice.[167] Meth A cells injected subcutaneously into CB6F$_1$ mice formed a tumor which then fully regressed when the animals were administered MuTNF. Subsequently, a second injection of Meth A cells was rejected by these mice, whereas other chemically induced BALB/c sarcomas including CMS4, CMS5, and CMS21 that are antigenically unrelated to Meth A sarcoma,[168] were not rejected.[167]

X. CONCLUDING REMARKS

TNF-α and TNF-β, two cytokines produced by macrophages and lymphocytes respectively, were originally isolated on the basis of their cytotoxicity to tumor cells and are related to each other both structurally and functionally. Using purified preparations obtained primarily by recombinant DNA methodology, a wide variety of new biological activities have recently been assigned to TNF-α and TNF-β. This has raised new questions regarding the true physiological role of TNFs. Based on their antipathogenic actions in vivo, their action on neutrophils and endothelial cells in vitro, their ability to induce IL-1 release and cell surface major histocompatibility antigen expression, and their similarity to the actions of IL-1, it is clear that TNFs are a potent immunomodulators and probably mediators of inflammation in vivo. Except during parasitic infections, or endotoxin administration, TNFs have not been detected in vivo. It is possible that they are produced locally at the site of injury/inflammation, although this remains to be demonstrated. Also, it is not clear why there are two distinct proteins, viz., TNF-α and TNF-β, with identical functions. More extensive investigation may reveal differences in the functions of the two proteins. It is possible that physiologically either their production is controlled by different stimuli or they have quite different roles.

In conclusion, it is interesting to note that the activities of TNF-α and -β are intimately related to the activities of other cytokines found in the immune system. Thus, TNF augments the actions of IFNs (Section VIII.J.2), mimics the actions of IL-1 (Table 4), and possibly inhibits the action of CSF (Section VIII.G). Elucidating the mechanism by which these responses occur will be a major step toward increasing our understanding of how the immune system works.

ACKNOWLEDGMENTS

The authors would like to thank Drs. J. Ramachandran, M. Shepard, T. Aune, and G. Wong for their helpful suggestions and critically reviewing this paper; and C. Morita, W. Anstine, and S. Cuisia for preparation of the manuscript.

LIST OF ABBREVIATIONS

ADCC	antibody dependent cellular cytotoxicity
Ad-2	Adenovirus-2
BCG	Bacillus Calmette-Guerrin
BFU-E	burst forming units-erythroid
CB6F$_1$	F$_1$ mice obtained from BALB/c × C57BL/6
cDNA	complementary DNA
CFU-GEMM	colony forming units-granulocyte erythroid myeloid monocyte
CFU-GM	colony forming units-granulocyte monocyte
Con A	concanavalin A
CP	corynebacterium parvum
CPG	controlled pore glass
DNA	deoxyribonucleic acid
EGF	epidermal growth factor
EMCV	encephalo myocarditis virus
FPLC	fast protein liquid chromatography
GM-CSF	granulocyte monocyte-colony stimulating factor
HPLC	high performance liquid chromatography
HuIFN	human interferon
HuTNF	human TNF
HSV-2	Herpes simplex virus type II
IFN	interferon
IL-1	interleukin-1
IL-2	interleukin-2
Kd	dissociation constant
kD	kilo dalton
LPS	lipopolysaccharide/endotoxin
LT	lymphotoxin
MHC	major histocompatibility complex
mRNA	messenger RNA
MuTNF	murine TNF
OAF	osteoclast activating factor
PBL	peripheral blood leukocytes
PBMC	peripheral blood mononuclear cells
PBS-BSA	Phosphate buffered saline containing bovine serum albumin
PGE$_2$	prostaglandin E$_2$
PMN	polymorphonuclear neutrophils
polyA	polyadenylate
RNA	ribonucleic acid
rHuTNF	recombinant human TNF
rMUTNF	recombinant murine TNF
rTNF	recombinant TNF
SDS-PAGE	sodium dodecylsulfate polyacrylamide gel electrophoresis
SRBC	sheep red blood cells
TNF	tumor necrosis factor
TNS	tumor necrosis serum
VSV	vesicular stomatitis virus

REFERENCES

1. **Busch,** Verhand lungen Artzlicher Gesellschaften, *Berl. Klin. Wchnschr.,* 5, 137, 1868.
2. **Bruns, P.,** Die Heilwirkung des Erysipels auf Geschwulste, *Beitr. Klin. Chir.,* 3, 443, 1868.
3. **Coley, W. B.,** Contribution to the knowledge of sarcoma, *Ann. Surg.,* 14, 199, 1891.
4. **Rosenrauch, C.,** A propos de l'erysipele salutaire et de son action therapeutique sur les tumeurs malignes, *Clinique, Paris,* 28, 324, 1933.
5. **Sakharov, G., and Rossiisky, D.,** Essai de traitment du cancer par l'organotherapie, *Acta medica URSS,* 2, 145, 1939.
6. **Shear, M. J. and Turner, F. C.,** Chemical treatment of tumors. V. Isolation of the hemorrhage-producing fraction from *Serratia marcescens* (*Bacillus prodigiosus*) culture filtrate, *J. Natl. Cancer Inst.,* 4, 81, 1943.
7. **Algire, G. H., Legallaies, F. Y., and Anderson, B. F.,** Vascular reactions of normal and malignant tissues *in vivo.* V. The role of hypotension in the action of a bacterial polysaccharide on tumors, *J. Natl. Cancer Inst.,* 12, 1279, 1952.
8. **O'Malley, W. E., Achinstein, B., and Shear, M. J.** Action of bacterial polysaccharide on tumors. II. Damage of Sarcoma 37 by serum of mice treated with *Serratia marcescens* polysaccharide, and induced tolerance, *J. Natl. Cancer Inst.,* 29, 1169, 1962.
9. **Carswell, E., Old, L. J., Kassel, R. L., Green, S., Fiore, N., and Williamson B.,** An endotoxin-induced serum factor that causes necrosis of tumors, *Proc. Natl. Acad. Sci.,* 72, 3666, 1975.
10. **Beutler, B. A., Milsark, I. W., and Cerami, A.,** Cachetin/tumor necrosis factor: production, distribution and metabolic fate *in vivo. J. Immunol.,* 135, 3972, 1985.
11. **Aggarwal, B. B., Kohr, W. J., Hass, P. E., Moffat, B., Spencer, S. A., Henzel, W. J., Bringman, T. S., Nedwin, G. E., Goeddel, D. V., and Harkins, R. N.,** Human tumor necrosis factor: Production, purification and characterization, *J. Biol. Chem.,* 260, 2345, 1985.
12. **Aggarwal, B. B., Moffat, B., and Harkins, R. N.,** Human lymphotoxin, *J. Biol. Chem.,* 259, 686, 1984.
13. **Aggarwal, B. B., Henzel, W. J., Moffat, B., Kohr, W. J., and Harkins, R. N.,** Primary structure of human lymphotoxin derived from 1788 lymphoblastoid cell line, *J. Biol. Chem.,* 260, 2334, 1985.
14. **Gray, P. W., Aggarwal, B. B., Benton, C. V., Bringman, T. S., Henzel, W. J., Jarrett, J. A., Leung, D. W., Moffat, B., Ng, P., Svedersky, L. P., Palladino, M. A., and Nedwin, G. E.,** Cloning and expression of cDNA for human lymphotoxin, a lymphokine with tumor necrosis activity, *Nature,* 322, 721, 1984.
15. **Pennica, D., Nedwin, G. E., Hayflick, J. S., Seeburg, P. H., Derynck, R., Palladino, M. A., Kohr, W. J., Aggarwal, B. B., and Goeddel, D. V.,** Human tumor necrosis factor: precursor structure, expression, and homology to lymphotoxin, *Nature,* 313, 803, 1984.
16. **Shirai, T., Yamaguchi, H., Ito, H., Todd, C. S., and Wallace, R. B.,** Cloning and expression in *Escherichia coli* of the gene for human tumour necrosis factor, *Nature,* 313, 803, 1985.
17. **Wang, A. M., Creasey, A. A., Ladner, M. B., Lin, L. S., Strickler, J., Van Arsdell, J. N., Yamamoto, R., and Mark D. F.,** Molecular cloning of the complementary DNA for human tumor necrosis factor, *Science,* 221, 149, 1985.
18. **Fransen, L., Muller, R., Marmemout, A., Tavernier, J., Van der Heyden, J., Kawashiura, E., Challet, A., Tizard, R., Van Heuverswyn, H., Van Vliet, A., Ruysschaert, M.-R., and Friers, W.,** Molecular cloning of mouse tumor necrosis factor cDNA and its eukaryotic expression, *Nucl. Acids. Res.,* 13, 4417, 1985.
19. **Pennica, D., Hayflick, J. S., Bringman, T. S., Palladino, M. A., and Goeddel, D. V.,** Cloning and expression in *Escherichia coli* of the cDNA for murine tumor necrosis factor, *Proc. Natl. Acad. Sci.,* 82, 6060, 1985.
20. **Marmenoit, A., Fransen, L., Tavernier, J., Van der Heyden, U., Tizard, R., Kawashima, E., Shaw, A., Johnson, M.-J., Semon, D., Muller, R., Ruysschaert, M.-R., Van Vliet, A., and Fiers, W.,** Molecular cloning and expression of human tumor necrosis factor and comparison with mouse tumor necrosis factor, *Eur. J. Biochem.,* 152, 515, 1985.
21. **Yamada, Y., Furutani, Y., Notake, M., Yamagishi, J., Yamayoshi, M., Fukui, T., Nomura, H., Komiya, M., Kuwashima, J., Nakano, K., Sohmura, Y., and Nakamura, S.,** Efficient production of human tumour necrosis factor in Escherichia coli, *J. Biotechnol.,* 3, 141, 1985.
22. **Helson, L., Green, S., Carswell, S., and Old, L. J.,** Effect of tumor necrosis factor on cultured human melanoma cells, *Nature,* 258, 731, 1975.
23. **Sugarman, B. J., Aggarwal, B. B., Hass, P. E., Figari, I. S., Palladino, M. A., Jr., and Shepard, H. M.,** Recombinant human tumor necrosis factor-α effects on proliferation of normal and transformed cells *in vitro, Science,* 230, 943, 1985.
24. **Granger, G. A. and Williams, T. W.,** Lymphocyte cytotoxicity *in vitro.* Activation and release of a cytotoxic factor, *Nature,* 218, 1253, 1968.
25. **Mannel, D. N., Falk, W., and Meltzer, M. S.,** Inhibition of non-specific tumoricidal activity by activated macrophages with antiserum against a soluble cytotoxic factor, *Infect. Immunity,* 33, 156, 1981.

26. **Helson, L., Helson, C., and Green, S.** Effects of murine tumor necrosis factor on heterotransplanted human tumors, *Expl. Cell Biol.*, 47, 53, 1979.
27. **Haranaka, K., Satomi, N., and Sakurai, A.**, Antitumor activity of murine tumor necrosis factor (TNF) against transplanted murine tumors and heterotransplanted human tumors in nude mice, *Int. J. Cancer*, 34, 263, 1984.
28. **Kull, F. C., Jr. and Cuatrecasas, P.**, Necrosin: Purification and properties of a cytotoxin derived from a murine macrophage-like cell line, *Proc. Natl. Acad. Sci.*, 81, 7932, 1984.
29. **Suyama, K., Goldstein, J., and Green, S.**, Effects of murine tumor necrosis factor on Friend erythroleukemic cells, *Expl. Cell Biol.*, 53, 85, 1985.
30. **Hammerstrom, J.**, Soluble cytostatic factor(s) released from human monocytes. I. Production and effect on normal and transformed human target cells, *Scand. J. Immunol.*, 15, 311, 1982.
31. **Mathews, N.**, Effect on human monocyte killing of tumour cells of antibody raised against an extracellular monocyte cytotoxin, *Immunology*, 48, 321, 1983.
32. **Fransen, L., van der Heyden, J., Ruysschaert, R., and Fiers, W.**, Recombinant tumor necrosis factor: its effect and its synergism with interferon-γ on a variety of normal and transformed human cell lines, *Eur. J. Cancer Clin. Oncol.*, 22, 419, 1986.
33. **Unsgaard, G., Hammerstrom, J., and Lamvik, J.**, Cytostatic effect on tumour cells induced in human monocytes by mediators from BCG-stimulated lymphocytes and MLC, *Acta Path. Microbiol Scand.*, Sect. C., 87, 159, 1979.
34. **Mathews, N.**, Anti-tumour cytotoxin from macrophages: no correlation between cytotoxin adsorption by tumour cell lines and their cytotoxin susceptibility, *Immunology*, 53, 537, 1984.
35. **Vilcek, J., Palombella, V. J., Henriksen-Destefano, D., Swenson, C., Feinman, R., Hirai, M., and Tsumimoto, M.**, Fibroblast growth enhancing activity of tumor necrosis factor and its relationship to other polypeptide growth factors, *J. Exp. Med.*, 163, 632, 1986.
36. **Spofford, B. T., Daynes, R. A., and Granger, G. A.**, Cell mediated immunity *in vitro*: a highly sensitive assay for human lymphotoxin, *J. Immunol.*, 112, 2111, 1974.
37. **Aggarwal, B. B., Moffat, B., Lee, S. H., and Harkins, R. N.**, Chemical and biological properties of human lymphotoxin, in *Thymic Hormones and Lymphokines*, Goldstein, A. L., Ed., Plenum Press, New York, 1985, chap. 21, 235.
38. **Walker, S. M. and Lucas, Z. J.**, Cytotoxic activity of lymphocytes. I. Assay for cytotoxicity by rubidium exchange at isotopic equilibrium, *J. Immunol.*, 109, 1223, 1972.
39. **Ruddle, N. H. and Waksman, B. H.**, Cytotoxicity mediated by soluble antigen and lymphocytes in delayed hypersensitivity. III. Analysis of mechanism, *J. Exp. Med.*, 128, 1267, 1968.
40. **Devlin, J. J., Klostergaard, J., Orr, S. L., Yamamoto, R. S., Masunaka, I. K., Plunkett, J. M., and Granger, G. A.**, Lymphotoxins: after fifteen years of research, *Lymphokines*, 9, 313, 1984.
41. **Wright, S. C. and Bonavida, B.**, Release of cytotoxic factors specific for NK-sensitive target cells (NKCF) during co-culture of NK effector cells with NK target cells, *J. Immunol.*, 129, 433, 1982.
42. **Uchida, A.**, Anti-tumor monocyte cytotoxic factors (MCF) produced by human blood monocytes: production, characterization, and biological significance, in *Leukolysins and Cancer*, Ransom, J. and Ortaldo, J. R., Eds., Humana Press, Clifton, N. J., in press.
43. **Ransom, J. H., Evans, C. H., McCabe, R. P., Pomato, N., Heinbaugh, J. A., Chin, M., and Hanna, M. G., Jr.**, Leukoregulin, a direct-acting anticancer immunological hormone that is distinct from lymphotoxin and intereron, *Cancer Res.*, 45, 851, 1985.
44. **Wallach, D.**, Preparations of lymphotoxin induce resistance to their own cytotoxic effect, *J. Immunol.*, 132, 2464, 1984.
45. **Green, L. M., Stern, M. L., Haviland, D. L., Mills, B. J., and Ware, C. F.**, Cytotoxic lymphokines produced by cloned human cytotoxic lymphocytes, I. Cytotoxins produced by antigen-specific and natural killer-like CTL and dissimilar to classical lymphotoxins, *J. Immunol.*, 135, 4034, 1985.
46. **Hahn, T., Toker, L., Budilovsky, S., Aderka, D., Eshhar, Z., and Wallach, D.**, Use of monoclonal antibodies to a human cytotoxin for its isolation and for examining the self-induction of resistance to this protein, *Proc. Natl. Acad. Sci. USA*, 82, 3814, 1985.
47. **Shalaby, M. R., Aggarwal, B. B., Rinderknecht, E., Svedersky, L. P., Finkle, B. S., and Palladino, M. A.**, Letter to Editor, *J. Immunol.*, 136, 2336, 1986.
48. **Aderka, D., Hoffmann, H., Toker, L., Hahn, T., and Wallach, D.**, Tumor necrosis factor induction by Sendai virus, *J. Immunol.*, 136, 2938, 1986.
49. **Beutler, B., Greenwald, D., Hulmes, J. D., Chang, M., Pan, Y. C., Mathison, J., Ulevitch, R., and Cerami, A.**, Identity of tumour necrosis factor and the macrophage-secreted factor cachetin, *Nature*, 316, 552, 1985.
50. **Rubin, B. Y., Anderson, S. L., Sullivan, S. A., Williamson, B. D., Carswell, E. A., and Old, L. J.**, Purification and characterization of a human tumor necrosis factor from LuKII cell line, *Proc. Natl. Acad. Sci. USA*, 82, 6637, 1985.

51. **Hibbs, J. B., Jr.**, Discrimination between neoplastic and non-neoplastic cells *in vitro* by activated macrophages, *J. Natl. Cancer Inst.*, 53, 1487, 1974.
52. **Urban, J. L., Shepard, H. M., Rothstein, J. L., Sugarman, B. J., and Schreiber, H.**, Tumor necrosis factor: A potent effector molecule for tumor cell killing by activated macrophages, *Proc. Natl. Acad. Sci. USA*, 83, 5233, 1986.
53. **Phillip, R. and Epstein, L. B.**, Tumour necrosis factor as immunomodulator and mediator of monocyte cytotoxicity induced by itself, γ-interferon and interleukin-1, *Nature*, 323, 86, 1986.
54. **Hoffmann, M. K., Oettgen, H. F., Old, L. J., Mitler, R. S., and Hammerling, U.**, Induction and immunological properties of tumor necrosis factor, *J. Reticuloendothel. Soc.*, 23, 307, 1978.
55. **Svedersky, L. P., Nedwin, G. E., Goeddel, D. V., and Palladino, M. A.**, Interferon-γ enhances induction of lymphotoxin in recombinant interleukin 2-stimulated peripheral blood mononuclear cells, *J. Immunol.*, 134, 1604, 1985.
56. **Nedwin, G. E., Svedersky, L. P., Bringman, T. S., Palladino, M. A., Jr., and Goeddel, D. V.**, Effect of interleukin-2, interferon-gamma, and mitogens on the production of tumor necrosis factors alpha and beta, *J. Immunol.*, 135, 2492, 1985.
57. **Wong, G. H. W. and Goeddel, D. V.**, Interferon-γ induces the expression of tumor necrosis factor/lymphotoxin and vice versa. Sixth International Congress of Immunology, Abstract No. 3.33.43, p. 365, 1986.
58. **Chroboczek-Kelker, H., Oppenheim, D. J., Stone-Wolff, D. S., Henriksen-De Stefano, D., Aggarwal, B. B., Stevenson, H. C., and Vilcek, J.**, Characterization of human tumor necrosis factor produced by peripheral blood monocytes and its separation from lymphotoxin, *Int. J. Cancer*, 36, 69, 1985.
59. **Peters, P. M., Ortaldo, J. R., Shalaby, M. R., Svedersky, L. P., Nedwin, G. E., Bringman, T. S., Hass, P. E., Aggarwal, B. B., Herberman, R. B., Goeddel, D. V., and Palladino, Jr., M. A.**, Natural killer-sensitive targets stimulate production of TNF-α but not TNF-β (lymphotoxin) by highly purified human peripheral blood large granular lymphocytes, *J. Immunol.*, 137, 2592, 1986.
60. **Sone, S., Lopez-Berestein, G., and Fidler, I. J.**, Potentiation of direct antitumor cytotoxicity and production of tumor cytolytic factors in human blood monocytes by human recombinant interferon-gamma and muramyl dipeptide derivatives, *Cancer Immunol. Immunother.*, 21, 93, 1986.
61. **Satoh, M., Inagawa, H., Minagawa, H., Kajikawa, T., Oshima, H., Abe, S., Yamazaki, M., and Mizuno, D.**, Endogenous production of TNF in mice with immune complex as a primer, *J. Biol. Response Modifiers*, 5, 140, 1986.
62. **Yamamoto, A., Nagamuta, M., Usami, H., Sugawara, Y., Watanabe, N., Niitsu, Y., and Urushizaki, I.**, Production of cytotoxic factor into mouse peritoneal fluid by OK-432, a streptococcal preparation, *Immunol. Lett.*, 11, 83, 1986.
63. **Mannel, D. N., Meltzer, M. S., and Mergenhagan, S. E.**, Generation and characterization of a lipopolysaccharide-induced and serum-derived cytotoxic factor for tumor cells, *Infect. Immun.*, 28, 204, 1980.
64. **Green, S., Dobrjansky, A., Carswell, E. A., Kassel, R. L., Old, L. J., Fiore, N., and Schwartz, M. K.**, Partial purification of a serum factor that causes necrosis of tumors, *Proc. Natl. Acad. Sci. USA*, 73, 381, 1976.
65. **Green, S., Dobrjansky, A., and Chiasson, M. A.**, Murine tumor necrosis-inducing factor: Purification and effects on myelomonocytic leukemia cells, *J. Natl. Cancer Inst.*, 68, 997, 1982.
66. **Ruff, M. R. and Gifford, G. E.**, Purification and physiochemical characterization of rabbit tumor necrosis factor, *J. Immunol.*, 125, 1671, 1980.
67. **Mathews, N., Ryley, H. C., and Neale, M. L.**, Tumour-necrosis factor from the rabbit. IV. Purification and chemical characterization, *Br. J. Cancer*, 42, 416, 1980.
68. **Nissen-Meyer, J. and Hammerstrom, J.**, Physicochemical characterization of cytostatic factors released from human monocytes, *Infect. Immun.*, 38, 67, 1982.
69. **Russell, S. W., Rosenau, W., Goldberg, M. L., and Kunitomi, G.**, Purification of human lymphotoxin, *J. Immunol.*, 109, 784, 1972.
70. **Boulos, G. N., Rosenau, W., and Goldberg, M. L.**, Comparison and yield of antigen- or mitogen-induced human lymphotoxins, *J. Immunol.*, 112, 1347, 1974.
71. **Peters, J. B., Stratton, J. A., Stempel, K. E., Yu, D., and Cardin, C.**, Characteristics of a cytotoxin ("lymphotoxin") produced by stimulation of human lymphoid tissue, *J. Immunol.*, 111, 770, 1973.
72. **Granger, G. A., Laserna, E. C., Kolb, W. P., and Chapman, F.**, Human lymphotoxin: Purification and some properties, *Proc. Natl. Acad. Sci. USA*, 70, 27, 1973.
73. **Klostergaard, J., Yamamoto, R. S., and Granger, G. A.**, Human and murine lymphotoxins as a multicomponent system: Progress in the purification of the human αL component, *Mol. Immunol.*, 17, 613, 1980.
74. **Klostergaard, J. and Granger, G. A.**, Human lymphotoxin: Purification to electrophoretic homogeneity of the αh receptor bearing class, *Mol. Immunol.*, 18, 455, 1982.
75. **Klostergaard, J., Long, S., and Granger, G. A.**, Purification of human alpha light class lymphotoxin to electrophoretic homogeneity, *Mol. Immunol.*, 18, 1049, 1981.

76. **Johnson, D. L., Yamamoto, R. S., Plunkett, J. M., Masunaka, I. K., and Granger, G. A.**, Purification to electrophoretic homogeneity of human alpha lymphotoxin from a cloned continuous lymphoblastoid cell line IR 3.4, *Mol. Immunol.*, 20, 1241, 1983.
77. **Yamamoto, R. S., Johnson, D. L., Masunaka, I. K., and Granger, G. A.**, Phorbol myristate acetate induction of lymphotoxins from continuous human B lymphoid cell lines *in vitro*, *J. Biol. Resp. Modifiers*, 3, 76, 1984.
78. **Haranaka, K., Satomi, N., Sakurai, A., and Nariuchi, H.**, Purification and partial amino acid sequence of rabbit tumor necrosis factor, *J. Int. Cancer*, 36, 395, 1985.
79. **Abe, S., Gatanaga, T., Yamozaki, M., Soma, G. and Mizuno, P.**, Purification of rabbit tumor necrosis factor, *FEBS Lett.*, 180, 203, 1985.
80. **Inagawa, H., Oshima, H., Abe, S., Gatanaga, T., Yamazaki, M., Soma, G., and Mizumo, D.**, Preparation of highly purified rabbit TNF by affinity chromatography with monoclonal antibody, submitted.
81. **Haranaka, K., Carswell, E. A., Williamson, B. D., Prendergast, J. S., Satomi, N., and Old, L. J.**, Purification, characterization, and antitumor activity of nonrecombinant mouse tumor necrosis factor, *Proc. Natl. Acad. Sci. USA*, 83, 3949, 1986.
82. **Aggarwal, B. B.**, Human lymphotoxin, *Meth. Enzymol.*, 16, 441, 1985.
83. **Aggarwal, B. B. and Kohr, W. J.**, Human tumor necrosis factor, *Meth. Enzymol.*, 116, 448, 1985.
84. **Nedwin, G. E., Naylor, S. L., Sakaguchi, A. Y., Smith, D., Jarret-Nedwin, J., Pennica, D., Goeddel, D. V., and Gray, P. W.**, Human lymphotoxin and tumor necrosis factor genes: structure, homology and chromosomal localization, *Nucleic Acids Res.*, 13, 6361, 1985.
85. **Nedwin, G. E., Jarrett-Nedwin, J., Smith, D. H., Naylor, S. L., Sakaguchi, A. Y., Goeddel, D. V., and Gray, P. W.**, Structure and chromosomal localization of the human lymphotoxin gene, *J. Cell. Biochem.*, 29, 171, 1985.
86. **Halpern, B., Fray, A., and Crepin, Y., Platica, O., Lorinet, A. M., Rabourdin, A., Sparrows, L., and Isaac, R.**, *Corynebacterium parvum:* A potent immunostimulant in experimental infections and in malignancies, *Ciba Found. Symp.*, 18(new series), 217, 1973.
87. **Old, L. J., Clark, D. A., Benacerraf, B., and Goldsmith, M.**, The reticuloendothelial system and the neoplastic process, *Ann. N.Y. Acad. Sci.*, 88, 264, 1960.
88. **Ribi, E. E., Granger, D. L., Milner, K. C., and Strain, S. M.**, Tumor regression caused by endotoxins and mycobacterial fractions, *J. Natl. Cancer Inst.*, 55, 1253, 1975.
89. **Balkwill, F. R., Lee, A., Aldam, G., Moodie, E., Thomas, J. A., Tavernier, J., and Fiers, W.**, Human tumor xenografts treated with recombinant human tumor necrosis factor alone or in combination with interferons, *Cancer Res.*, 46, 3990, 1986.
90. **Granger, G. A., Kobayashi, M., Orr, S. L., Masunaka, I., Plunkett, M., and Yamamoto, R. S.**, Human Lymphotoxins: A multicomponent family of proteins with selectivity for transformed cells *in vitro* and *in vivo*. in *Recent Advances in Chemotherapy*, Ishigami, J., Ed., University of Tokyo Press, 1985, 86.
91. **Williams, T. W. and Bellanti, J. A.**, *In vitro* synergism between interferons and human lymphotoxin: enhancement of lymphotoxin-induced target cell killing, *J. Immunol.*, 130, 518, 1983.
92. **Williamson, B. D., Carswell, E. A., Rubin, B. Y., Prendergast, J. S., and Old, L. J.**, Human tumor necrosis factor produced by human B-cell lines: Synergistic cytotoxic interaction with human interferon, *Proc. Natl. Acad. Sci. USA*, 80, 5397, 1983.
93. **Williams, T. W.**, *In vitro* synergistic effects of interferon on human lymphotoxin activity: A new property of interferon in lymphocyte-mediated target cell killing, *Lymphokine Res.*, 3, 113, 1984.
94. **Lee, S. H., Aggarwal, B. B., Rinderknecht, E., Assisi, F., and Chiu, H.**, The synergistic anti-proliferative effect of γ-interferon and human lymphotoxin, *J. Immunol.*, 133, 1083, 1984.
95. **Ruggiero, V., Tavernier, J., Fiers, W., and Baglioni, C.**, Induction of the synthesis of tumor necrosis factor receptors by interferon-γ, *J. Immunol.*, 136, 2445, 1986.
96. **Kohase, M., Henriksen-DeStefano, D., May, L. T., Vilcek, J., and Sehgal, P. B.**, Induction of β_2-interferon by tumor necrosis factor: A homeostatic mechanism in the control of cell proliferation, *Cell*, 45, 1986.
97. **Nawroth, P. P., Bank, I., Handley, D., Cassimeris, J., Chess, L., and Stern, D.**, Tumor necrosis factor/cachetin interacts with endothelial cell receptors to induce release of interleukin-1, *J. Exp. Med.*, 163, 1363, 1986.
98. **Dinarello, C. A., Cannon, J. G., Wolff, S. M., Bernheim, H. A., Beutler, B., Cerami, A., Figari, I. S., Palladino, Jr., M. A., and O'Connor, J. V.**, Tumor necrosis factor (cachetin) is an endogenous pyrogen and induces production of interleukin 1, *J. Exp. Med.*, 163, 1433, 1986.
99. **Bashwich, P. R., Chensue, S. W., Larrick, J. W., and Kunkel, S. W.**, Tumor necrosis factor stimulates interleukin-1 and prostaglandin E_2 production in resting macrophages, *Biochem. Biophys. Res. Commun.*, 136, 94, 1986.
100. **Kirstein, M. and Baglioni, C.**, Tumor necrosis factor induces synthesis of two proteins in human fibroblasts, *J. Biol. Chem.*, 261, 9565, 1986.

101. **Roberts, A. B., Anzano, M. A., Wakefield, L. M., Roche, N. S., Stern, D. F., and Sporn, M. B.**, Type B transforming growth factor: A bifunctional regulator of cellular growth, *Proc. Natl. Acad. Sci. USA*, 82, 119, 1985.
102. **Torti, F. M., Dieckmann, B., Beutler, B., Cerami, A., and Ringold, G. M.**, A macrophage factor inhibits adipocyte gene expression: An *in vitro* model of cachexia, *Science*, 229, 867, 1985.
103. **Beutler, B., Milsark, I. W., and Cerami, A. C.**, Passive immunization against cachetin/tumor necrosis factor protects mice from lethal effect of endotoxin, *Science*, 229, 869, 1985.
104. **Beutler, B. A. and Cerami, A.**, Recombinant interleukin 1 suppresses lipoprotein lipase activity in 3T3 L1 cells, *J. Immunol.*, 135, 3969, 1985.
105. **Keay, S. and Grossberg, S. E.**, Interferon inhibits the conversion of 3T3 L1 fibroblasts into adipocytes, *Proc. Natl. Acad. Sci. USA*, 77, 4099, 1980.
106. **Patton, J. S., Shepard, H. M., Wilking, H., Lewis, G., Aggarwal, B. B., Eessalu, T. E., Gavin, L. A., and Grunfeld, C.**, Interferons and tumor necrosis factors have similar catabolic effects on 3T3 L1 cells, *Proc. Natl. Acad. Sci., U.S.A.*, 83, 8313, 1986.
107. **Parant, M.**, Antimicrobial resistance enhancing activity of tumor necrosis serum factor induced by endotoxin in BCG-treated mice, *Recent Results Cancer Res.*, 75, 213, 1980.
108. **Hardaris, C. G., Haynes, J. D., Meltzer, M. S., and Allison, A. C.**, Serum containing tumor necrosis factor is cytotoxic for the human malaria parasite *Plasmodium falciparum*, *Infect. Immunity*, 42, 385, 1983.
109. **Taverne, J., Matthews, N., Depledge, P., and Playfair, J. H. L.**, Malarial parasites and tumor cells are killed by the same component of tumor necrosis serum, *Clin. Exp. Immunol.*, 57, 293, 1984.
110. **Silberstein, D. and David, J. R.**, Tumor necrosis factor enhances eosinophil toxicity to *Schistosoma mansoni* larvae, *Proc. Natl. Acad. Sci. USA*, 83, 1055, 1986.
111. **Mestan, J., Digel, W., Jacobsen, H., Hillen, H., Blohm, D., Moller, A., and Kirchner, H.**, In vitro antiviral effects of recombinant tumor necrosis factor, *Nature*, 323, 816, 1986.
112. **Wong, G. C. and Goeddel, D. V.**, Tumour necrosis factors-α and -β inhibit DNA and RNA virus replication and synergize with interferons, *Nature*, 323, 819, 1986.
113. **Shalaby, M. R., Aggarwal, B. B., Rinderknecht, E., Svedersky, L. P., Finkle, B. S., and Palladino, M. A., Jr.**, Activation of human polymorphonuclear neutrophil functions by interferon-gamma and tumor necrosis factor, *J. Immunol.*, 135, 2069, 1985.
114. **Klebanoff, S. J., Vadas, M. A., Harlan, J. M., Sparks, L. H., Gamble, J. R., Agosti, J. M., and Waltersdorph, A. M.**, Stimulation of neutrophils by tumor necrosis factor, *J. Immunol.*, 136, 4220, 1986.
115. **Harlan, J. M., Killen, P. D., Senecal, F. M., Schwartz, B. R., Yee, E. K., Taylor, R. F., Beatty, P. G., Price, T. H., and Ochs, H. D.**, The role of neutrophil membrane glycoprotein GP 150 in neutrophil adherence to endothelium *in vitro*, *Blood*, 66, 167, 1985.
116. **Gamble, J. R., Harlan, J. M., Klebanoff, S. J., and Vadas, M. A.**, Stimulation of the adherence of neutrophils to umbilical vein endothelium by human recombinant tumor necrosis factor, *Proc. Natl. Acad. Sci. USA*, 82, 8667, 1985.
117. **Pohlman, T. H., Stanness, K. A., Beatty, P. G., Ochs, H. D., and Harlan, J. M.**, An endothelial cell surface factor(s) induced *in vitro* by lipopolysaccharide, interleukin 1, and tumor necrosis factor-α increases neutrophil adherence by a CDW18-dependent mechanism, *J. Immunol.*, 136, 4548, 1986.
118. **Collins, T., Lapierre, L. A., Fiers, W., Strominger, J. L., and Pober, J. S.**, Recombinant human tumor necrosis factor increases mRNA levels and surface expression of HLA-A,B antigens in vascular endothelial cells and dermal fibroblasts *in vitro*, *Proc. Natl. Acad. Sci. USA*, 83, 446, 1985.
119. **Nawroth, P. P. and Stern, D. M.**, Modulation of endothelial cell hemostatic properties by tumor necrosis factor, *J. Exp. Med.*, 164, 740, 1986.
120. **Bach, R., Nemerson, Y., and Konigsberg, W.**, Purification and characterization of bovine tissue factor, *J. Biol. Chem.*, 256, 8324, 1981.
121. **Stern, D. M., Nawroth, P., Handley, D., and Kisiel, W.**, An endothelial cell dependent pathway of coagulation, *Proc. Natl. Acad. Sci. USA*, 82, 2523, 1985.
122. **Esmon, N., Owen, W., and Esmon, C.**, Isolation of a membrane-bound cofactor for thrombin-catalyzed activation of protein C, *J. Biol. Chem.*, 257, 859, 1982.
123. **Stolpen, A. H., Guinan, E. C., Fiers, W., and Pober, J. S.**, Recombinant tumor necrosis factor and immune interferon act singly and in combination to reorganize human vascular endothelial cell monolayers, *Am. J. Pathol.*, 123, 16, 1986.
124. **Stern, D. M., Bank, I., Nawroth, P. P., Cassimeris, J., Kisiel, W., Fenton, J. W., Dinarello, C., Chess, L., and Jaffe, E. A.**, Self-regulation of procoagulant events on the endothelial cell surface, *J. Exp. Med.*, 162, 1223, 1985.
125. **Degliatoni, G., Murphy, M., Kobayashi, M., Francis, M. K., Perussia, B., and Trinchieri, G.**, Natural killer (NK) cell-derived hematopoietic colony-inhibiting activity and NK cytotoxic factor. Relationship with tumor necrosis factor and synergism with immune interferon, *J. Exp. Med.*, 162, 1512, 1985.

126. **Broxmeyer, H. E., Williams, D. E., Lu, L., Cooper, S., Anderson, S. L., Beyer, G. S., Hoffman, R., and Rubin, B. Y.**, The suppressive influence of human tumor necrosis factors on bone marrow hematopoietic progenitor cells from normal donors and patients with leukemia: synergism of tumor necrosis factor and interferon-gamma, *J. Immunol.*, 136, 448, 1986.
127. **Murphy, M., Loudon, R., Kobayashi, M., and Trinchieri, G.**, γ-Interferon and lymphotoxin, released by activated T cells, synergize to inhibit granulocyte/monocyte colony formation, *J. Exp. Med.*, 164, 263, 1986.
128. **Bertolini, D. R., Nedwin, G. E., Bringman, T. S., Smith, D. D., and Mundy, G. R.**, Stimulation of bone resorption and inhibition of bone formation *in vitro* by human tumour necrosis factors, *Nature*, 319, 516, 1986.
129. **Chambers, T. J. and Magnus, C. T.**, Calcitonin alters behaviour of isolated osteoclasts, *J. Pathol.*, 136, 27, 1982.
130. **Majeska, R. J., Rodan, S. B., and Rodan, G. A.**, Parathyroid hormone-responsive clonal cell lines from rat osteosarcoma, *Endocrinology*, 107, 1494, 1980.
131. **Dominquez, J. H. and Mundy, G. R.**, Monocytes mediate osteoclastic bone resorption by prostaglandin production, *Calcif. Tissue Int.*, 31, 29, 1980.
132. **Gowen, M., Wood, D. D., Ihrie, E. J., McGuire, M. K. B., and Russell, R. G. G.**, An interleukin 1 like factor stimulates bone resorption *in vitro*, *Nature*, 306, 378, 1983.
133. **Pujol, J. P., Penfornis, H., Arenzana-Seisdedos, F., Bocquet, J., Farjanel, J., Rattner, A., Brisset, M., Virelizier, J. L., Beliard, R., and Loyau, G.**, Mononuclear cell-mediated modulation of synovial cell metabolism. I. Collagen Synthesis, *Exp. Cell Res.*, 158, 63, 1985.
134. **Dayer, J.-M., Beutler, B., and Cerami, A.**, Cachetin/tumor necrosis factor stimulates synovial cells and fibroblasts to produce collagenase and prostaglandin E_2, *J. Exp. Med.*, 162, 2163, 1985.
135. **Gowen, M., Nedwin, G. E., and Mundy, G. R.**, Preferential inhibition of cytokine-stimulated bond resorption by recombinant interferon gamma, *J. Immunol.*, 136, 1986.
136. **Saklatvala, J.**, Tumour necrosis factor-α stimulates resorption and inhibits synthesis of proteoglycan in cartilage, *Nature*, 322, 547, 1986.
137. **Schmid, D. S., Tite, J. P., and Ruddle, N. H.**, DNA fragmentation: Manifestation of target cell destruction mediated by cytotoxic T-cell lines, lymphotoxin-secreting helper T-cell clones, and cell-free lymphotoxin-containing supernatant, *Proc. Natl. Acad. Sci. USA*, 83, 1881, 1986.
138. **Schmid, D. S., Hornung, R., McGrath, K. M., Paul, N., and Ruddle, N. H.**, Target cell DNA fragmentation is mediated by the soluble cytotoxic mediators lymphotoxin and tumor necrosis factor, *Lymphokine Res.*, 6, 195, 1987.
139. **Friedman, R. M. and Vogel, S. N.**, Interferons with special emphasis on the immune system, *Adv. Immunol.*, 34, 97, 1983.
140. **Matsushima, K., Durum, S. K., Kimball, E. S., and Oppenheim, J. J.**, Purification of human interleukin-1 and identity of thymocyte co-mitogenic factor, fibroblast proliferation, acute phase inducing factor and endogenous pyrogen, *Cell. Immunol.*, 29, 290, 1985.
141. **Onozaki, K., Matsushima, K., Aggarwal, B. B., and Oppenheim, J. J.**, Human interleukin-1 is a cytocidal factor for several tumor cell lines, *J. Immunol.*, 135, 3962, 1985.
142. **Lovett, D., Kazan, B., Hadam, M., Resch, K., and Gemsa, D.**, Macrophage cytotoxicity: Interleukin 1 as a mediator of tumor cytostasis, *J. Immunol.*, 136, 340, 1986.
143. **Hass, P. E., Hotchkiss, A., Mohler, M., and Aggarwal, B. B.**, Characterization of specific high affinity receptors for human tumor necrosis factor on mouse fibroblasts, *J. Biol. Chem.*, 260, 12214, 1985.
144. **Aggarwal, B. B., Eessalu, T. E., and Hass, P. E.**, Characterization of receptors for human tumour necrosis factor and their regulation by gamma-interferon, *Nature*, 318, 665, 1985.
145. **Aggarwal, B. B., Traquina, P. R., and Eessalu, T. E.**, Modulation of receptors and cytotoxic response of tumor necrosis factor-α by various lectins, *J. Biol. Chem.*, 261, 3652, 1986.
146. **Tsujimoto, M., Yip, Y. K., and Vilcek, J.**, Tumor necrosis factor: specific binding and internalization in sensitive and resistant cells, *Proc. Natl. Acad. Sci. USA*, 82, 7626, 1985.
147. **Tsujimoto, M., Yip, Y. K., and Vilcek, J.**, IFN-gamma enhances expression of cellular receptors for tumor necrosis factor, *J. Immunol.*, 136, 2441, 1986.
148. **Tsujimoto, M. and Vilcek, J.**, Tumor necrosis factor receptors in HeLa cells and their regulation by interferon-γ. *J. Biol. Chem.*, 261, 5384, 1986.
149. **Baglioni, C., McCandless, S., Tavernier, J., and Fiers, W.**, Binding of human tumor necrosis factor to high affinity receptors on HeLa and lymphoblastoid cells sensitive to growth inhibition, *J. Biol. Chem.*, 260, 13395, 1985.
150. **Kull, F. C., Jr., Jacobs, S., and Cuatrecasas, P.**, Cellular receptor for ^{125}I-labeled tumor necrosis factor: specific binding, affinity labeling, and relationship to sensitivity, *Proc. Natl. Acad. Sci. USA*, 82, 5756, 1985.

151. **Beutler, B., Mahoney, J., Trang, N. L., Pekala, P., and Cerami, A.,** Purification of cachectin, a lipoprotein lipase-suppressing hormone secreted by endotoxin-induced RAW 264.7 cells, *J. Exp. Med.,* 161, 984, 1985.
152. **Rubin, B. Y., Anderson, S. L., Sullivan, S. A., Williamson, B. D., Carswell, E. A., and Old, L. J.,** High affinity binding of ^{125}I-labeled human tumor necrosis factor (LuKII) to specific cell surface receptors, *J. Exp. Med.,* 162, 1099, 1985.
153. **Scheurich, P., Ucer, U., Kronke, M., and Pfizenmaier, K.,** Quantification and characterization of high-affinity membrane receptors for tumor necrosis factor on human leukemic cell lines, *Int. J. Cancer,* 38, 122, 1986.
154. **Tsujimoto, M., Feinman, R., Kohase, M., and Vilcek, J.,** Characterization and affinity crosslinking of receptors for tumor necrosis factor on human cells, *Arch. Biochem. Biophys.,* 249, 563, 1986.
155. **Munker, R., Gasson, J., Ogawa, M., and Koeffler, H. P.,** Recombinant human TNF induces production of granulocyte-monocyte colony-stimulating factor, *Nature,* 323, 79, 1986.
156. **Darlington, G. J., Wilson, D. R., Lachman, L. B.,** Monocyte-conditioned medium, interleukin-1, and tumor necrosis factor stimulate the acute phase response in human hepatoma cells *in vitro, J. Cell Biol.,* 103, 787, 1986.
157. **Ghezzi, P., Saccardo, B., and Bianchi, M.,** Recombinant tumor necrosis factor depresses cytochrome P450-dependent microsomal drug metabolism in mice, *Biochem. Biophys. Res. Commun.,* 136, 316, 1986.
158. **Ruff, M. R. and Gifford, G. E.,** Rabbit tumor necrosis factor: Mechanism of action, *Infect. Immun.,* 31, 380, 1981.
159. **Ruff, M. R. and Gifford, G. E.,** Tumor Necrosis Factor, in *Lymphokines,* Vol. 2, Academic Press, 1981, 235.
160. **Kull, Jr., F. C. and Cuatrecasas, P.,** Possible requirement of internalization in the mechanism of *in vitro* cytotoxicity in tumor necrosis serum, *Cancer Res.,* 41, 4885, 1981.
161. **Niitsu, Y., Watanabe, N., Sone, H., Neda, H., Yamauchi, N., and Urushizaki, I.,** Mechanism of the cytotoxic effect of tumor necrosis factor, *Jpn. J. Cancer Res. (Gann),* 76, 1193, 1985.
162. **Podack, E. R.,** The molecular mechanism of lymphocyte-mediated tumor cell lysis, *Immunol. Today,* 6, 21, 1985.
163. **Young, J. D.-E., Hengartner, H., Podack, E. R., and Cohn, Z. A.,** Purification and characterization of a cytolytic pore-forming protein from granules of cloned lymphocytes with natural killer activity, *Cell,* 44, 849, 1986.
164. **Yamada, M., Yamayoshi, M., Furuta, R., Kotani, H., Asaka, Y., Nakata, K., Yoshida, H., Kashimoto, S., and Nakamura, S.,** Biochemical and biological properties of recombinant human interleukin-1 alpha, *Sixth International Congress of Immunology,* Abstract No. 3.31.7, p. 344, 1986.
165. **Hirai, Y., Nakai, S., Nishino, N., Nishida, T., Yanagihara, Y., and Kikumoto, Y.,** Anti-tumor effect of recombinant human GIF-α/IL-1β, *Sixth International Congress of Immunology,* Abstract No. 3.31.40, p. 349, 1986.
166. **Nakai, S., Kikumoto, Y., Kaneta, M., Hong, Y., Takegata, S., Kawai, K., and Hirai, Y.,** IL-1 as a potential anti-tumor factor, *Sixth International Congress of Immunology,* Abstract No. 3.31.39, p. 349, 1986.
167. **Palladino, M. A., Shalaby, M. R., Kramer, S. M., Ferraiolo, B. L., Baughman, R. A., DeLeo, A. B., Crase, D., Marafino, B., Aggarwal, B. B., Figari, I. S., Liggit, D., and Patton, J. S.,** Characterization of the antitumor activities of human tumor necrosis factor-alpha and the comparison with other cytokines: induction of tumor specific immunity, *J. Immunol.,* 138, 4023, 1987.
168. **Deleo, A. B., Shiku, H., Takahashi, T., John, M., and Old, L. J.,** Cell surface antigens of chemically induced sarcomas of the mouse. I. Murine leukemia virus related antigens and alloantigens on cultured fibroblasts and sarcoma cells: description of a unique antigen on BALB/c Meth A sarcoma, *J. Exp. Med.,* 146, 720, 1977.
169. **Kramer, S. M. and Carver, M. E.,** Serum-free *in vitro* bioassay for the detection of tumor necrosis factor, *J. Immunol. Methods,* in press.
170. **Matsunaga, K. and Mashiba, H.,** Augmentation of *in vitro* cytotoxicity and *in vivo* tumor-inhibition by combined use of lymphotoxin-containing supernatants and antitumor drugs, *Cancer Lett.,* 20, 21, 1983.
171. **Yamamoto, R. S., Plunkett, J. M., Masunaka, I. K., Yamamoto, R. S., and Granger, G. A.,** Purification and functional studies of LT and "TNF-like" Lt forms from a continuous human T Cell line, *J. Immunol.,* 137, 1885, 1986.
172. **Yamamoto, R. S., Ware, C. F., and Granger, G. A.,** Identification of LT and TNF-like forms from stimulated natural killers, specific and nonspecific cytotoxic human T Cells *in vitro, J. Immunol.,* 137, 1878, 1986.

Section III: Therapeutic Applications

Chapter 22

ANTIBODY CONJUGATES WITH COBRA VENOM FACTOR AS SELECTIVE AGENTS FOR TUMOR CELL KILLING

Carl-Wilhelm Vogel

TABLE OF CONTENTS

I.	Introduction	136
II.	Synthesis and Biochemical Characterization	136
III.	In Vitro Cytotoxic Activity	141
IV.	In Vivo Studies	146
V.	Conclusion	146
	Note Added In Proof	148
	Acknowledgments	148
	References	149

I. INTRODUCTION

Cobra venom factor (CVF) is the complement-activating protein in cobra venom. It is a glycoprotein of $M_r = 136,000$[1,2] that structurally resembles C3 and its physiological activation products C3b and C3c.[3,45] In mammalian serum, CVF functions like C3b, which is physiologically formed during the activation of the alternative complement pathway (for review see Reid and Porter[4] and Pangburn and Müller-Eberhard[5]). Like C3b, CVF binds in serum to Factor B.[46] When in complex with CVF, Factor B is cleaved by Factor D (EC 3.4.21.46) into Bb which remains bound to CVF, and Ba which is released.[6,7] The bimolecular complex CVF,Bb is a C3/C5 convertase (EC 3.4.21.47). The catalytic site resides in the Bb subunit of the enzyme which cleaves the alpha chains of C3 and C5 at positions 77 (Arg-Ser) and 74 (Arg-Leu), respectively.

The molecular architecture of the enzyme CVF,Bb was elucidated by high resolution transmission electronmicroscopy.[8] It was shown that the Bb fragment consists of two globular domains connected by a short linker piece, and that one of the two domains of Bb binds to one end of the ellipsoidal CVF molecule. The analogous complex formed with C3b during activation of the alternative pathway (C3b,Bb) shares with CVF,Bb the catalytic specificity and the molecular architecture.[9] However, the two enzymes differ in several important properties. While both enzymes exhibit spontaneous decay-dissociation into the two respective subunits, the half-life of this decay-dissociation at 37°C is 1.5 min for C3b,Bb[10] and is 7 hr for CVF,Bb.[11] C3b,Bb is disassembled by Factor H,[12] and C3b is inactivated by the combined action of Factor H and Factor I (EC 3.4.21.45).[13] In contrast, CVF,Bb is resistant to these regulatory complement proteins.[14,15] C3b,Bb requires additional C3b to act on C5[16,17] while CVF,Bb can cleave C5 directly.[18,19] Due to these properties, the CVF,Bb enzyme continuously activates C3 and C5. For this reason, CVF is commonly used in immunological research to decomplement laboratory animals.[20-22]

The physicochemical stability of the CVF,Bb enzyme and its resistance to the regulatory complement proteins Factor H and Factor I were the rationale for conjugating CVF to monoclonal antibodies with specificity for cellular surface antigens. The antibody should target the CVF to the cell surface. In the presence of complement, the CVF-dependent C3/C5 convertase should form which, through exhaustive and uncontrollable activation of C3 and C5, should induce complement-mediated killing of the target cell. In the absence of complement, conjugates of CVF and monoclonal antibodies should be devoid of cytotoxic effects since CVF, despite it occurrence in cobra venom, is a nontoxic protein. The biological function of CVF in the cobra venom is believed to facilitate the entry of the toxic venom components into the blood stream. This is achieved by complement activation causing release of the anaphylatoxins C3a and C5a which increase the vascular permeability.

II. SYNTHESIS AND BIOCHEMICAL CHARACTERIZATION

Heterobifunctional cross-linking reagents are commonly used for the synthesis of antibody-CVF conjugates as well as other immunoconjugates (for review see Vogel[23]). These cross-linking agents introduce sulfhydryl-reactive groups into proteins which subsequently react with free sulfhydryl groups in the other protein. If both proteins have no free sulfhydryl groups — as in the case of IgG antibodies and CVF — heterobifunctional cross-linking reagents can also be used to introduce free sulfhydryl groups into one of the two proteins to be coupled. Since the derivatization of the proteins with heterobifunctional cross-linking reagents is random and usually results in an average substitution of several groups per protein molecule, a mixture of conjugates of different compositions is obtained. Figure 1 shows that a typical reaction mixture of antibody and CVF contains dimers (Ab-CVF), trimers (Ab-CVF$_2$, Ab$_2$-CVF), tetramers (Ab-CVF$_3$, Ab$_2$-CVF$_2$, Ab$_3$-CVF), and higher oligomers in addition to nonreacted free antibody and CVF.[47] With increasing degrees of substitution

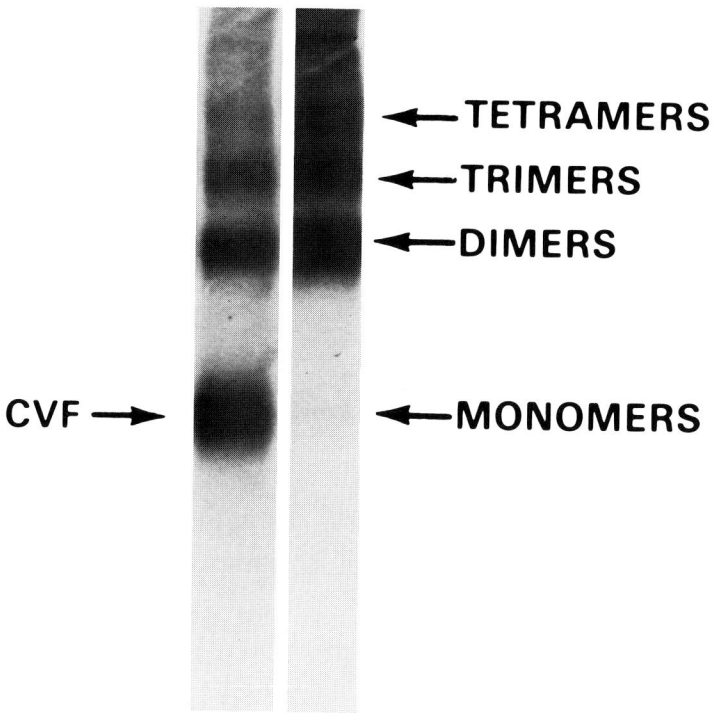

FIGURE 1. Occurrence of antibody-CVF conjugates of different antibody-CVF ratio. Shown is an autoradiograph after SDS gradient polyacrylamide gel electrophoresis under nonreducing conditions of a typical reaction mixture before (left) and after (right) gel permeation chromatography. The reaction mixture contains dimers (Ab-CVF), trimers (Ab-CVF$_2$, Ab$_2$-CVF), tetramers (Ab-CVF$_3$, Ab$_2$-CVF$_2$, Ab$_3$-CVF), and some higher oligomeric conjugates. In addition, the reaction mixture contains free monomeric CVF and antibody which are successfully removed by the gel permeation chromatography.[47] (Free antibody is not visible since the ^{125}I radiolabel was only in the CVF.)

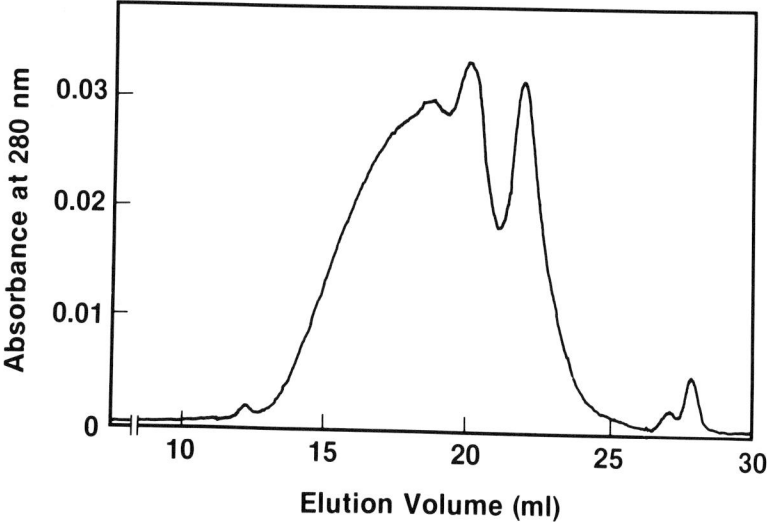

FIGURE 2. Removal of free IgG antibody and CVF and partial separation of antibody-CVF conjugates of different composition by gel permeation chromatography. Shown is an elution profile of a typical reaction mixture using a TSK-4000 HPLC column. The peak at 22 mℓ elution volume contains free antibody and CVF, at 20 mℓ elution volume contains dimeric conjugates, and at 18 mℓ elution volume contains trimeric conjugates virtually unresolved from higher oligomeric conjugates.[47]

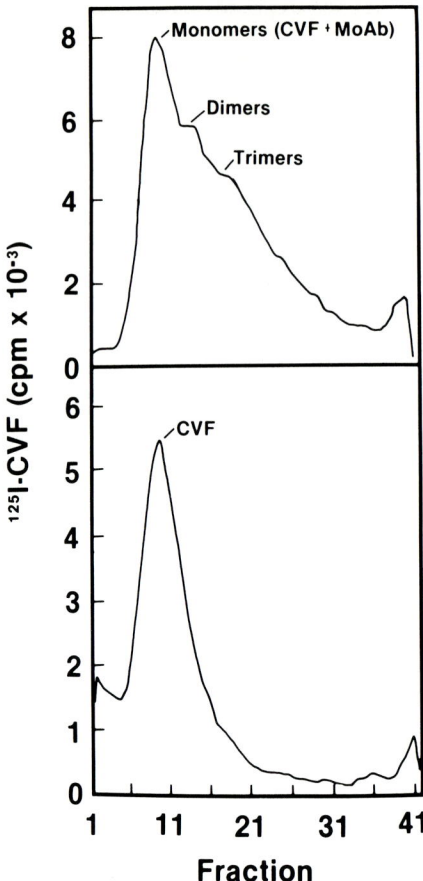

FIGURE 3. Sucrose gradient ultracentrifugation of a reaction mixture of antibody-CVF conjugates. Shown are the radioactive profiles after centrifugation for 16 hr through a 10 to 30% sucrose gradient of a reaction mixture (upper panel) and of a purified CVF (lower panel). The bottom of the centrifugation tubes is to the right. The positions of free monoclonal antibody and CVF and of dimeric and trimeric conjugates are indicated. (From Petrella, E. C. et al., *J. Immunol. Meth.*, 1987, in press. With permission.)

of the two proteins and with increasing protein concentration in the reaction mixture a shift to higher oligomeric conjugates with a concomitant decrease of non-reacted monomeric antibody and CVF occurs. We usually aim to adjust our reaction conditions such as to obtain predominantly dimeric conjugates. As shown in Figure 2, free antibody and CVF can be removed by gel permeation chromatography. Due to the molecular weight differences, the separation of different oligomeric antibody-CVF conjugates is not or only partially possible.

Since the concept of targeting proteins by covalent coupling to antibodies is an immunological one, most laboratories have predominantly characterized their immunoconjugates with regard to cytotoxicity and selectivity for antigen-positive target cells. Very little work has been reported on the biochemical characterization of immunoconjugates. However, from a biochemical point of view, immunoconjugates represent an interesting new class of semi-synthetic bio-organic macromolecules. We therefore have started to biochemically characterize antibody-CVF conjugates in order to reveal structure-function relationships that may be helpful in the future design of effective immunoconjugates.

Our initial biochemical characterization included the determination of sedimentation coefficients.[47] As shown in Figure 3 and 4, dimeric ($s_{20,w} = 10.0$ S) and trimeric ($s_{20,w} = 12.5$ S) antibody-CVF conjugates have sedimentation coefficients similar to those reported for IgG dimers ($s_{20,w} = 9.7$ S) and IgG trimers ($s_{20,w} = 11.4$ S).[24] The antibody-CVF conjugates

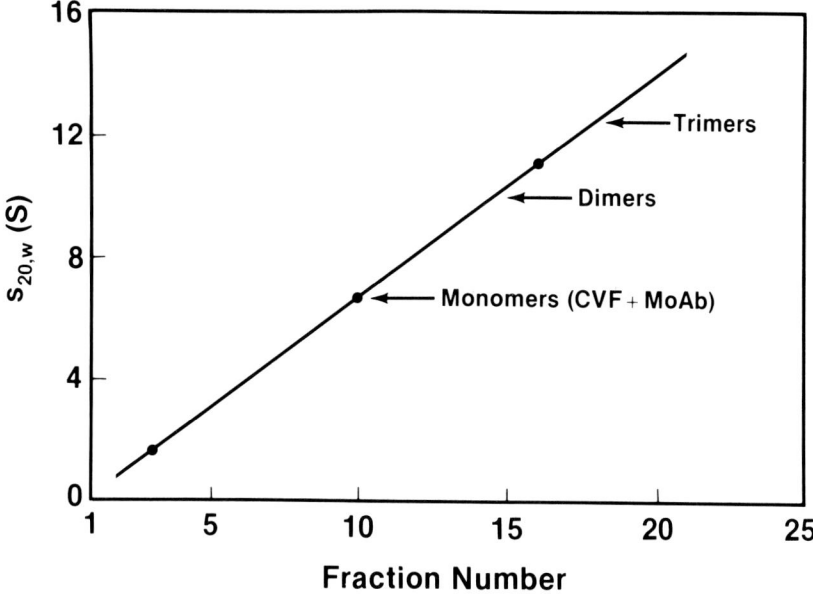

FIGURE 4. Determination of the sedimentation coefficients for dimeric and trimeric antibody-CVF conjugates. Shown is a calibration curve derived from sucrose gradient ultracentrifugation of internal and external standards (●) (cytochrome c, 1.7 S; purified CVF, 6.7 S; complement component C1q, 11.1 S). The sedimentation positions for free monoclonal antibody and CVF and for dimeric and trimeric antibody-CVF conjugates are indicated. (From Petrella, E. C. et al., *J. Immunol. Meth.*, 1987, in press. With permission.)

were also subjected to high resolution transmission electron microscopy (Figure 5).[47] The typical IgG structure and the ellipsoidal CVF molecule can be identified in images of the hybrids. Screening of many images revealed that no preferential orientation of the two molecules to each other occurred, indicating that the derivatization with the cross-linking reagent and the subsequent coupling were random. Figure 6 shows the far UV circular dichroism spectra of CVF, of the IgG antibody, and of antibody-CVF conjugates. The secondary structures as determined from the circular dichroism spectra by the method of Provencher and Glöckner[26] are shown in Table 1. Assuming an average composition of the conjugates of CVF and antibody of 1:1, the predicted secondary structure of the conjugates was within experimental error of the secondary structure determined from the circular dichroism spectrum, indicating that the conjugation of the proteins did not lead to major structural changes.[47]

The effect of derivatization and coupling on the activity of CVF and the antibody is shown in Figures 7 and 8. The derivatization of CVF with the heterobifunctional cross-linking reagent N-succinimidyl-3-(2-pyridyldithio)-propionate (SPDP) results in a concentration-dependent inhibition of its hemolytic activity. An average substitution of seven SPDP residues per CVF molecule caused approximately a $1/3$ reduction of the hemolytic activity (Figure 7). The subsequent coupling of CVF to an IgG antibody further reduces the activity of CVF to approximately $1/4$ of the initial hemolytic activity remaining (Figure 7).[47]

The effect of derivatization and conjugation is less pronounced on the binding activity of an IgG antibody. Figure 8 demonstrates that the binding of an antibody-CVF conjugate to its target cells is only minimally reduced compared to the native antibody.[47] The lesser effect of derivatization and conjugation on the binding activity of the antibody is most likely due to the fact that each antibody molecule has two antigen binding sides, thereby reducing the chance of interfering with the binding by chemical modification of the binding side with the cross-linker or by steric hindrance due to an attached CVF molecule.

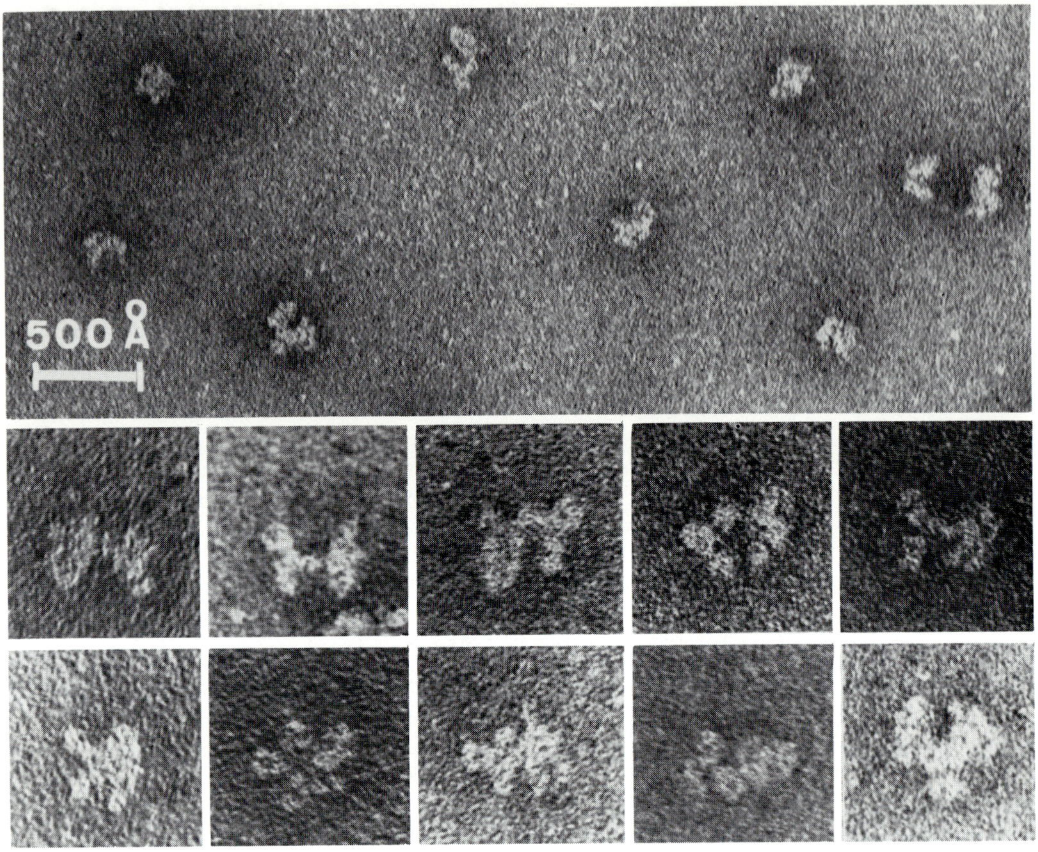

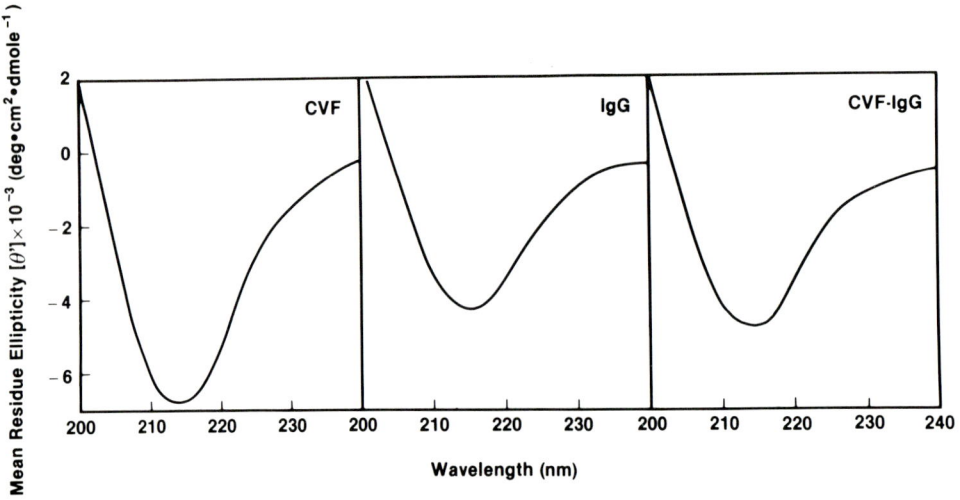

FIGURE 5. High resolution transmission electron microscopy of antibody-CVF conjugates. Shown are a field view (upper panel, magnification approximately 300,000 ×) and selected images (magnification approximately 600,000 ×) of dimeric conjugates. The center image shows particularly clearly the ellipsoidal CVF molecule bound to an Fab portion of the IgG antibody. The lower right panel shows a trimeric conjugate consisting of two CVF molecules bound to one IgG molecule. The micrographs were taken after negative staining with the pleated sheet method of Smith and Seegan.[25] (From Petrella, E. C. et al., *J. Immunol. Meth.*, 1987, in press. With permission.)

FIGURE 6. Far UV circular dichroism spectra of CVF, IgG monoclonal antibody, and antibody-CVF conjugates. (From Petrella, E. C. et al., *J. Immunol. Meth.*, 1987, in press. With permission.)

Table 1
SECONDARY STRUCTURES OF CVF, IgG, AND CVF-IgG FROM FAR UV CIRCULAR DICHROISM SPECTRA

Protein	α-Helix (%)	β-Sheet (%)	β-Turn (%)	Remainder (%)
CVF	11	47	18	24
IgG	5	51	18	26
CVF-IgG (expected)	8	49	18	25
CVF-IgG (found)	8	51	16	25

From Petrella, E. C. et al., *J. Immunol. Meth.*, 1987, in press. With permission.

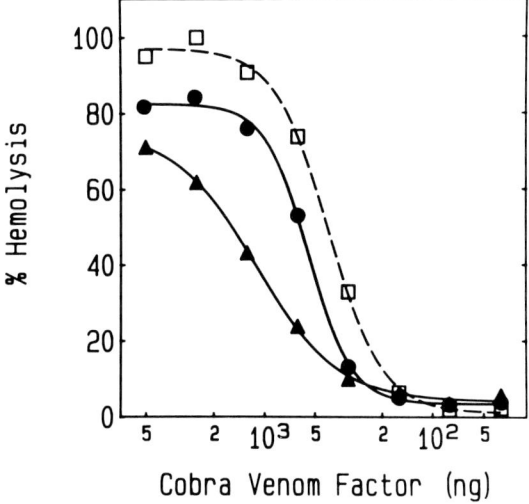

FIGURE 7. Effect of derivatization and conjugation of CVF on hemolytic activity. Shown are the hemolytic activities of native CVF (□), of CVF derivatized with SPDP (●) and of the SPDP-derivatized CVF after conjugation to a monoclonal antibody (▲). The hemolytic test is according to Vogel and Müller-Eberhard.[1] (From Petrella, E. C. et al., *J. Immunol. Meth.*, 1987, in press. With permission.)

III. IN VITRO CYTOTOXIC ACTIVITY

In a first model system, CVF was linked to the 9.2.27 monoclonal antibody to human melanoma[27] using the heterobifunctional cross-linking reagent N-succinimidyl-3-(2-pyridyldithio)-propionate (SPDP).[28] While the unconjugated 9.2.27 antibody was devoid of complement cytotoxic activity, its conjugates with CVF caused complement-dependent killing of human melanoma cells. Antibody-CVF conjugates were also cytotoxic in the presence of C4-deficient serum (Figure 9). This result demonstrates that the killing does not depend on the antibody portion of the conjugates and the classical pathway but that it proceeds through activation of the alternative pathway by the CVF. The cytotoxic effect of antibody-CVF conjugates was also selective. The killing of antigen-positive melanoma cells proceeded in the presence of antigen-negative bystander cells that remained unharmed.[28] Antigen-positive melanoma cells were unaffected by the antibody-CVF conjugates in the absence of serum indicating that the conjugates do not exert direct, complement-independent cytotoxic effects. Figure 10 demonstrates the morphological changes of human melanoma cells during killing by antibody-CVF conjugates and complement as seen by scanning electron microscopy.

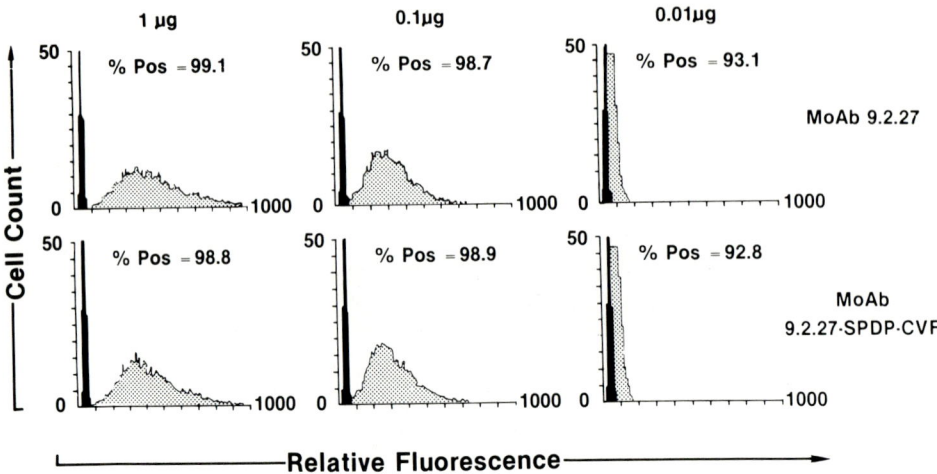

FIGURE 8. Flow cytofluorometric analysis of binding to human FMX-MET II melanoma cells of the 9.2.27 monoclonal antibody and its SPDP-linked conjugate with CVF. Shown are the flow cytofluorometric profiles of a constant number of cells incubated with either 1.0 μg, 0.1 μg, or 0.01 μg of native antibody or antibody-CVF conjugate after staining with FITC-conjugated goat anti-mouse IgG. The profiles obtained with a negative control antibody of the same subclass are also indicated. (From Petrella, E. C. et al., *J. Immunol. Meth.*, 1987, in press. With permission.)

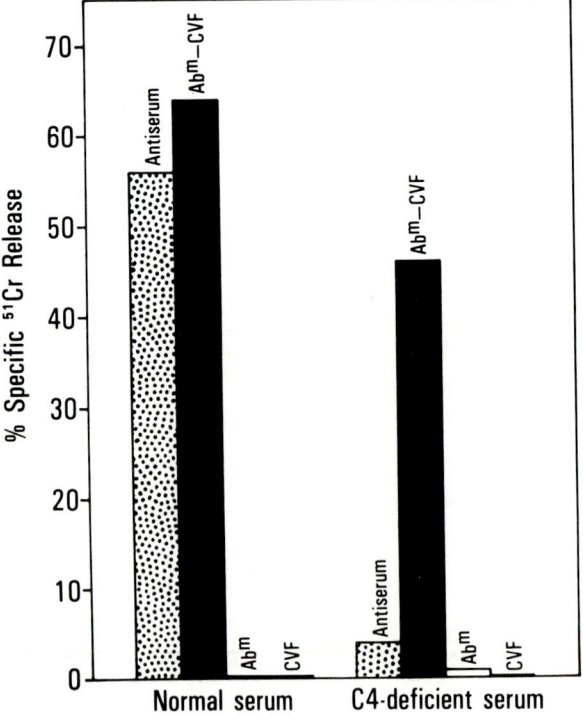

FIGURE 9. Killing of human M21 melanoma cells by conjugates of CVF with the 9.2.27 monoclonal antibody. Shown are the results of a ^{51}Cr-release test performed with the conjugates, a polyclonal rabbit anti-melanoma antiserum, the unconjugated monoclonal antibody (Ab^m), and purified CVF in the presence of normal (left) and C4-deficient (right) guinea pig serum. (From Vogel, C.-W. and Müller-Eberhard, H. J., *Proc. Natl. Acad. Sci. USA*, 78, 7707, 1981. With permission.)

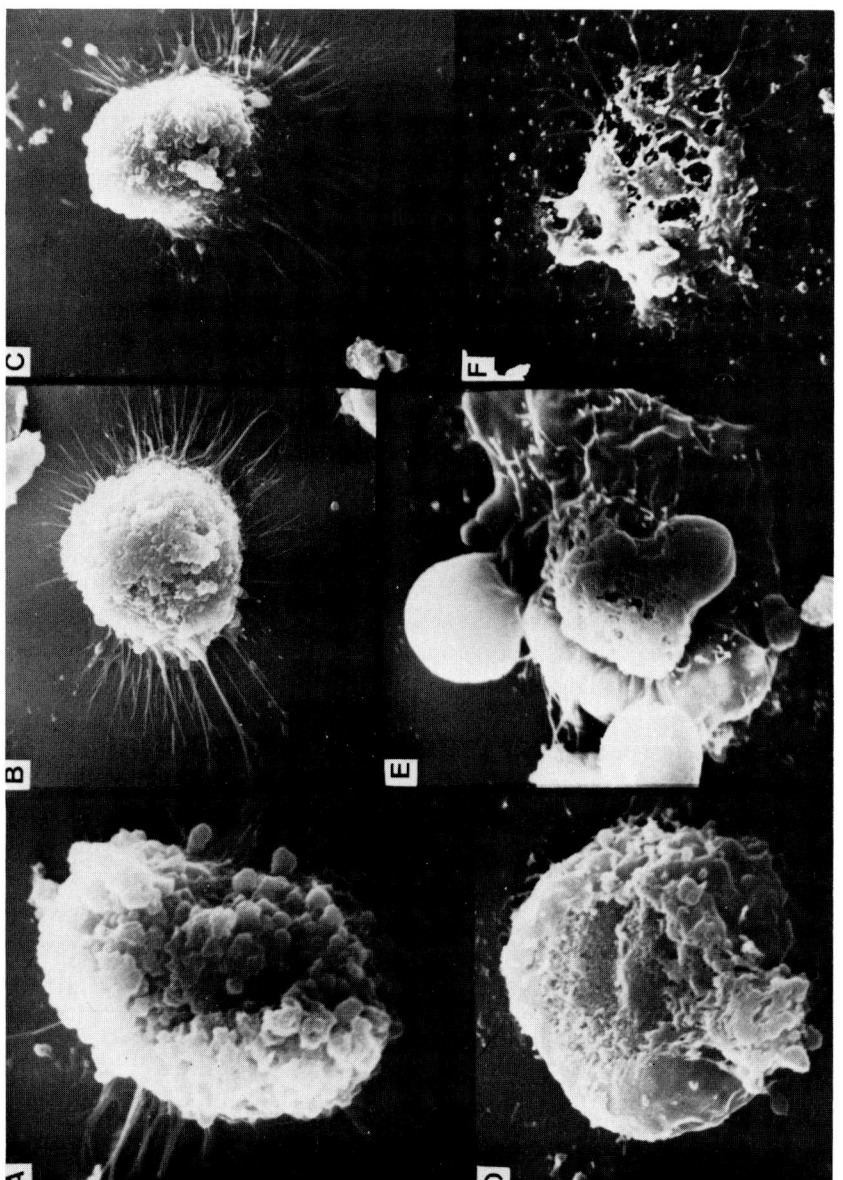

FIGURE 10. Scanning electron microscopy of M21 human melanoma cells before and after treatment with 9.2.27-CVF conjugates and complement. Panels A to C show viable M21 melanoma cells. Panels D to F show treated melanoma cells with different degrees of cytopathological changes. (From Vogel, C.-W. and Müller-Eberhard, H. J., *Proc. Natl. Acad. Sci. U.S.A.*, 78, 7707, 1981. With permission.)

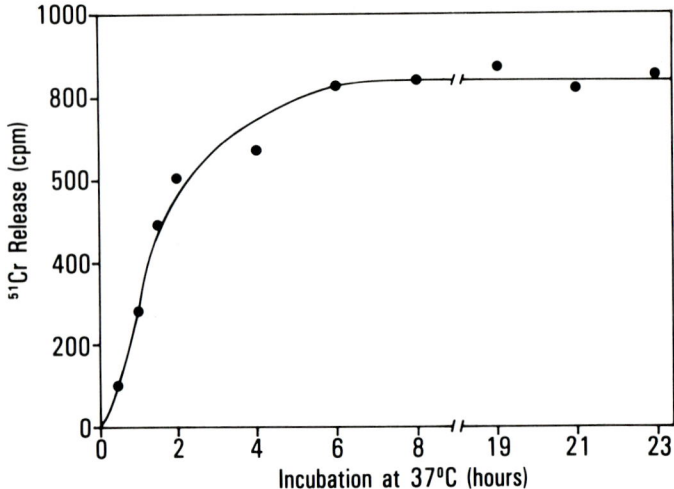

FIGURE 11. Kinetics of killing of M21 melanoma cells by CVF conjugates of the 9.2.27 monoclonal antibody and complement. Shown are the results of a ^{51}Cr-release assay (From Vogel, C.-W. and Müller-Eberhard, H. J., *Proc. Natl. Acad. Sci. USA*, 78, 7707, 1981. With permission.)

Figure 11 shows the kinetics of killing of human melanoma cells by antibody-CVF conjugates. Half-maximal killing was reached after approximately 1.5 hr of incubation. This was substantially faster than killing of Raji cells by alternative pathway activation, which was shown to require 10 hr for half-maximal killing.[29] The different kinetics of cell killing may be due to differences in the ability of the different target cells to defend themselves against the complement attack. Alternatively, the observed differences may be due to differences in the activation of the cytolytic alternative pathway in the two systems compared. In the case of Raji cells, the activation of the alternative pathway is due to surface properties of the cells which render the cells activators of that pathway, while in the case of the melanoma cells the activation of the alternative pathway is achieved by the CVF portion of the antibody-CVF conjugates.

An important factor in determining the rate of target cell death seems to be the extent of C5b-6 formation. As shown in Figure 12, antibody-CVF conjugates do not require native C3 for the cytotoxic effect since they initiate melanoma cell killing in the presence of serum containing only C5 through C9 activity. This result suggests that the C5 convertase activity of the CVF,Bb enzyme is of particular importance in the cytotoxic efficiency of antibody-CVF conjugates. This observation may also explain the faster cytotoxicity by antibody-CVF conjugates than by regular activation of the alternative pathway. Consistent with this hypothesis is the observation by Podack and Müller-Eberhard[30] that cell death of Raji cells occurs within several minutes if they are attacked by preformed C5b-6.

Another interesting observation is that melanoma cells susceptible to killing by conjugates of the 9.2.27 monoclonal antibody and CVF cannot be killed by a polyclonal antiserum recognizing the same high molecular weight antigen as the 9.2.27 monoclonal antibody.[31] This observation demonstrates that the lack of cytotoxicity of a monoclonal antibody may not be due to an inherent inability of that antibody to activate complement, but that it may be due to the nature or the local environment of the cell surface antigen recognized by the antibody. This result further demonstrates that coupling of CVF to a monoclonal antibody may not only provide that antibody with a "lost" effector function but may — as in the case of the 9.2.27 antibody — provide for a more efficient way of activating complement.

CVF was also coupled to the murine IgG3 monoclonal antibody against the G_{D3} antigen

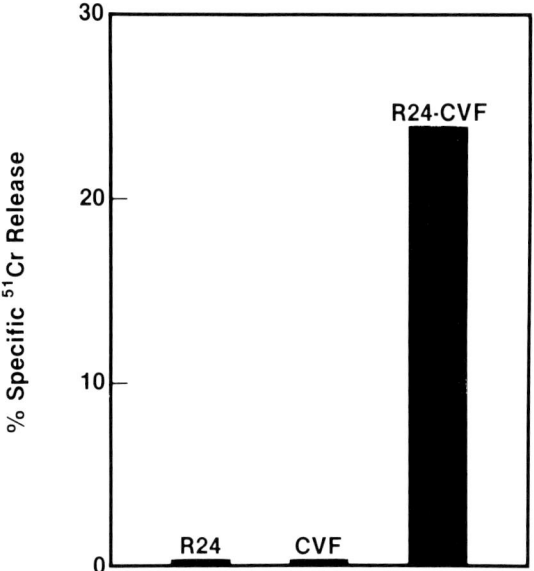

FIGURE 12. The cytotoxic activity of antibody-CVF conjugates does not require native C3. Shown are results of a ^{51}Cr-release assay with SK-MEL-93-2 human melanoma cells and conjugates of the R24 monoclonal antibody with CVF, the native complement-activating R24 antibody, and purified CVF in the presence of serum containing active C5 through C9 but no native C3.

of human melanoma cells, designated R24.[32,33] In contrast to the 9.2.27 antibody, the R24 antibody is an efficient activator of complement.[21,48] In order to demonstrate the activity of the CVF portion of the R24-CVF conjugates we employed genetically C4-deficient guinea pig serum or C4-depleted human serum. In both C4-deficient reagents, the unconjugated R24 antibody was unable to kill antigen-positive melanoma cells while the R24-CVF conjugates remained cytotoxic, indicating that the CVF in the conjugates was active and induced killing utilizing the proteins of the alternative complement pathway.[31]

We also coupled CVF to monoclonal antibodies directed against human renal cancer, human myeloic leukemia, and guinea pig hepatocarcinoma (Vogel and Old, unpublished). All conjugates exhibited no or only insignificant cytotoxic activities against their various target cells, although the conjugates bound to the cells and the CVF-portion was active when assayed for in a hemolytic test. These observations indicate that not every system of antibody and target cell is suitable for antibody-CVF conjugates. The reasons for the resistance to killing by antibody-CVF conjugates may be due to cellular properties such as defense mechanisms or density and local environment of the antigen recognized by the antibody. In addition, CVF from different *Naja naja* subspecies has recently been shown to exhibit structural and functional differences[34] which may account for activity differences observed with antibody-CVF conjugates.

Conjugates of antibodies with CVF were also prepared by other investigators. Ganu et al.[35] coupled CVF to a monoclonal antibody directed against human C3b. These authors report that their conjugates were functionally active with respect to antibody binding and C3/C5 convertase activity as judged by the induction of hemolysis of sheep erythrocytes coated with human C3b. Similarly, Parker and White[36] coupled CVF to an antibody to human erythrocytes. They report that both constituents of their conjugates retained their functional activity. Their conjugates deposited C3 onto human erythrocytes with human serum in the presence of Mg-EGTA while the same cells were lysed with rabbit serum in the presence of Mg-EGTA.

Müller and Müller-Ruchholtz[37] prepared conjugates of CVF with the IgG fraction of a rabbit antiserum to human lymphoid cells. They report that their conjugates were active in killing several antigen-positive cell lines using human complement in the presence of Mg-EGTA. In the presence of calcium, where simultaneous activation of the classical pathway by the antibody portion of the conjugates occurs, cytolysis by antibody-CVF conjugates was slower than by unconjugated antibody, but the overall cytotoxic activity of the antibody-CVF conjugates was 2.5-fold higher. (See ''Note Added in Proof''.)

IV. IN VIVO STUDIES

Initial in vivo experiments were performed in nude mice with human melanoma transplants to determine the immunotherapeutic potential of antibody-CVF conjugates. Our first model system consisted of nude mice receiving 5×10^7 human melanoma cells i.p. The animals were subsequently treated with a single injection of conjugates of the 9.2.27 monoclonal antibody with CVF or of the unconjugated 9.2.27 antibody. The tumor growth was delayed by 2 weeks in animals receiving the antibody-CVF conjugates compared to animals receiving the unconjugated antibody or saline.[38]

Before embarking on further immunotherapeutic experiments we decided to first study the pharmacokinetics and biodistribution of antibody-CVF conjugates and their stability in vivo.[38,39,49] These investigations are not only of interest to antibody conjugates with CVF but are likely to be pertinent for other immunoconjugate approaches. However, antibody conjugates with CVF represent a particularly convenient model system for these in vivo studies because of the lack of toxicity of CVF.

We synthesized conjugates with several different heterobifunctional cross-linking reagents differing in their sulfhydryl-reactive groups and in their resulting intermolecular cross-links. Figure 13 demonstrates that conjugates prepared with SPDP (N-succinimidyl-3-(2-pyridyl-dithio)-propionate), SMCC (succinimidyl-4-(N-maleimidomethyl)-cyclohexane-1-carboxylate), or IAHS (iodoacetyl-N-hydroxysuccinimide ester) exhibited plasma half-times in normal mice of 23 to 25 hr, while conjugates prepared with MBS (m-maleimidobenzoyl-hydroxysuccinimide ester) were rapidly removed from the circulation with a half-time of 3.5 hr.[38,39] Preliminary results indicate that the aromatic benzene ring or the benzene ring adjacent to the maleimide structure in MBS and in a similar cross-linker (succinimidyl-4-(p-maleimidophenyl)-butyrate, SMPB) is responsible for the rapid removal of conjugates prepared with MBS or SMPB from the circulation.[31,40,41,49]

Another concern of investigators in the immunoconjugate field is the potential instability of intermolecular cross-links containing a disulfide bond. Figure 14 shows that antibody-CVF conjugates prepared with SPDP, a cross-linking reagent that results in a disulfide bond-containing cross-link, are indeed subject to degradation in vivo. However, the extent of cleavage is moderate; even after 4 days in circulation the majority of the material is in the form of intact conjugates (Figure 14).[49]

These results taken together indicate that heterobifunctional cross-linking reagents used for the synthesis of immunoconjugates can have major effects on the pharmacokinetics of the resulting conjugates. This observation may also explain the apparent discrepancy between the in vitro and in vivo cytotoxic activities of immunoconjugates. So far we could not identify an optimal cross-linker. Consequently, work has to continue to develop new cross-linking methods which allow the synthesis of immunoconjugates without adverse effects on the activity or in vivo properties of the resulting hybrids.

V. CONCLUSION

The concept of targeting CVF is a particularly attractive one since the molecule is devoid of direct cytotoxic effects. CVF is, therefore, an example of a biological response modifier.

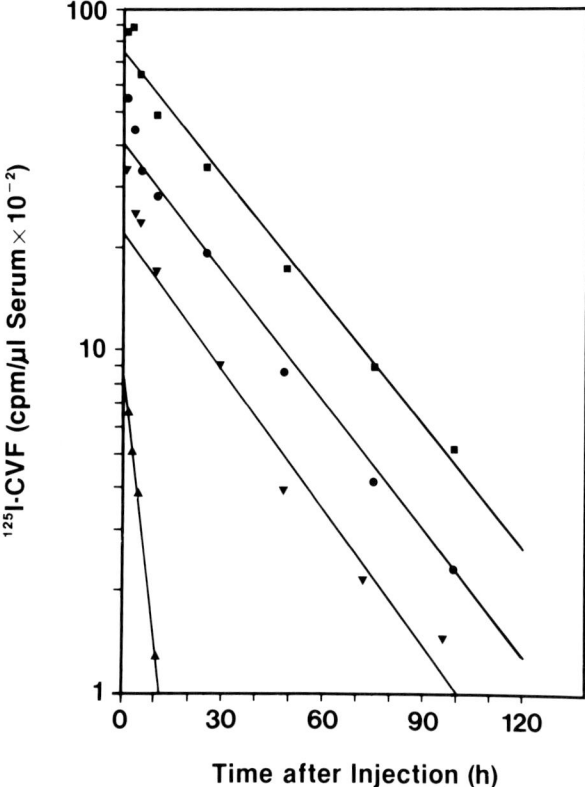

FIGURE 13. Plasma half-times of antibody-CVF conjugates. Radiolabeled conjugates prepared with IAHS (■), SPDP (●), SMCC (▼), and MBS (▲) were injected i.v. into BALB/c mice. At time intervals as indicated, blood samples were taken and the plasma was counted for radioactivity. (From Wilkie, S. D., Grier, A. H., Petrella, E. C., and Vogel, C. -W., submitted.)

In contrast, antibody conjugates containing protein toxins such as ricin (immunotoxins) or low molecular weight chemotherapeutic drugs such as adriamycin (chemoimmunoconjugates) are toxic, causing side effects by the same mechanisms that are responsible for the antitumor effects.[23] The site of action of CVF is the cell surface. There is no need for internalization and resistance to intracellular degradation in order to become effective. In addition, CVF can be reused to form a C3/C5 convertase with a new molecule of Factor B once the CVF,Bb enzyme has decayed, since the interaction of CVF with its "receptor" Factor B does not lead to inactivation or degradation of the CVF molecule. It is likely that CVF exerts its in vivo antitumor effect not only through the direct cytolytic action of the membrane attack complex but also through the production of localized inflammation by releasing the complement-derived phlogogenic peptides C3a, C5a, and Bb, thereby attracting additional effector systems of host defense to the tumor site. However, CVF is immunogenic for mammalian organisms. Nevertheless, the C3b-like function of CVF offers the theoretical possibility of reducing or even preventing an immune response by replacing CVF with an appropriately modified human C3 derivative that would function like CVF. While such a "human CVF" has not been obtained yet, we have been able to generate a novel fragment of human C3, named C3o, by use of a newly discovered protease in cobra venom.[42] This new cleavage product C3o structurally resembles CVF and is able to form a convertase with human Factor B.[43,44,50] While the concept of targeting CVF and the current experimental results are encouraging, it remains to be seen whether antibody-CVF conjugates will become clinically useful agents for therapy of cancer.

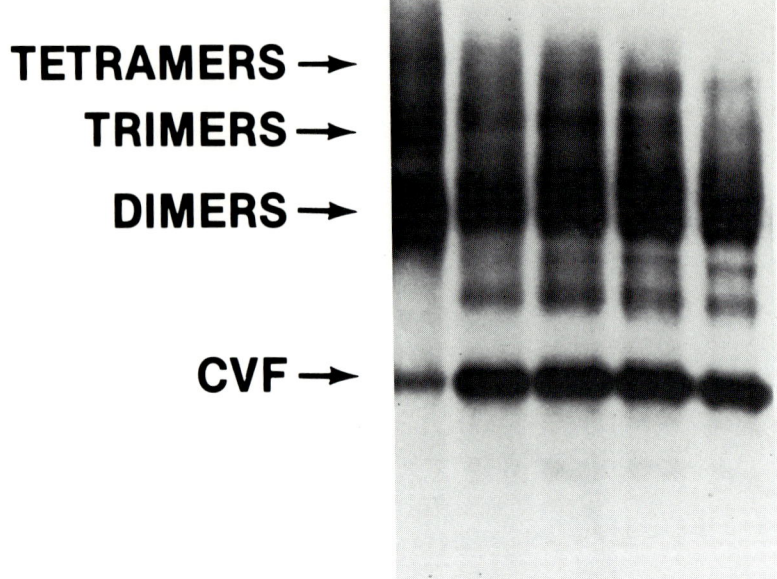

FIGURE 14. *In vivo* stability of antibody-CVF conjugate prepared with SPDP. The antibody conjugate was prepared with ^{125}I-CVF and was injected i.v. into BALB/c mice. At time intervals as indicated, blood samples were taken, and the plasma was subjected to SDS gradient polyacrylamide gel electrophoresis and autoradiography. The control lane (C) shows the composition of the injected material. (From Wilkie, S. D., Grier, A. H., Petrella, E. C., and Vogel, C. -W., submitted.)

NOTE ADDED IN PROOF

Since this manuscript was written, Müller-Ruchholtz and co-workers have continued their work characterizing antibody conjugates with CVF as specific cytotoxic agents for lymphocytes and leukemia cells.[51,52,53] They found that monoclonal antibodies coupled to CVF allow the selective lysis of their target cells using complement from several species, including human. The authors also compared the selectivity and potency of antibody-CVF conjugates with antibody-ricin conjugates. They found that the number of antibody conjugates required for optimal cytotoxicity is somewhat lower for antibody-ricin conjugates but that these conjugates exhibit nonspecific toxicity for antigen-negative cells. In contrast, antibody-CVF conjugates were devoid of any nonspecific toxicity for antigen-negative cells, a property that may render antibody-CVF conjugates superior for bone marrow purging.

ACKNOWLEDGMENTS

I would like to acknowledge the important contributions of my co-workers and collaborators as evident from the authorship of cited publications. Work performed in my laboratory was supported by NIH Grants CA 35525 and HL 29523 and by Research Career Development

Award CA 01039 from the National Cancer Institute, Department of Health and Human Services.

REFERENCES

1. **Vogel, C.-W. and Müller-Eberhard, H. J.**, Cobra venom factor: improved method for purification and biochemical characterization, *J. Immunol. Meth.*, 73, 203, 1984.
2. **Eggersten, G., Lind, P., and Sjöquist, J.**, Molecular characterization of the complement activating protein in the venom of the indian cobra *(Naja n. siamensis), Mol. Immunol.*, 18, 125, 1981.
3. **Vogel, C.-W., Smith, C. A., and Müller-Eberhard, H. J.**, Cobra venom factor: structural homology with the third component of human complement, *J. Immunol.*, 133, 3235, 1984.
4. **Reid, K. B. M. and Porter, R. R.**, The proteolytic activation systems of complement, *Ann. Rev. Biochem.*, 50, 433, 1981.
5. **Pangburn, M. K. and Müller-Eberhard, H. J.**, The alternative pathway of Complement, *Springer Semin. Immunopathol.*, 7, 163, 1984.
6. **Vogt, W., Dieminger, L., Lynen, R., and Schmidt, G.**, Alternative pathway for the activation of complement in human serum. Formation and composition of the complex with cobra venom factor that cleaves the third component of complement, *Hoppe-Seyler's Z. Physiol. Chem.*, 355, 171, 1974.
7. **Lesavre, P. H., Hugli, T. E., Esser, A. F., and Müller-Eberhard, H. J.**, The alternative pathway C3/C5 convertase: chemical basis of factor B activation, *J. Immunol.* 123, 529, 1979.
8. **Smith, C. A., Vogel, C.-W., and Müller-Eberhard, H. J.**, Ultrastructure of cobra venom factor-dependent C3/C5 convertase and its zymogen, factor B of human complement, *J. Biol. Chem.*, 257, 9879, 1982.
9. **Smith, C. A., Vogel, C.-W., and Müller-Eberhard, H. J.**, MHC class III products: an electron microscopic study of the C3 convertases of human complement, *J. Exp. Med.*, 159, 324, 1984.
10. **Medicus, R. G., Götze, O., and Müller-Eberhard, H. J.**, Alternative pathway of complement: recruitment of precursor properdin by the labile C3/C5 convertase and the potentiation of the pathway, *J. Exp. Med.*, 144, 1076, 1976.
11. **Vogel, C.-W. and Müller-Eberhard, H. J.**, The cobra venom factor-dependent C3 convertase of human complement. A kinetic and thermodynamic analysis of a protease acting on its natural high molecular weight substrate, *J. Biol. Chem.*, 257, 8292, 1982.
12. **Whaley, K. and Ruddy, S.**, Modulation of the alternative complement pathway by beta-1H globulin, *J. Exp. Med.*, 144, 1147, 1976.
13. **Pangburn, M. K., Schreiber, R. D., and Müller-Eberhard, H. J.**, Human complement C3b inactivator: isolation, characterization, and demonstration of an absolute requirement for the serum protein beta-1H for cleavage of C3b and C4b in solution, *J. Exp. Med.*, 146, 257, 1977.
14. **Lachmann, P. J. and Halbwachs, L.**, The influence of C3b inactivator (KAF) concentration on the ability of serum to support complement activation, *Clin. Exp. Immunol.*, 21, 109, 1975.
15. **Nagaki, K., Iida, K., Okubo, M., and Inai, S.**, Reaction mechanisms of beta-1H globulin, *Int. Archs. Allergy Appl. Immunol.*, 57, 221, 1978.
16. **Daha, M. R., Fearon, D. T., and Austen, K. F.**, C3 requirements for formation of alternative pathway C5 convertase, *J. Immunol.*, 117, 630, 1976.
17. **Medicus, R. G., Götze, O., and Müller-Eberhard, H. J.**, The serine protease nature of the C3 and C5 convertases of the classical and alternative complement pathways, *Scand. J. Immunol.*, 5, 1049, 1976.
18. **von Zabern, I., Hinsch, B., Przyklenk, H., Schmidt, G., and Vogt, W.**, Comparison of *Naja n. naja* and *Naja h. haje* cobra venom factors: correlation between binding affinity for the fifth component of complement and Mediation of its cleavage, *Immunobiology*, 157, 499, 1980.
19. **Miyama, A., Kato, T., Horai, S., Yokoo, J., and Kashiba, S.**, Trypsin-activated complex of human factor B with cobra venom factor (CVF), cleaving C3 and C5 and generating a lytic factor for unsensitized guinea pig erythrocytes. I. Generation of the activated complex, *Biken J.*, 18, 193, 1975.
20. **Cochrane, C. G., Müller-Eberhard, H. J., and Aikin, B. S.**, Depletion of plasma complement in vivo by a protein of cobra venom: its effects on various immunologic reactions, *J. Immunol.* 105, 55, 1970.
21. **Vogel, C.-W., Welt, S., Carswell, E. A., Old, L. J., and Müller-Eberhard, H. J.**, A murine IgG3 monoclonal antibody to a melanoma antigen that activates complement in vitro and in vivo, *Immunobiology*, 164, 309, 1983.
22. **Ryan, A. F., Catanzaro, A., Wasserman, S. I., Harris, J. A., and Vogel, C.-W.**, Complement depletion reduces immunologically mediated middle ear effusion and Inflammation, *Clin. Immunol. Immunopathol.*, 40, 410, 1986.

23. **Vogel, C.-W.**, Ed., *Immunoconjugates. Antibody Conjugates in Radioimaging and Therapy of Cancer*, Oxford University Press, New York, 1987.
24. **Schumaker, V. N., Seegan, G. W., Smith, C. A., Ma, S. K., Rodwell, J. D., and Schumaker, M. F.**, The free energy of angular position of the Fab arms of IgG antibody, *Mol. Immunol.*, 17, 413, 1980.
25. **Smith, C. A. and Seegan, G. W.**, The pleated sheet: an unusual negative-staining method for transmission electron microscopy of biological macromolecules, *J. Ultrastruc. Res.*, 89, 111, 1984.
26. **Provencher, S. W. and Glöckner, J.**, Estimation of globular protein secondary structure from circular dichroism, *Biochemistry*, 20, 33, 1981.
27. **Morgan, Jr., A. C., Galloway, D. R., and Reisfeld, R. A.**, Production and characterization of monoclonal antibody to a melanoma specific glycoprotein, *Hybridoma*, 1, 27, 1981.
28. **Vogel, C.-W. and Müller-Eberhard, H. J.**, Induction of immune cytolysis: tumor-cell killing by complement is initiated by covalent complex of monoclonal antibody and stable C3/C5 convertase, *Proc. Natl. Acad. Sci. USA*, 78, 7707, 1981.
29. **Schreiber, R. D., Pangburn, M. K., Medicus, R. G., and Müller-Eberhard, H. J.**, Raji cell injury and subsequent lysis by the purified cytolytic alternative pathway of human complement, *Clin. Immunol. Immunopathol.*, 15, 384, 1980.
30. **Podack, E. R., and Müller-Eberhard, H. J.**, Complement mediated membrane injury of tumor cells: release of membrane fragments by C5b-9, *Fed. Proc.*, 40, 359, 1981.
31. **Vogel, C.-W.**, Antibody conjugates without inherent toxicity: the targeting of cobra venom factor and other biological response modifiers, in *Immunoconjugates. Antibody Conjugates in Radioimaging and Therapy of Cancer*, Vogel C.-W., Ed., Oxford University Press, New York, 1987, 170.
32. **Dippold, W. G., Lloyd, K. O., Li, L. T. C., Ikeda, H., Oettgen, H. F., and Old, L. J.**, Cell surface antigens of human malignant melanoma: definition of six antigenic systems with mouse monoclonal antibodies, *Proc. Natl. Acad. Sci. USA*, 77, 6114, 1980.
33. **Pukel, C. S., Lloyd, K. O., Travassos, L. R., Dippold, W. G., Oettgen, H. F., and Old, L. J.**, G_{D3}, a prominent ganglioside of human melanoma. Detection and characterization by mouse monoclonal antibody, *J. Exp. Med.*, 155, 1133, 1982.
34. **Petrella, E. C. and Vogel, C.-W.**, Cobra venom factor from different *Naja naja* subspecies exhibits structural and functional differences, *Fed. Proc.*, 45, 1942, 1986.
35. **Ganu, V., Fernandez-Cruz, E., and Müller-Eberhard, H. J.**, Synthesis and properties of a monoclonal antibody-cobra venom factor complex which is stable in vivo, *Fed. Proc.*, 43, 1772, 1984.
36. **Parker, C. J. and White, V. F.**, Site-specific activation of the alternative pathway of complement (APC): creation of a hybrid molecule consisting of antibody and cobra venom factor (CoF), *Complement*, 2, 61, 1985.
37. **Müller, B. and Müller-Ruchholtz, W.**, Antibody (Ab)/cobra venom factor (CVF) conjugates supplement the classical human serum complement pathway with alternate pathway cytolysis, *Complement*, 2, 56, 1985.
38. **Vogel, C.-W., Wilkie, S. D., and Morgan, A. C.**, In vivo studies with covalent conjugates of cobra venom factor and monoclonal antibodies to human tumors, in *Modern Trends in Human Leukemia*, VI, Neth, R., Gallo, R. C., Greaves, M. F., and Janka, G., Eds., Springer Verlag, Berlin, Heidelberg, 1985, 514.
39. **Wilkie, S. D. and Vogel, C.-W.**, The effect of different heterobifunctional crosslinking reagents on the in vivo stability of antibody-cobra venom factor conjugates, *Fed. Proc.*, 43, 1971, 1984.
40. **Petrella, E. C., Wilkie, S. D., Grier, A. H., and Vogel, C.-W.**, Covalent conjugates of cobra venom factor (CVF) with monoclonal antibodies: effect of different heterobifunctional reagents on activity and in vivo properties, *Complement*, 2, 63, 1985.
41. **Petrella, E. C., Wilkie, S. D., Grier, A. H., and Vogel, C.-W.**, Effect of different heterobifunctional crosslinkers on activity and pharmacokinetics of antibody conjugates with cobra venom factor, *J. Cell. Biochem. (Suppl.)*, 10B, 97, 1986.
42. **O'Keefe, M. C., Vogel, C.-W., and Caporale, L. H.**, Characterization of a protease from cobra venom that cleaves the human complement component C3, *Fed. Proc.*, 43, 1956, 1984.
43. **Caporale, L. H., O'Keefe, M. C., and Vogel, C.-W.**, C3o, A new cleavage product of human C3 generated by a protease from cobra venom, *Fed. Proc.*, 43, 1448, 1984.
44. **O'Keefe, M. C., Caporale, L. H., and Vogel, C.-W.**, Structural and functional characterization of a human analog of cobra venom factor, *Complement*, 2, 58, 1985.
45. **Grier, A. H., Schultz, M., and Vogel, C.-W.**, Cobra venom factor and human C3 share carbohydrate antigenic determinants, *J. Immunol.*, 139, 1245, 1987.
46. **Hensley, P., O'Keefe, M. C., Spangler, C. J., Osborne, Jr., J. C., and Vogel, C. -W.**, The effects of metal ions and temperature on the interaction of cobra venom factor and human complement factor B, *J. Biol. Chem.*, 261, 11038, 1986.

47. **Petrella, E. C., Wilkie, S. D., Smith, C. A., Morgan, Jr., A. C., and Vogel, C. -W.**, Antibody conjugates with cobra venom factor. Synthesis and biochemical characterization, *J. Immunol. Meth.*, 1987, in press.
48. **Welt, S., Carswell, E. A., Vogel, C. -W., Oettgen, H. F., and Old, L. J.**, Immune and non-immune effector functions of IgG3 mouse monoclonal antibody R24 detecting the disialoganglioside GD3 on the surface of melanoma cells, *Clin. Immunol. Immunopathol.*, 45, 214, 1987.
49. **Wilkie, S. D., Grier, A. H., Petrella, E. C., and Vogel, C. -W.**, Effect of different heterobifunctional crosslinking reagents on the pharmacokinetics of antibody conjugates with cobra venom factor, submitted.
50. **O'Keefe, M. C., Caporale, L. H., and Vogel, C. -W.**, Comparison of the alpha chain fragments of C3o, C3c and CVF: implications for C3 convertase formation, *Complement*, 4, 204, 1987.
51. **Müller, B., Harpprecht, H., Anderson, M. J. D., and Müller-Ruchholtz, W.**, Activation of human complement by covalent conjugates of mouse monoclonal antibodies and cobra venom factors, *Br. J. Cancer*, 54, 537, 1986.
52. **Müller, B. and Müller-Ruchholtz, W.**, In vitro killing of target cells by antibody/ricin or antibody/cobra venom factor conjugates: comparison of selectivity and potency, *Immunobiology*, 173, 195, 1986.
53. **Müller, B. and Müller-Ruchholtz, W.**, Covalent conjugates of monoclonal antibody and cobra venom factor mediate specific cytotoxicity via alternative pathway of human complement activation, *Leukemia Res.*, 11, 461, 1987.

Chapter 23

A FUNCTION FOR NK CELLS IN ACUTE BONE MARROW ALLOGRAFT REJECTION*

Gunther Dennert

TABLE OF CONTENTS

I.	Introduction	154
II.	The Bone Marrow Transplantation Model	154
III.	Cloned NK Cells Cause Specific Bone Marrow Graft Rejection	154
IV.	The Ability to Reject Bone Marrow Grafts Can Be Transferred by Serum	155
V.	The Serum Component Responsible for Marrow Graft Rejection is Antibody	156
VI.	Serum from Responder Mice Induces a Specific Antibody Dependent Cell Mediated Cytotoxic Reaction	157
VII.	H-2 Specific Monoclonal Antibody is Able to Convert Nonresponder into Responder Recipients	157
VIII.	Conclusion	158
References		159

---

* This work was supported by Public Health service grants CA 37706, CA 39501, and CA 39623.

I. INTRODUCTION

The murine model of bone marrow transplantation has provided an interesting tool to examine the mechanism of marrow graft rejection. Grafts of normal or neoplastic hemopoietic cells fail to grow in certain strains of irradiated allogeneic or semiallogeneic mice, a phenomenon which has been referred to as natural resistance.[1-4] The antigenic determinants recognized on hemopoietic tissues and therefore responsible for the rejection are controlled by hemopoietic histocompatibility (Hh) loci which can be associated with or closely linked to the major histocompatibility gene complex.[4-8] Understanding the nature of marrow graft rejection has been complicated by both the unorthodox non-codominant inheritance of Hh genes[4] as well as the unusual characteristics of the effector mechanism.

Marrow allograft rejection is caused by an effector mechanism that is relatively radiation-resistant, matures late in ontogeny, exhibits exquisite immunogenetic specificity and appears to be independent of conventional immune responses. Moreover, graft rejection occurs within 12 to 24 hrs;[1] therefore, the effectors must be functional at the time of marrow transplantion. These observations as well as the finding that mice with the beige mutation[9,10] and which are deficient in natural killer (NK) activity do not reject marrow grafts, have pointed to the possibility that marrow graft rejection may be a function of NK cells.[11-15] NK cells do not exhibit H-2 specific cytotoxicity in vitro; therefore, if they indeed play a role in bone marrow graft rejection, the mechanism by which they perform this specific function must be explained. In this chapter, we will discuss experiments that show that NK cells likely are responsible for marrow graft rejection and explain why this rejection shows Hh specificity.

II. THE BONE MARROW TRANSPLANTATION MODEL

Mice to be transplanted with bone marrow have to be lethally irradiated by α or x-ray source. The transplant is obtained from the femur of donor mice and is injected i.v. into sex- and age-matched recipients. Proliferation of transplanted bone marrow stem cells is assayed in the spleen 5 to 12 days after injection by either counting spleen colonies (CFUS = colony forming units; spleen) or by assessing cell proliferation by measuring ^{125}I-IUDR incorporation into the spleen.[1-3] The dose of transplanted marrow is varied between 0.5 to 2×10^6 cells depending on the strain combination. This dose range gives rise to about 200 to 300 CFUS in the syngeneic situation and results in approximately 1% incorporation of injected radioactivity into the spleen. For each experiment syngeneic growth controls are set arbitrarily at 100 growth units and the values in the experimental groups are calculated accordingly. Fifty to one hundred units reflect uninhibited growth, 10 to 50 units partial growth, and less than 10 units no growth.

III. CLONED NK CELLS CAUSE SPECIFIC BONE MARROW GRAFT REJECTION

One of the arguments for the involvement of NK cells in marrow graft rejection is the finding that NK deficient C57BL/6 mice carrying the homozygous beige mutation (Table 1 and References 9, 10, 16) or that were made NK deficient by 4 weekly doses of 200 rads (data not shown, References 17-21) fail to reject H-2^d marrow grafts. In contrast, C57BL/6 mice which are wild type or heterozygous for the beige mutation and therefore express NK activity reject marrow grafts of H-2^d haplotype (Table 1). The specificity of graft rejection in normal or beige heterozygous C57BL/6 mice is controlled predominantly by genes close to or in the H-2D region (Table 1). When NK-deficient C57BL/6 mice are injected i.v. with 2×10^6 syngeneic cloned NK cells[19,20] marrow transplants of H-2^d genotype are rejected (Table 1). Graft rejection in these mice is again specific for determinants encoded in the H-

Table 1
GENETIC SPECIFICITY OF NK-MEDIATED BONE MARROW ALLOGRAFT REJECTION

Donor bone marrow		Irradiated recipient[a]	Donor bone marrow growth[b]
Strain	H-2 K I S D		
B10	b b b b	bg/+	100 ± 10
B10.D2	d d d d	bg/+	1 ± 1
B10.A (18R)	b b b d	bg/+	8 ± 2
D2.GD	d d b b	bg/+	30 ± 3
B10	b b b b	bg/bg	68 ± 10
B10.D2	d d d d	bg/bg	70 ± 5
B10.A (18R)	b b b d	bg/bg	64 ± 3
D2.GD	d d b b	bg/bg	90 ± 12
B10	b b b b	bg/bg + NK[c]	70 ± 8
B10.D2	d d d d	bg/bg + NK	2 ± 1
B10.A (18R)	b b b d	bg/bg + NK	6 ± 1
D2.GD	d d b b	bg/bg + NK	26 ± 2

[a] Lethally irradiated 57BL/6 (H-2^b) recipients were injected with 1 × 10^6 donor bone marrow cells.
[b] Values relative to syngeneic growth controls were arbitrarily set at 100 units.
[c] Injected with 2 × 10^6 cloned NK cells (NKB61B10) 4 days before transplantation.

2D region. Thus B10.A (18R) marrow grafts are strongly rejected while D2.GD grafts show weaker rejection (Table 1). Hence the specificity of graft rejection in beige recipients injected with NK cells is identical to that of normal mice or mice which are heterozygous for the beige mutation (Table 1). These results show two important points, one is that NK cells indeed cause marrow graft rejection and the other is that rejection is specific for antigens coded for by genes close to or in the H-2D region.

IV. THE ABILITY TO REJECT BONE MARROW GRAFTS CAN BE TRANSFERRED BY SERUM

The observation that NK clones cause specific marrow graft rejection in vivo is unexpected because NK cells do not express H-2 specificity in in vitro cytolytic assays.[19-21] However, NK cells had been previously suggested to function in antibody dependent cell mediated lysis of nucleated targets.[22,24] It is therefore possible that the specificity of cloned NK cells in vivo is due to target specific antibody in the recipient able to reject a particular marrow graft. To test this possibility, sera from mice able to reject marrow grafts were transferred to recipients not able to reject the respective marrow graft. BALB/c (H-2^d) bone marrow grafts are rejected by C57BL/6 (H-2^b), but not by 129/SvJ (H-2^b) mice; therefore serum from C57BL/6 mice was transferred into 129/SvJ mice and the recipient mice assayed for rejection of BALB/c grafts. Results showed (Table 2) that serum transfer from C57BL/6 mice into 129/SvJ mice results in rejection of H-2^d marrow grafts. The rejection was again specific for determinants expressed on the donor marrow encoded in the H-2D region (Table 2). Thus, B10.A (18R) grafts are much better rejected than D2.GD grafts (Table 2). These results demonstrate that specific marrow graft rejection can be transferred from responder to nonresponder mice by serum.

Table 2
GENETIC SPECIFICITY OF BONE MARROW GRAFT REJECTION FOLLOWING TRANSFER OF SERUM FROM RESPONDER MICE

Donor Bone Marrow			
Strain	H-2 K I S D	Irradiated recipient[a]	Donor bone marrow growth[b]
B10	b b b b	C57BL/6J	90 ± 4
B10.D2	d d d d	C57BL/6J	7 ± 2
B10.A (18R)	b b b d	C57BL/6J	13 ± 3
D2.GD	d d b b	C57BL/6J	82 ± 10
B10	b b b b	129/SvJ	100 ± 13
B10.D2	d d d d	129/SvJ	100 ± 4
B10.A (18R)	b b b d	129/SvJ	98 ± 10
D2.GD	d d b b	129/SvJ	100 ± 15
B10	b b b b	129/SvJ + C57BL/6 serum[c]	120 ± 18
B10.D2	d d d d	129/SvJ + C57BL/6 serum	9 ± 3
B10.A (18R)	b b b d	129/SvJ + C57BL/6 serum	18 ± 2
D2.GD	d d b b	129/SvJ + C57BL/6 serum	91 ± 15

[a] Lethally irradiated H-2^b recipients were transplanted with 1×10^6 donor bone marrow cells and marrow growth assayed 6 days later.
[b] Values relative to syngeneic growth control of 100 units.
[c] Irradiated recipient mice were injected with a mixture of donor bone marrow and serum (1:4) collected from C57BL/6J mice.

Table 3
IMMUNOGLOBULIN-DEPLETED SERUM DOES NOT INDUCE MARROW GRAFT REJECTION

Marrow recipient	C57BL/6 Serum given to recipient[a]	Marrow[b] growth
C57BL/6	None	7 ± 2
129/SvJ	None	100 ± 14
129/SvJ	Normal	9 ± 3
129/SvJ	Ig depleted	97 ± 9
129/SvJ	Ig fraction	8 ± 1

[a] BALB/c bone marrow cells were injected with either normal C57BL/6 serum, C57BL/6 serum which was Ig depleted by affinity chromatography, or the Ig fraction of C57BL/6 serum which was bound and acid-eluted from an affinity column.
[b] Irradiated recipient mice were transplanted with 1×10^6 BALB/c (H-2^d) bone marrow cells and assayed 6 days later for marrow growth.

V. THE SERUM COMPONENT RESPONSIBLE FOR MARROW GRAFT REJECTION IS ANTIBODY

The finding that serum transfers the ability to induce specific bone marrow graft rejection points to the possibility that specific antibody is responsible for the effect. If this were the case, then depletion of immunoglobulin (Ig) from responder serum should eliminate its ability to induce marrow graft rejection in nonresponder mice. C57BL/6 serum was run over a rabbit anti-mouse Ig agarose-coupled affinity column, and the adsorbed and nonadsorbed materials were tested for their ability to induce marrow graft rejection. Table 3 shows that both the unfractionated C57BL/6 serum and the eluted column-bound material (i.e., Ig) but

Table 4
SPECIFICITY OF SERUM IN THE ADCC REACTION

Mouse serum or monoclonal antibody	ADCC (% lysis) of tumor targets[a]		
	C1.18.4 (H-2^k)	RAW 253 (H-2^d)	EL4 (H-2^b)
None	<1	<1	<1
129/SvJ serum[b]	9 ± 1	<1	<1
C57BL/6 serum[c]	<1	11 ± 2	<1
11-4-1 (Anti-H-2^k)[d]	24 ± 2	<1	<1
34-5-8 (Anti-H-2^d)[d]	<1	13 ± 2	<1

[a] Percent ^{51}Cr-release using C57BL/6 effector splenocytes in an 8 hr assay. Effector:target cell ratio was 100:1, and the final serum dilution and monoclonal antibody dilution was 1:5 and 1:10, respectively.
[b] 129/SvJ mice reject H-2^k but not H-2^d or H-2^b bone marrow.
[c] C57BL/6 mice reject H-2^d but not H-2^k or H-2^b bone marrow.
[d] 11-4-1 and 34-5-8 are monoclonal anti H-2^k and anti H-2^d antibodies.

not the Ig depleted serum induce BALB/c marrow graft rejection in otherwise nonresponsive 129/SvJ mice. This result convincingly demonstrates that Ig is indeed responsible for the specific rejection of bone marrow in mice transplanted with allogeneic marrow transplants.

VI. SERUM FROM RESPONDER MICE INDUCES A SPECIFIC ANTIBODY DEPENDENT CELL MEDIATED CYTOTOXIC REACTION

To collect further evidence for the conclusion that antibody is responsible for specific bone marrow graft rejection, we examined whether sera from responder mice are able to induce a specific cell mediated cytotoxic reaction in vitro. Sera from 129/SvJ mice that reject H-2^k but not H-2^d bone marrow were tested for their ability to induce C57BL/6 NK cells to lyse H-2^k, H-2^d, and H-2^b targets respectively. Sera from C57BL/6 mice that reject H-2^d but not H-2^k marrow grafts were also tested by using the same effectors and the same targets. Results in Table 4 show that the sera induce lysis of the respective targets as expected, demonstrating that sera from responder mice not only induce specific marrow graft rejection in vivo but also a specific ADCC reaction in vitro.

VII. H-2 SPECIFIC MONOCLONAL ANTIBODY IS ABLE TO CONVERT NONRESPONDER INTO RESPONDER RECIPIENTS

Since antibody in responder mice appears to induce NK cells for specific bone marrow graft rejection it was interesting to find out whether nonresponder marrow graft recipients could be converted into responder recipients by injection of antibody. C57BL/6 mice were transplanted with a C3H marrow graft and also injected with either of the two monoclonal antibodies 11-4-1 or 12-2-2S both of which are H-2^k specific. Results in Table 5 show that 11-4-1 induces strong graft rejection but 12-2-2S does not. This result suggests that antibody of IgG isotype is able to induce marrow graft rejection, while antibody of IgM isotype is not. Since both antibodies fix complement but only IgG induces ADCC, it is very likely that antibody-induced marrow graft rejection is independent of complement and is cell mediated. The cell type responsible for antibody induced C3H marrow graft rejection in C57BL/6 mice is likely a NK cell since split dose γ-irradiation which efficiently eliminates NK activity completely inhibits antibody induced graft rejection (Table 5).

Table 5
INDUCTION OF BONE MARROW GRAFT REJECTION IN NONRESPONDER RECIPIENTS BY MONOCLONAL ANTIBODY

Bone marrow recipient	Bone marrow donor	Antibody given to recipient	Antibody specificity	Antibody isotype	Bone marrow growth
C57BL/6 normal	C3H	—	—	—	100 ± 21
C57BL/6 normal	C3H	11-4-1	K^k	IgG2a	4 ± 1
C57BL/6 normal	C3H	12-2-2S	K^kD^k	IgM	105 ± 22
C57BL/6 4x-200r[a]	C3H	11-4-1	K^k	IgG2a	84 ± 1

[a] Mice were made NK-deficient by split dose γ-irradiation.

VIII. CONCLUSION

In this chapter evidence is presented for the hypothesis that acute bone marrow allograft rejection is mediated by NK effector cells and specific antibody. The hypothesis is supported by several observations. One is that NK deficient mice, that either carry the beige mutation or received split dose irradiation, fail to acutely reject bone marrow allografts,[17,18] whereas nude mice that are devoid of T cells but possess NK activity reject marrow grafts. Another one is that cloned cell lines with NK activity injected into NK deficient mice cause the rejection of bone marrow allografts.[17,18] Marrow graft rejection induced by cloned NK cells shows the same specificity as that by normal mice, pointing to the participation of specificity-mediating components in the rejection. NK cells are very likely identical to K cell, i.e., to those cells that mediate in vitro cytolysis of nucleated targets.[22,25] A possible explanation for the in vivo specificity of NK cells therefore could be that they acquire specificity in vivo by interaction with antibody. Several approaches aimed at examining this hypothesis are presented. In one it is shown that sera from normal C57BL/6 mice that are able to reject $H-2^d$ marrow grafts induce rejection of $H-2^d$ marrow in strain 129/SvJ mice. The serum-induced graft rejection has the same specificity as that seen in normal C57BL/6 mice. It is likely that antibody is responsible for this effect, because removal of Ig from the serum voids its ability to induce graft rejection. Moreover the serum is also able to induce a specific ADCC in vitro. Taken together, these observations provide overwhelming evidence that marrow graft rejection in this model is indeed due to NK cells and specific antibody.

To further prove this hypothesis, it was examined whether monoclonal antibody is able to convert nonresponder into responder mice. Results showed that antibody of IgG, but not of IgM isotype, induces marrow graft rejection. This suggested that the mechanism by which antibody causes graft rejection involves a cell-mediated, rather than complement-mediated, reaction since both IgG and IgM fix complement. Support for this conclusion comes from the finding that antibody is not able to cause graft rejection in split-dose irradiated NK deficient mice.

An interesting question is whether, besides this NK mediated ADCC type reaction, other mechanisms of marrow graft rejection could also play a role in acute marrow graft rejection. The observation that thymus-deficient nude mice reject marrow grafts and that rejection takes place in lethally irradiated mice would a priori exclude the participation of sensitized T cells in the process of graft rejection. On the other hand, it is obvious that T cells may react with allogeneic histocompatibility antigens expressed on bone marrow cells. In instances, therefore, in which there are functional T cells in the transplant recipient (e.g., in sublethally irradiated recipients or in a situation in which a marrow graft has not been rejected acutely) the participation of sensitized T cells during the rejection could well play a role.

In fact we have recently shown that C57BL/6 mice that do not acutely reject a C3H marrow graft are able to do so once T killer cells are sensitized to H-2^k histocompatibility antigens.[26] It is therefore clear that while NK cells are the primary effectors in acute marrow allograft rejection, T killer cells may play an equally important effector function during the secondary phase of the rejection.

Antibody-dependent marrow allograft rejection by NK cells is the first demonstration of its kind in vivo. The question therefore is justified of how efficient this mechanism of transplant rejection may be. In a recent communication we reported that human melanoma tumors that grow progressively in immunodeficient mice can be rejected with the help of NK cells and target-specific monoclonal antibody.[27] Taken together, these results suggest that NK-dependent antibody-mediated transplant rejection is sufficiently potent to play a role in clinical transplant rejection and could be of therapeutic value in the treatment of neoplasia.

REFERENCES

1. **Cudkowicz, G. and Bennett, M.**, Peculiar immunobiology of bone marrow allografts. I. Graft rejection by irradiated responder mice, *J. Exp. Med.*, 134, 83, 1971.
2. **Cudkowicz, G. and Stimpfling, J. H.**, Induction of immunity and of unresponsiveness to parental marrow grafts in adult F1 hybrid mice, *Nature (London)*, 204, 450, 1964.
3. **Cudkowicz, G. and Bennett, M.**, Peculiar immunobiology of bone marrow allografts. II. Rejection of parental grafts by resistant F1 hybrid mice, *J. Exp. Med.*, 134, 1513, 1971.
4. **Cudkowicz, G.**, Hybrid resistance to parental grafts of hemopoietic and lymphoma cells, in *The Proliferation and Spread of Neoplastic Cells*, Williams & Wilkins, Baltimore, 1968, 661.
5. **Cudkowicz, G.**, Genetic control of resistance to allogeneic and xenogenic bone marrow grafts in mice, *Transplant Proc.*, 7, 155, 1975.
6. **Cudkowicz, G., and Lotzova, E.**, Hemopoietic cell-defined components of the major histocompatibility complex of mice. Identification of responsive and unresponsive recipients to bone marrow transplants, *Transplant Proc.*, 5, 1399, 1973.
7. **Cudkowicz, G. and Warner, J. F.**, Natural resistance of irradiated 129-strain mice to bone marrow allografts: genetic control by the H-2K region, *Immunogenetics*, 8, 13, 1979.
8. **Cudkowicz, G.**, Genetic control of bone marrow graft rejection. I. Determinant specific difference of reactivity in two pairs of inbred mouse strains, *J. Cell. Med.*, 134, 281, 1971.
9. **Roder, J. C., and Duwe, A. K.**, The beige mutation in the mouse selectively impairs natural killer cell function, *Nature*, 278, 451, 1979.
10. **Roder, J. C., Lohmann-Matthes, M. L., Domzig, W., and Wigzell, H.**, The beige mutation in the mouse. II. Selectivity of the natural killer cell defect, *J. Immunol.*, 123, 2174, 1979.
11. **Kiessling, R., Hochman, P. S., Haller, O., Shearer, G. M., Wigzell, H., and Cudkowicz, G.**, Evidence for a similar or common mechanism for natural killer cell activity and resistance to hemopoietic grafts, *Eur. J. Immunol.*, 7, 655, 1977.
12. **Trentin, J. J., Kiessling, R., Wigzell, H., Gallagher, M. T., Dalta, S. K., and S. S. Kulkarni**, Bone marrow transplantation immunology, in *Experimental Hematology Today*, Baum, S. J. and Ledney, G. D., Eds., Springer-Verlag, New York, 1977, 179.
13. **Cudkowicz, G., Landy, M., and Shearer, G. M., Eds.**, Natural Resistance Against Foreign Cells, Tumors and Microbes, Academic Press, New York, 1978.
14. **Okumura, K., Habu, S., and Shimamura, K.**, The role of asialo Gm1$^+$ cells in the resistance to transplants of bone marrow or other tissues, in *NK Cells and Other Natural Effector Cells*, Herberman, R. B., Ed., Academic Press, New York, 1982, 1527.
15. **Lotzova, E., Savary, C. A., and Pollack, S. B.**, Prevention of rejection of allogenic bone marrow transplants by NK1.1 antiserum, *Transplantation*, 35, 490, 1983.
16. **Kaminsky, S. and Cudkowicz, G.**, Natural killing resistance to marrow grafts: correlations in four beige mutant mouse lines, *Fed. Proc.*, 39, 466 (abstr)., 1980.
17. **Warner, J. F. and Dennert, G.**, Effects of a cloned cell line with NK activity on bone marrow transplants, tumor development and metastasis *in vivo*, *Nature*, 300, 31, 1982.

18. **Warner, J. F. and Dennert, G.,** Effects of a cloned cell line with NK activity on *in vivo* marrow grafts and tumor development, in *Normal and Neoplastic Hematopoiesis,* UCLA Symposia on Molecular and Cellular Biology. New Series. Vol. 9., Golde, D. W. and Marks, P. A., Eds., Alan R. Liss, New York, 1983, 567.
19. **Dennert, G.,** Cloned lines of natural killer cells, *Nature,* 287, 47, 1980.
20. **Dennert, G., Yogeeswaran, G., and Yamagata, S.,** Cloned cell lines with natural killer activity. Specificity, function and cell surface markers, *J. Exp. Med.,* 153, 545, 1981.
21. **Warner, J. F. and Dennert, G.,** Establishment and cloning of cell lines with natural killer activity in lymphokine-containing media. in *Lymphokines,* Vol. 6, Mizel, S., Ed., Academic Press, New York, 1982, 165.
22. **Klein, M., Roder, J., Haliotis, T., Kores, S., Jett, J. R., Heberman, R. B., Katz, P., and Fauci, A. S.,** Chediak-Higashi gene in humans. II. The selectivity of the defect in natural killer and antibody-dependent and cell-mediated cytotoxicity function, *J. Exp. Med.,* 151, 1049, 1980.
23. **Warner, J. F., and G. Dennert,** Bone marrow graft rejection as a function of antibody-directed natural killer cells, *J. Exp. Med.,* 161, 563, 1985.
24. **Bradley, T. P., and B. Bonavida,** Mechanism of cell mediated cytotoxicity at the single cell level. Natural killing and antibody-dependent cellular cytotoxicity can be mediated by the same human effector cell as determined by the two-target conjugate assay, *J. Immunol.,* 129, 2260, 1982.
25. **Roder, J. C.,** The beige mutation in the mouse. I. A stem cell predetermined impairment in natural killer cell function, *J. Immunol.,* 123, 2168, 1979.
26. **Dennert, G., Anderson, C. G., and Warner, J. F.,** T killer cells play a role in allogeneic bone marrow graft rejection but not in hybrid resistance, *J. Immunol.,* in press.
27. **Schulz, G., Staffileno, L. K., Reisfeld, R. A., and Dennert, G.,** Eradication of established human melanoma tumors in nude mice by antibody-directed effector cells, *J. Exp. Med.,* 161, 1315, 1985.

Chapter 24

CYTOLYTIC T LYMPHOCYTE CLONES IN ANTI-VIRAL IMMUNITY: EFFECTOR FUNCTION IN VIVO AND MECHANISM OF ACTION*

T. J. Braciale, A. E. Lukacher, M. T. Sweetser, and V. L. Braciale

TABLE OF CONTENTS

I.	Introduction	162
II.	Influenza Virus Recognition by Class I MHC Restricted CTL	162
III.	In Vivo Effector Activity of Class I MHC Restricted CTL	163
IV.	Viral Antigen Recognition and In Vivo Effector Activity	166
V.	In Vivo Effector Function of Class II MHC Restricted CTL	168
VI.	Mechanism of CTL Action In Vivo	169
VII.	Discussion and Future Proposals	171
References		172

---

* Supported in part by U.S.P.H.S. grants AI-15608, HL-33391, and AI-15353 and Medical Scientist Training Program Grant 5T32 GM-07200 (A.E.L. and M.T.S.).

I. INTRODUCTION

Both antigen-specific and nonspecific host defense mechanisms play an important role in antiviral immunity.[1] While "nonspecific" cell-mediated effector mechanisms, like natural killer cell lysis, have only recently been appreciated for their inhibitory role in viral infection,[2] a role for virus-specific T lymphocytes in anti-viral immunity has been appreciated for over a decade.[3-5] In most instances, T lymphocytes have been postulated to play a positive role in recovery from experimental viral infection,[5] but in certain circumstances activated virus-specific T lymphocytes have been found to be the primary mediator of pathology.[6] In spite of the wealth of information on T lymphocyte function in viral infection, fundamental questions remain unresolved. Notably, what is the role of T lymphocytes of different subsets as promoters of recovery from infection and as mediators of injury? What is (are) the mechanism by which T lymphocytes eliminate infectious virus and promote recovery in vivo? Is the expression of anti-viral immunity associated with the recognition of particular viral gene products by T lymphocytes? Similarly, do particular viral antigens serve as triggers for immune mediated injury?

Important recent advances in the field of cellular immunology have opened up these and other questions to detailed analysis. Notable among these advances is the development of techniques to isolate, expand, and maintain in continuous culture cloned populations of functional T lymphocytes.[7] In addition to its obvious impact on the elucidation of the T cell receptor,[8,9] this technology has allowed investigators to identify and characterize homogeneous populations of "cytolytic" T lymphocytes (CTL) and "helper" T lymphocytes with precisely defined antigenic specificity.[7] The availability of cloned T lymphocyte populations have allowed the initial characterization of the soluble cytokines produced by T lymphocytes of different functional subsets[10] and the determination of the relationship of effector activity to the expression of T lymphocyte specific cell surface differentiation markers.[11]

In this report we will review studies on T lymphocyte function in anti-viral immunity, emphasizing observations made with cloned virus-specific T lymphocyte populations. For the most part, we will focus on recent results from this laboratory where cloned populations of class I and class II MHC restricted influenza virus-specific T lymphocytes have been used to analyze T lymphocyte function in recovery from lethal murine influenza infection.

II. INFLUENZA VIRUS RECOGNITION BY CLASS I MHC RESTRICTED CTL

Innoculation of mice with infectious type A influenza virus stimulates a vigorous CTL response which shows a high degree of cross-reactivity for type A influenza strains of serologically distinct subtypes.[12-14] There is also heterogeneity in the anti-viral fine specificity of this anti-viral CTL response. The extent of heterogeneity is evident when this response is examined at the clonal level.[15] Table 1 shows the cytolytic specificity in a conventional ^{51}Cr release cytotoxicity assay of two CTL clones of BALB/c (H-2^d) origin directed against the prototype A/JAPAN/57 type A influenza virus strain of the H2N2 virus subtype. Clone A7 shows cross-reactivity for target cells infected with influenza strains of the major human type A influenza subtypes, i.e. H1N2, H2N2, and H3N2, represented in the table by the A/MEL/35, A/JAP/57, and A/HK/68 strains respectively. The broad cross-reactivity of this clone reflects the cross-reactivity observed in the CTL response to type A influenza viruses in vivo in the mouse and the human.[16] Clone A4, on the other hand, shows a narrower range of target cell recognition which is restricted to virus strains of the immunizing H2N2

Table 1
INFLUENZA VIRUS SPECIFICITY OF CTL CLONES

CTL clone	Effector: target ratio[b]	Percent specific ^{51}Cr release from target cells[a]					
		Uninfected	A/JAP/57 (H2N2)	A/AA/67 (H2N2)	A/MEL/35 (H1N1)	A/HK/68 (H3N2)	B/Lee
A4	0.5:1	0	48	35	0	1	0
	1:1	0	66	52	2	2	1
	2:1	0	84	67	2	2	1
A7	0.5:1	0	52	58	57	43	0
	1:1	0	76	76	77	54	0
	2:1	0	85	88	89	62	1

Note: CTL lines were examined for cytotoxic activity on uninfected and infected ^{51}Cr-labeled target cells 5 days after routine subculturing in the presence of 10% TCGF-supplemental medium and A/JAP/57 virus-infected irradiated BALB/c splenocytes.

[a] Values are the means from 4 replicate wells with spontaneous release subtracted. Spontaneous release from all target groups was <13%. SEM are <5% of mean values and are omitted.

[b] One × 10^4 P815 (H-2^d) target cells were added per well.

From Lukacher, A. E., Braciale, V. L., and Braciale, T. J., *J. Exp. Med.*, 160, 814, 1984. With permission of the Rockefeller University Press.

subtype represented in Table 1 by target cells infected with the A/JAP/57 and the A/AA/67 strains. This subtype-specific recognition had also been inferred from cold target inhibition studies carried out with heterogeneous CTL populations generated in vivo.[12,14] Thus, the antigenic specificities defined by CTL clones isolated and maintained in vitro, is reflected in the spectrum of anti-viral specificities of the CTL response in the mouse in vivo. Not surprisingly, CTL with a wide range of anti-viral specificities have been detected at the clonal level.[15-17] As discussed below, CTL specificities can be correlated with the recognition of specific influenza viral polypeptides. Among the issues raised by this heterogeneity in CTL recognition of influenza virus is whether anti-viral effector activity is linked to the expression of a particular viral specificity by the CTL population. This is a question that is readily addressed by analysis with cloned CTL populations.

III. IN VIVO EFFECTOR ACTIVITY OF CLASS I MHC RESTRICTED CTL

T lymphocytes have been postulated to play an important role in recovery from viral infection.[1] In the case of experimental influenza infection, studies by Yap, Ada and co-workers,[18,19] and Wells and co-workers[20] have implicated Thy-1$^+$ Lyt 2$^+$ class I MHC restricted CTL as important mediators of anti-viral immunity. In these studies, influenza immune cell populations enriched for CTL activity could effectively reduce pulmonary virus titers and prolong survival after adoptive transfer of these cells into mice with influenza pneumonia. Since heterogeneous populations of immunocytes were employed in these analyses, the precise role of CTL in eliminating virus could not be determined. This point has been definitively answered by studies with cloned CTL populations.

Lin and Askonas first reported that a cloned population of H-2 restricted influenza specific CTL maintained in continuous in vitro culture in the presence of interleukin-2[21] could, upon in vivo adoptive transfer, reduce pulmonary virus titers and prolong survival of influenza infected mice.[22] This important observation not only directly affirmed that CTL could exhibit an antiviral effect in vivo, but also implied that an antigen-specific T lymphocyte population cultured in vitro for an extended period was functionally active in vivo.

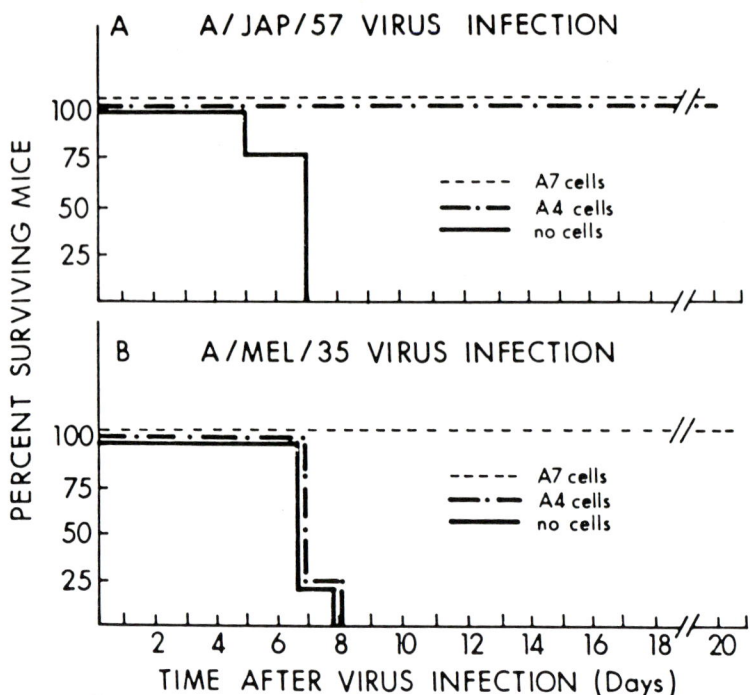

FIGURE 1. Viral antigenic specificity of in vivo anti-viral activity expressed by CTL clones A4 and A7. BALB/c mice were innoculated intranasally with 10 LD_{50} units of A/JAP/57 virus (A) or A/MEL/35 virus (B). Within 1 hr of infection, groups of 4 mice each received either 1×10^7 cells of clone A7 (---), 1×10^7 cells of clone A4 (-·-), or were left untreated (—). Cumulative mortality was tabulated over 20 days. (From Lukacker, A. E., Braciale, V. L., and Braciale, T. J., *J. Exp. Med.*, 160, 814, 1984. With permission of the Rockefeller University Press.)

Although there have been numerous reports of the expression of in vivo functional activity by T lymphocyte clones,[23-25] such success has not been encountered by all investigators.[26,27] Factors ranging from aberrant in vivo trafficking in the vascular compartment of in vitro propagated clones to rapid death of interleukin-2 dependent cloned cells after in vitro transfusion have been implicated as causes for the failure of clones to function in vivo.[26,27] As discussed below, neither aberrant in vivo trafficking nor the interleukin-2 dependence of in vitro cell propagation can fully account for the failure of cloned CTL to express effector function in vivo.

Our studies on the in vivo effector activity of cloned influenza-specific CTL were prompted by a long-term interest in understanding the mechanism of action of CTL in vivo. Our immediate interest was to determine if in vitro propagated CTL clones could, upon in vivo adoptive transfer, alter the outcome of lethal infection and to ascertain if the fine specificity exhibited by a CTL clone in vitro was reflected in its in vivo activity. For this purpose, the H-2^d restricted CTL clones A4 and A7 were infused i.v. into BALB/c mice which had been lethally infected with either A/JAP/57 (H2N2) or A/MEL/35 (H1N1) virus. As Figure 1 demonstrates, control mice lethally infected with A/JAP/57 virus died rapidly. Autopsy revealed massive bilateral pulmonary consolidation consistent with viral pneumonia (not shown). Recipients of either the subtype-specific A4 clone or the cross-reactive A7 clone were protected from A/JAP/57 virus-lethal infection (Figure 1A). In contrast, clone A4, which failed to recognize target cells infected with A/MEL/35 (H1N1) virus in the in vitro cytotoxicity assay (Table 1), also failed to protect mice lethally infected with this H1N1 subtype virus. The type A cross-reactive, A7 clone, on the other hand, effectively protected

Table 2
SPECIFICITY OF PULMONARY VIRUS REDUCTION BY CTL CLONE A4

	Recipients	
Cloned CTL transferred[a]	Virus instilled intranasally[b]	Virus titer in lungs[c]
None	A/JAP/57 (H2N2)	$(1.61 \pm 0.30) \times 10^6$
A4	A/JAP/57	<100
None	A/MEL/35 (H1N1)	$(2.07 \pm 0.52) \times 10^6$
A4	A/MEL/35	$(2.00 \pm 0.45) \times 10^6$

[a] One $\times$ 10^7 of cloned CTL line A4 were injected i.v. into each BALB/c recipient at the same time as virus infection. Control infected mice received 0.5 mℓ medium i.v.

[b] Recipient mice were inoculated i.n. with 10 LD$_{50}$ of the indicated influenza type A virus strain. Virus subtype appears in parentheses.

[c] Expressed as mean PFU/mℓ $\pm$ SEM of lung extracts from three individual mice at day 5 after infection, as assayed by plaque formation on MDCK cell monolayer.

From Lukacher, A. E., Braciale, V. L., and Braciale, T. J., *J. Exp. Med.*, 160, 814, 1984. With permission of the Rockefeller University Press.

Table 3
H-2 RESTRICTION OF RECOVERY MEDIATED BY CLONE A7

	Percent survival of A/JAP-infected recipient mice[a]		
Cells transferred	BALB/c (H-2)^d	C57BL/6 (H-2)^b	C3H/He (H-2)^k
None	0 (<7d)[b]	0 (<9d)	0 (<4d)
A7[c]	100 (>21d)	0 (<8d)	0 (<4d)

[a] Groups of 4 to 6 mice of the indicated strain received 10 LD$_{50}$ units of A/JAP/57 virus i.v. Animals received 10^7 clone A7 cells within 2 hr of lethal injection.

[b] Values in parentheses are the mean survival time in days.

[c] Clone A7 is restricted by H-2L^d.

A/MEL/35 infected mice (Figure 1B). The in vitro protective function of these cloned cells correlated with their capacity to eliminate infectious virus from the lungs of lethally infected recipient mice. As Table 2 demonstrates, clone A4 reduced pulmonary virus titers at day 5 after infection in an antigen-specific manner. This effect on virus titer paralleled the in vitro antigenic specificity of the clone and the specificity of its protective effect in vivo. Recovered mice showed no gross evidence of residual pulmonary pathology when lungs were examined at 21 to 28 days after infection. Thus, these cloned CTL which had been maintained in continuous in vitro culture for up to a year could reduce pulmonary virus titers and promote recovery from lethal infection in a fashion analogous to conventional heterogeneous CTL populations.

Other features of the in vitro effector activity of these virus-specific CTL clones have been examined. The in vivo antiviral effector activity of these clones is H-2 restricted. That is, these H-2^d restricted CTL clones will promote recovery only when adoptively transferred into mice of the H-2^d haplotype (Table 3). Not surprisingly, the size of the cell innoculum required to eliminate infectious virus from the lungs of T cell clone recipients is dependent upon the virus dose administered intranasally. We have been able to protect mice infected with a minimal lethal dose, i.e., 2 LD_{50}, with as little as 1 to 2 × 10^5 cloned CTL cells per recipient. We have not as yet examined virus clearance from the lungs of mice receiving sublethal viral infections, but based on available data, much less than 10^4 transferred cells of a given clone might be anticipated to control infection in sublethally infected mice.

T cell clone proliferation in vivo appears not to be a requisite for effector activity of the class I MHC restricted CTL. In preliminary studies, cloned CTL cells which had received 5000 rads of gamma irradiation could promote recovery from lethal infection. When the minimum cell dose required for recovery was titrated, however, irradiated cells were less efficient per cell than untreated cells (A. Lukacher, unpublished observations). This raises the possibility that clonal proliferation in vivo and/or clonal viability after adoptive transfer may be important factors in recovery. In this connection, preliminary studies on the effect of cloned T cells administered prophylactically indicate that cells can be transferred in vivo 1 week and possibly up to 2 weeks prior to lethal infection and still promote recovery (A. Lukacher and M. Sweetser, unpublished observations). Likewise, we have found that clones can be administered up to 4 days after lethal infection and still promote recovery. The efficiency of these clones in promoting recovery when administered late after infection depends on both the virus dose to infect the recipients and the size of cell innoculum administered.

In most instances, class I MHC restricted Lyt 2^+ CTL clones have been shown to require an exogenous source of IL-2 in order to support their proliferation and continuous cultivation in vitro.[28] Several groups have reported the isolation of class I MHC restricted or class I MHC alloreactive CTL clones[29-31] which can proliferate in response to antigen in the absence of exogenous IL-2. These CTL clones most likely proliferate in response to an antigenic stimulus by an autocrine mechanism where endogenous IL-2 is utilized to drive cellular proliferation in vitro.[32] Although early results of Engers et al.[31] raised the possibility that only these exogenous IL-2 independent CTL clones could exhibit in vivo effector function, this appears not to be the case. In our hands both IL-2 dependent CTL clones like A4 and A7 (Figure 1) and autonomous influenza-specific CTL clones (not shown) can function in vivo to promote recovery from lethal viral infection.

IV. VIRAL ANTIGEN RECOGNITION AND IN VIVO EFFECTOR ACTIVITY

Influenza is a negative-stranded RNA virus with a segmented genome consisting of eight gene segments, each of which encodes at least one viral polypeptide.[33] As mentioned above, early studies on the fine specificity of CTL directed to type A influenza viruses revealed a high degree of cross-reactivity among serologically distinct type A influenza strains at the level of CTL recognition.[12-14] Recently, it has been possible to correlate CTL fine specificity with recognition of specific viral polypeptides, including the virion surface hemagglutinin (HA) glycoprotein[34-36] and the nucleocapsid protein (NP).[36,37] In view of the recent evidence implicating the nucleocapsid protein as an important target antigen for class I MHC restricted CTL in the mouse,[36,37] it was of interest to ascertain if CTL directed to the nucleocapsid protein can exhibit anti-viral activity in vivo. Figure 2 shows an analysis of the in vivo antiviral effect of two cross-reactive CTL clones, A7 and 14-13, after transfer into mice lethally infected with A/JAP/57, A/MEL/35, or the unrelated B/Lee virus. The results indicate that both of these cross-reactive clones can efficiently promote recovery from lethal infection with type A influenza strains of different subtypes. Furthermore, as Table 4 shows, clone 14-13 is directed to nucleocapsid protein as defined by its capacity to recognize target cells infected with a recombinant vaccinia virus expression vector containing the gene for the nucleocapsid protein. Clone A7, on the other hand, fails to recognize either the NP or the HA gene product expressed via the recombinant vaccinia viruses while the protective clone A4 (Figure 1) can be mapped to the hemagglutinin (Table 4). We have now analyzed more

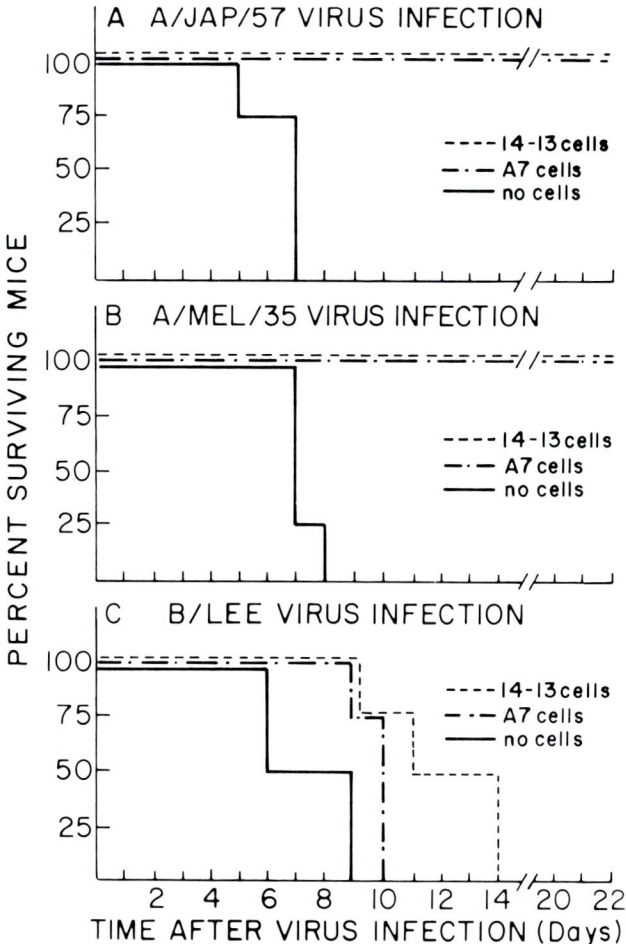

FIGURE 2. Specificity of in vivo anti-viral effector activity of the cross-reactive NP-specific CTL clone 14-13 and the NP-nonreactive CTL clone A7. One × 10^7 cells of either clone 14-13 (---) or clone A7 (-·-) were injected intranasally with 10 LD_{50} units of A/JAP/57 virus (A), A/MEL/35 virus (B) or B/LEE virus (C). Control mice received medium with no cells (—). Cumulative mortality was tabulated over 21 days.

Table 4
RECOGNITION OF DISTINCT INFLUENZA POLYPEPTIDES BY CLONED CTL

CTL clone	Percent specific ^{51}Cr release from indicated infected target cells[a]				
	A/JAP/57	(HA)VV	(NP)VV	VV	B/LEE
14-13	39	2	22	1	7
A7	68	2	1	2	11
A4	44	65	0	1	5

[a] P815 target cells were infected with the indicated influenza strain (A/JAP/57, B/LEE), the parental WR vaccinia virus strain (VV), or with recombinant vaccinia viruses containing the gene for the A/JAP/57 hemagglutinin ((HA)VV) or the gene for the nucleocapsid protein, ((NP) VV). Assay times were 6 hr at an effector to target ratio of 5:1.

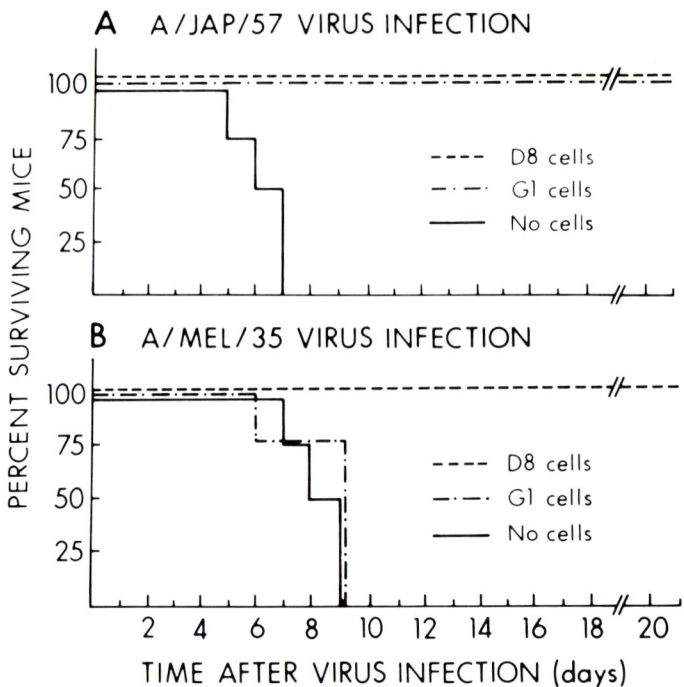

FIGURE 3. Viral antigenic specificity of in vivo antiviral effector activity of class II MHC restricted CTL clones D8 and G1. BALB/c mice were inoculated intranasally with 10 LD_{50} units of either A/JAP/57 virus (A) or A/MEL/35 virus (B). Within 2 hr of infection, groups of 4 mice were injected i.v. with 1×10^7 cells of CTL clone D8 (---) or clone G1 (-··-) or were untreated (—). Cumulative mortality was assessed over 21 days.

than ten CTL clones of differing fine specificity directed to either the HA, NP, or other internal virion polypeptides and restricted by either the H-2K^d, H-2L^d, or H-2D^d locus product. All of these clones can promote recovery after in vivo transfer into lethally infected mice (A. E. Lukacher, manuscript in preparation).

V. IN VIVO EFFECTOR FUNCTION OF CLASS II MHC RESTRICTED CTL

Although CTL with specificity for class II MHC products, i.e., HLA-D locus products in man and H-2I region products in the mouse, have been well documented among alloreactive CTL,[38,39] H-2I/HLA-D region restricted CTL have only recently been documented at the clonal level in the recognition of non-MHC foreign antigens.[40-42] In the influenza system, we have described cloned populations of class II MHC restricted CTL in both mouse[43] and man.[40] In the mouse, these cloned CTL exhibit many of the properties of helper T lymphocytes, including expression of the L3T4 cell surface determinant and the capacity to provide nonspecific help to B lymphocytes upon specific antigenic stimulation.[43]

The finding that I region-restricted virus-specific T lymphocytes could express specific cytolytic activity raised the issue of the role of these T cells in recovery from viral infection. This was of particular interest in view of the observations of Leung and Ada who showed that heterogeneous populations of H-2I region-restricted Lyt-1$^+$2$^-$ influenza-specific effector T lymphocytes would, upon in vivo transfer into influenza infected mice, enhance mortality and pulmonary inflammation.[44] We have begun to analyze the in vivo effector activity of cloned class II MHC restricted CTL. Figure 3 shows the results of an analysis of the in vivo effector activity of CTL clones G1 and D8. Clone G1, which recognizes an epitope shared

Table 5
CLASS I AND CLASS II MHC RESTRICTED CTL CLONES RELEASE IFN

	Culture supernatant[a]		Titer
CTL clone	MHC restricted	Antigen	IFN released[b]
none	—	−	0
		+	0
A4	Class I	−	0
		+	126
A7	Class I	−	0
		+	100
D8	Class II	−	0
		+	316
G1	Class II	−	0
		+	126

[a] 48 hr supernatants were harvested from co-cultures of cells of the indicated CTL cloned line with irradiated uninfected (−) or A/JAP/57 virus-infected (+) A20-1.11 cells.

[b] Values are the reciprocal of the dilution of culture supernatant which provided 50% inhibition of cytopathic effect of VSV on L929 cells.

by HA of the H2 subtype and is restricted by I-E^d,[43] efficiently promotes recovery of T cell clone recipients from lethal infection with A/JAP/57 virus. Clone D8 exhibits cross-reactivity for both A/JAP/57 infected and A/MEL/35 infected target cells and is restricted by I-A^d in target cell recognition. This CTL clone promotes recovery from lethal infection with either A/JAP/57 or A/MEL/35 virus. A limited analysis of the in vivo activity of several other I-region restricted CTL clones also suggests that they act to promote recovery from viral infection.

VI. MECHANISM OF CTL ACTION IN VIVO

Cloned populations of antigen-specific T lymphocytes have been shown to release a variety of lymphokines[10] among which interferon-γ would be expected to play an important role in halting the spread of viral infection. Askonas and co-workers[45] first reported that interferon-γ is released by a cloned influenza virus specific class I MHC restricted CTL during the process of target cell recognition and lysis in vitro. Comparable findings have been reported by other investigators.[46]

We have examined a panel of virus-specific CTL clones for interferon-γ production in response to antigenic stimulation. As Table 5 shows, both class I MHC restricted clones (A4,A7) and class II MHC restricted CTL clones (G1,D8) can produce interferon-γ after stimulation with influenza-treated splenocyte stimulators. Both class I and class II MHC restricted CTL clones can induce footpad swelling in an antigen-specific fashion when introduced with virus locally in the footpads (Table 6). Induction of footpad swelling and other manifestations of delayed-type hypersensitivity have been previously reported both for class I and class II MHC restricted T lympocytes after local or systemic cell transfer.[5]

The fact that these cloned CTL populations can release soluble immune effector molecules raises the important issue of the mechanism by which these effector T lymphocytes exert their anti-viral effect in vivo. Available evidence suggests that the induction of effector activity by these T cells is antigen specific.[43] If in vivo effector activity is orchestrated by soluble lymphokines released after antigenic stimulation at sites of infection, then the expression of in vivo effector activity might be nonspecific. On the other hand, if in vivo effector

Table 6
CLASS I AND CLASS II MHC RESTRICTED CTL CLONES INDUCE LOCAL DTH REACTIONS[a]

Cloned CTL cells transferred[b]	Injection into footpad	Mean increase in footpad thickness (%)[c]
None	Virus	1.0 ± 0.6
A4	Cells	0
	Cells + virus	12.2 ± 0.6
A7	Cells	2.5 ± 2.5
	Cells + virus	14.3 ± 1.2
D8	Cells	0
	Cells + virus	29.7 ± 1.0
G1	Cells	0
	Cells + virus	17.4 ± 1.3

[a] Groups of three BALB/c mice were injected into the right hind footpad with cloned CTL cells (2 × 10^6 cells), A/JAP/57 virus (250 HAU), or a mixture of cloned CTL cells and virus in a total volume of 50 $\mu\ell$. The left hind footpad was injected with 50 $\mu\ell$ PBS only. Footpad thickness was measured 24 hr after injection.

[b] H-2 restriction by proliferation and by recognition of L cell transfectants expressing MHC gene products mapped restriction of clone A4 by K^d, clone A7 by L^d, and clones D8 and G1 by $I-E^d$.

[c] Values represent the percentage mean increase in footpad thickness, as calculated from the formula [right (experimental) — left (control) footpad]/left footpad ± SEM.

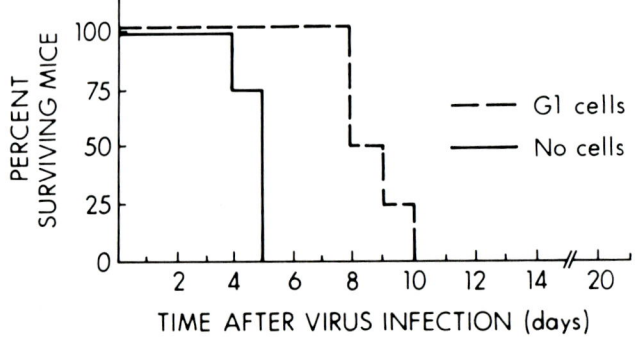

FIGURE 4. *In vivo* anti-viral effector activity of the class II MHC restricted CTL clone G1 in mice infected simultaneously with virus strains of two different type A influenza virus subtypes. One × 10^7 cells of CTL clone G1 (---) were injected i.v. into four BALB/c mice intranasally infected simultaneously with 10 LD_{50} units of A/JAP/57 virus and 10 LD_{50} units of A/MEL/35 virus. Control infected mice received no cells (—). Cumulative mortality was assessed over 21 days.

activity is mediated by a highly focused mechanism like direct lysis of infected cells, then these CTL would be highly specific both at the level of induction and expression of in vivo effector activity. To distinguish between these possibilities, mice were simultaneously infected with lethal doses of the antigenically distinct A/JAP/57 and A/MEL/35 viruses and transfused with a CTL clone specific for only one of the two viruses. As shown for the A/JAP/57 HA specific, I-region restricted CTL clone G1 (Figure 4) dually infected recipients of this T cell clone did not recover and died of overwhelming influenza infection. Examination of lungs of companion mice at day 5 post infection (Table 7) revealed that the transferred clone had markedly decreased the titer of A/JAP/57 virus in the lungs of T cell clone recipients. The titer of the unrecognized A/MEL/35 virus in the lungs of these mice was

Table 7
SPECIFICITY OF PULMONARY VIRUS REDUCTION BY CLASS II MHC RESTRICTED CTL CLONE G1

	Recipients[a]	
CTL clone transferred	Virus instilled intranasally[b]	Virus titer in lungs[c]
None	A/JAP/57 (H2N2)	$(1.2 \pm 0.2) \times 10^6$
G1	A/JAP/57	$(1.3 \pm 0.5) \times 10^3$
None	A/MEL/35 (H1N1)	$(3.6 \pm 0.2) \times 10^6$
G1	A/MEL/35	$(2.8 \pm 0.3) \times 10^6$

[a] 1×10^7 cells of CTL clone G1 were injected i.v. into each BALB/c recipient at the same time as virus infection. Control infected mice received 0.5 mℓ medium i.v.

[b] Recipient mice were inoculated intranasally with 10 LD_{50} of the indicated type A influenza virus strain. Subtype of virus strains appears in parentheses.

[c] Expressed as mean (PFU $\pm$ SEM)/mℓ of lung extracts from three individual mice at day 5 after infection as assayed by plaque formation on MDCK cell monolayers (Materials and Methods).

comparable to that of dually infected control mice. Thus, this A/JAP/57 specific I-region restricted CTL clone could efficiently eliminate A/JAP/57 virus from the lungs of these dually infected mice in the face of overwhelming infection with the A/MEL/35 virus. Similar results have been recently reported by us for class I MHC restricted murine CTL clones specific for type A influenza viruses.[47]

VII. DISCUSSION AND FUTURE PROPOSALS

This report has focused on recent studies from this laboratory dealing with the expression of in vivo effector activity by cloned virus specific-T lymphocyte populations maintained in long-term in vitro culture. It is evident from our studies and from the work of many other laboratories that these cloned T lymphocytes can function in vivo in an antigen-specific fashion and carry out a variety of efferent immune functions associated with T lymphocytes. These findings suggest that cloned continuous cell lines may be an important in vitro paradigm for the analysis of normal T lymphocyte function in vivo.

Our studies to date suggest that CTL with a range of different antigenic specificities can express in vivo effector activity in an antigen-specific manner. More importantly, CTL directed to molecules as diverse as the membrane-anchored influenza HA glycoprotein and the "soluble" nonglycosylated NP antigen can be triggered in vivo by these antigens to express anti-viral effector function. This point is particularly intriguing in light of recent evidence that H-2 K/D restricted NP-specific CTL might recognize processed forms, i.e., fragments, of the NP gene product expressed at the infected cell surface.[48] We, likewise, have recently reported[49] that class II MHC restricted, HA-specific CTL clones like G1 do not recognize the newly synthesized HA expressed on the infected cell surface, but rather recognize a processed form of the HA molecules introduced exogenously into target cells from the infectious virion inoculum. In spite of the apparent failure of these class II MHC restricted T lymphocytes to recognize newly synthesized viral polypeptides on the infected cell surface, the T cells efficiently eliminate virus from infected tissue (Table 7).

Recent studies have emphasized the importance of cytolytic granules in the expression of lytic activity by CTL.[50,51] Similarly, there is now evidence suggesting that CTL recognition of target cells is associated with an asymmetric redistribution of the CTL cytoplasmic organelles (and possibly membrane constituents).[52] Also, recent data indicates that engagement of the T lymphocyte receptor by antigen is sufficient to activate the CTL for target cytolysis without any need in the killing process on the target cell for direct recognition by the T cell receptor of membrane bound antigen.[53,54] These findings are beginning to reshape our view of the CTL-target cell interaction.

Our evidence from the adoptive transfer of CTL clones does suggest that these T cells mediate in vivo effector activity in a highly specific fashion. This most likely reflects direct cytolysis by these CTL clones in vivo. We cannot as yet rule out labile lymphokines, released by the T cells after specific antigenic stimulation, as the in vivo mediators of anti-viral activity. Of necessity these lymphokines would have to operate over an extremely short distance to account for our observations on the specificity of the in vivo effector activity of the CTL clones (Figure 4).[47] With the recent revelations on the mechanism of CTL killing[50,51] and the role of the T cell receptor in the killing process,[53,54] the arguments on the role of direct cytolysis vs. soluble lymphokines in CTL function in vivo may be reduced to semantic rather than mechanistic concerns.

Undoubtedly, the most exciting and important prospect raised by our findings and the results of many other investigators is the possibility that cloned continuous populations of human effector T lymphocytes could serve as therapeutic modalities in a clinical setting. The routine application of cloned T lymphocyte populations in the treatment of viral infections, malignancies, or disorders of immune regulation remains in the future. Studies carried out in model systems, such as influenza infection of mice, should provide a rational framework for such future studies.

REFERENCES

1. **Mim, C. A. and White, D. O.**, Viral Pathogenesis and Immunology, Blackwell Scientific, Oxford, 1984.
2. **Bukowski, J. F., Warner, J. F., Dennert, G., and Welsh, R. M.**, Adoptive transfer studies demonstrating the antiviral effect of natural killer cells in vivo, *J. Exp. Med.*, 161, 40, 1985.
3. **Blanden, R. V.**, T Cell response to viral and bacterial infection, *Transplant Rev.*, 19, 56, 1974.
4. **Doherty, P. C., Blanden, R. V., and Zinkernagel, R. M.**, Specificity of virus-immune effector T cells for H-2K or H-2D compatible interactions: Implications for H-antigen diversity, *Transplant Rev.*, 29, 89, 1976.
5. **Zinkernagel, R. M. and Doherty, P. C.**, MHC-restricted cytotoxic T cells: studies on the biological role of polymorphic major transplantation antigens determining T-cell restriction specificity function and responsiveness, *Adv. Immunol.*, 27, 51, 1979.
6. **Buchmeier, M. J., Welsh, R. M., Dutko, F. J., et al.**, The virology and immunobiology of lymphocytic choriomenigitis virus infection, *Adv. Immunol.*, 30, 275, 1980.
7. **Fathman, C. G. and Fitch, F. W., Eds.**, Isolation characterization and utilization of T lymphocytes, Academic Press, New York, 1982.
8. **Haskins, K., Kappler, J., and Marrack, P.**, The major histocompatability complex restricted antigen receptor on T cells, *Ann. Rev. Immunol.*, 2, 51, 1984.
9. **Meuer, S. C., Acuto, O., Hercend, T., Schlossmann, S. F., and Reinherz, E. L.**, The human T cell receptor, *Ann. Rev. Immunol.*, 2, 23, 1984.
10. **Prystowsky, M. B., Ely, J. M., Beller, D. I., Eisenberg, L., Goldman, J., Goldman, M., Goldwasser, E., Ihle, J., Quintans, J., Remold, H., Vogel, S. N., and Fitch, F. W.**, Alloreactive cloned T cell lines, *J. Immunol.*, 129, 2337, 1982.
11. **Swain, S. L.**, T cell subsets and the recognition of MHC class, *Immunol. Rev.*, 74, 129, 1983.
12. **Effros, R. B., Doherty, P. C., Gerhard, W., and Bennink, J.**, Generation of both cross-reactive and virus specific T cell populations after immunization with serologically distinct influenza A viruses, *J. Exp. Med.*, 145, 557, 1977.
13. **Zweerink, H. J., Courtneidge, S. A., Skehel, J. J., Crumpton, M. J., and Askonas, B. A.**, Cytotoxic T cells kill influenza virus-infected cells but do not distinguish between serologically distinct type A virus, *Nature (London)*, 267, 354, 1977.

14. **Braciale, T. J.**, Immunologic recognition of influenza virus-infected cells. I. Generation of a virus strain-specific and cross-reactive subpopulation of cytotoxic T cells in the response of type A influenza viruses of different subtypes, *Cell. Immunol.*, 33, 423, 1977.
15. **Braciale, T. J., Andrew, M. E., and Braciale, V. L.**, Heterogeneity and specificity of clone lines of influenza-virus-specific cytotoxic T lymphocytes, *J. Exp. Med.*, 153, 910, 1981.
16. **Townsend, A. R. M. and McMichael, A. J.**, Specificity of cytotoxic T lymphocytes stimulated with influenza virus. Studies in mice and humans, *Prog. Allergy*, 36, 10, 1985.
17. **Braciale, T. J., Lukacher, A. E., Morrison, L., Braciale, V. L., Smith, G., Moss, B., Gething, M.-J., and Sambrook, J.**, Influenza virus antigen recognition by class I and class II MHC restricted cytolytic T lymphocytes, in *Options for the Control of Influenza. UCLA Symposia on Molecular and Cellular Biology, New Series*, Vol. 36, Kendal, A. P. and Patriarca, P. A., Eds., Alan R. Liss, New York, 1986.
18. **Yap, K. L., Ada, G. L., and McKenzie, I. F. C.**, Transfer of specific cytotoxic T lymphocytes protects mice infected with influenza virus, *Nature (London)*, 273, 238, 1978.
19. **Ada, G. L., Leung, K. N., and Ertl, H.**, An analysis of effector T cell generation and function in mice exposed to influenza A or Sendai virus, *Immunol. Rev.*, 58, 5, 1981.
20. **Wells, M. A., Ennis, F. A., and Albrecht, P.**, Recovery from a viral respiratory tract infection II. Passive transfer of immune spleen cells to mice with influenza pneummonia, *J. Immunol.*, 126, 1042, 1981.
21. **Lin, L.-Y. and Askonas, B. A.**, Cross-reactivity for different type A influenza viruses of a cloned T killer cell line, *Nature (London)*, 288, 164, 1980.
22. **Lin, L.-Y. and Askonas, B. A.**, Biological properties of an influenza A virus specific killer T cell clone, *J. Exp. Med.*, 154, 225, 1981.
23. **Byrne, J. A. and Oldstone, M. B. A.**, Biology of cloned cytotoxic T lymphocytes specific for lymphocyte choriomeningitis virus: clearance of virus in vivo, *J. Virol.*, 51, 682, 1984.
24. **Sethi, K. K., Omata, Y., and Schneweis, K. E.**, Protection of mice from fatal herpes simplex virus type I infection by adoptive transfer of cloned virus-specific and H-2-restricted cytotoxic T lymphocytes, *J. Gen. Virol.*, 64, 443, 1983.
25. **Engers, H. D., Glasebrook, A. L., and Sorenson, G. D.**, Allogeneic tumor rejection induced by the intravenous injection of Lyt 2^+ cytolytic T lymphocyte clones, *J. Exp. Med.*, 156, 1280, 1982.
26. **Daily, M. O., Fathman, G. C., Butcher, E. G., Pillemer, E., and Weissman, I.**, Abnormal migration of T lymphocyte clones, *J. Immunol.*, 128, 2126, 1982.
27. **Taylor, D. A. and Askonas, B. A.**, Diversity in the biological properties of anti influenza cytotoxic T cell clones, *Eur. J. Immunol.*, 13, 707, 1985.
28. **Andrew, M. E. and Braciale, T. J.**, Antigen-dependent proliferation of cloned continuous lines of H-2 restricted influenza virus-specific cytotoxic T lymphocytes, *J. Immunol.*, 127, 1201, 1981.
29. **Widmer, M. B. and Bach, F. H.**, Antigen-driven helper cell independent cloned cytolytic T lymphocytes, *Nature (London)*, 294, 750, 1981.
30. **Glasebrook, A. L., Kelso, A., and MacDonald, H. R.**, Cytolytic T lymphocyte clones that proliferate autonomously to specific alloantigenic stimulation, *J. Immunol.*, 130, 1545, 1983.
31. **Engers, H. D., Lahaye, T., Sorenson, G. D., Glasebrook, A. L., Horvath, C., and Brunner, K. T.**, Functional activity in vivo of effector 1 cell populations, *J. Immunol.*, 133, 1665, 1984.
32. **Smith, K. A. and Cantrell, D. A.**, Interleukin 2 regulates its own receptors, *Proc. Natl. Acad. Sci. U.S.A.*, 82, 864, 1985.
33. **Lamb, R. A.**, The influenza virus RNA segments and their encoded proteins, in *Genetics of Influenza Viruses*, Palese, P. and Kingsbury, D. W., Eds., Springer, New York, 1983, 21.
34. **Braciale, T. J., Braciale, V. L., Henkel, T. J., Sambrook, J., and Gething, M. J.**, Cytotoxic T lymphocyte recognition of the influenza hemagglutinin gene product expressed by DNA-mediated gene transfer, *J. Exp. Med.*, 159, 341, 1984.
35. **Bennink, J., Yewdell, J. W., Smith, G. L., Moller, C., and Moss, B.**, Recombinant vaccinia virus primes and stimulates influenza hemagglutinin specific cytotoxic T cells, *Nature (London)*, 311, 578, 1984.
36. **Townsend, A. R. M., McMichael, A. J., Carter, M. P., Huddleston, J. A., and Brownlee, G. G.**, Cytotoxic T cell recognition of the influenza nucleoprotein and hemagglutinin expressed in transfected L cells, *Cell*, 39, 13, 1984.
37. **Yewdell, J. W., Bennink, J. R., Smith, G. L., and Moss, B.**, Influenza A virus nucleoprotein is a major target antigen for cross-reactive anti-influenza A virus cytotoxic T lymphocytes, *Proc. Natl. Acad. Sci. U.S.A.*, 1982, 1785, 1985.
38. **Feighery, C. and Stastny, P.**, HLA-D region associated determinants serve as targets for human cell-mediated lysis, *J. Exp. Med.*, 149, 485, 1979.
39. **Wagner, H., Starzinski-Powitz, A., Jung, H., and Rollinghoff, M.**, Induction of I region-restricted hapten-specific cytotoxic T lymphocytes, *J. Immunol.*, 119, 1365, 1977.
40. **Kaplan, D. R., Griffith, R., Braciale, V. L., and Braciale, T. J.**, Influenza virus-specific human cytotoxic T cell clones: heterogeneity in antigenic specificity and restriction by class II MHC products, *Cell. Immunol.*, 88, 193, 1984.

41. **Yasukawa, M. and Zarling, J. M.,** Human cytotoxic T cell clones directed against herpes simplex virus-infected cells. I. Lysis restricted by HLA class II MB and DR antigens, *J. Immunol.,* 133, 422, 1984.
42. **Jacobson, S., Richert, J. R., Biddison, W. E., Satinsky, A., Hartzman, R. J., and McFarland, H. F.,** Measles virus-specific T4$^+$ human cytotoxic T cell clones are restricted by class II HLA antigens, *J. Immunol.,* 133, 754, 1984.
43. **Lukacher, A. E., Morrison, L. A., Braciale, V. L., Malissen, B., and Braciale, T. J.,** Expression of specific cytolytic activity by H-2I region restricted influenza virus specific T lymphocyte clones, *J. Exp. Med.,* 162, 171, 1985.
44. **Leung, K. N. and Ada, G. L.,** Different functions of subsets of effector T cells in murine influenza virus infection, *Cell. Immunol.,* 67, 312, 1982.
45. **Morris, A. G., Lin, Y.-L. and Askonas, B. A.,** Immune interferon release when a cloned cytotoxic T cell line meets its correct influenza-infected target cell, *Nature (London),* 295, 150, 1982.
46. **Klein, J. R., Raulet, D. H., Pasternack, M. S., and Bevan, M. J.,** Cytolytic T lymphocytes produce immune interferon in response to antigen or mitogen, *J. Exp. Med.,* 155, 1198, 1982.
47. **Lukacher, A. E., Braciale, V. L., and Braciale, T. J.,** In vivo effector function of influenza virus-specific cytotoxic T lymphocyte clones is highly specific, *J. Exp. Med.,* 160, 814, 1984.
48. **Townsend, A. R. M., Gotch, F. M., and Davey, J.,** Cytotoxic T cells recognize fragments of the influenza nucleoprotein, *Cell,* 42, 457, 1985.
49. **Morrison, L. A., Lukacher, A. E., Braciale, V. L., Fan, D. P., and Braciale, T. J.,** Differences in viral antigen recognition by MHC class I and class II influenza virus specific CTL clones, *J. Exp. Med.,* 163, 903, 1986.
50. **Podack, E. R. and Konigsberg, P. J.,** Cytolytic T cell granules. Isolation structural biochemical and functional characterization, *J. Exp. Med.,* 160, 695, 1984.
51. **Henkart, P. A., Millard, P. J., Reynolds, C. W., and Henkart, M. D.,** Cytolytic activity of purified cytoplasmic granules from cytotoxic rat large granular lymphocyte tumors, *J. Exp. Med.,* 160, 75, 1984.
52. **Kupfer, A., Singer, S. J., and Dennert, G.,** On the mechanism of unidirectional killing in mixtures of two cytotoxic T lymphocytes, *J. Exp. Med.,* 163, 489, 1986.
53. **Lanzavecchia, A.,** Is the T-cell receptor involved in T-cell killing? *Nature (London),* 319, 778, 1986.
54. **Staerz, U. D. and Bevan, M. J.,** Cytotoxic T lymphocyte-mediated lysis via the F^c receptor of target cells, *Eur. J. Immunol.,* 15, 1172, 1985.

Chapter 25

INTERLEUKIN-2 ACTIVATED CYTOTOXIC LYMPHOCYTES (LAK CELLS) AS ANTIGEN NONSPECIFIC AMPLIFIERS OF THE IMMUNE RESPONSE: GENERAL CHARACTERISTICS AND CONSIDERATIONS FOR CANCER THERAPY

Elizabeth Ann Grimm

TABLE OF CONTENTS

I. Introduction 176

II. Methods Employed are Designed to Approximate In Vivo Conditions 176

III. LAK Activation and Maintenance Characteristics 177
    A. IL-2 Alone Directly Activates LAK 177
    B. No Accessory Requirements are Obvious for LAK Activation 178
    C. Presence of Tumor During Activation Can Be Inhibitory 179
    D. LAK Activation is Inhibited by Hydrocortisone, but Not Cyclosporine 179

IV. Specificity of LAK Lysis is Broad and Not Limited to Tumors 180
    A. Autologous and Allogeneic Tumors are Lysed Comparably by LAK and LAK Clones 180
    B. Human Oncogen-Transfected 3T3 Cells are Lysed by LAK 181
    C. Hapten Modification Confers LAK Sensitivity on Resistant PBL 182
    D. LAK Recognition of Target Cells Requires a Trypsin-Sensitive Protein 182

V. Relationship of LAK to Other Cytolytic Lymphocyte Systems 183
    A. The LAK Phenomenon is Unique 183
    B. LAK Precursor Cells are Not Well-Defined 185
    C. LAK Effectors are Heterogeneous 186

VI. Therapeutic Potential of LAK 187
    A. Studies in Progress 187
    B. Advantages and Disadvantages of the Current Approach 188
    C. Future Prospects 188

VII. Summary and Conclusions 188

References 189

I. INTRODUCTION

In 1982, the term lymphokine-activated killer (LAK) phenomenon was coined to describe a novel lymphocytotoxic system with many apparent characteristics distinct from the previously accepted natural killer (NK) and cytotoxic T lymphocyte (CTL) cells.[1] LAK were defined as interleukin-2 (IL-2) activated cytotoxic cells capable of lysing NK-resistant fresh human tumors.[2-4] The rapid acceptance of this system by the immunologic community was due in part to its easily reproducible methodology, but also because of previously reported compelling evidence for existence of a third distinct lymphocytotoxic system. Some of the names used previously are activated killers, activated NK cells, anomolous killers, and promiscuous killer cells (reviewed in Reference 1). The prior unavailability of purified IL-2 combined with the widespread use of cultured tumor, rather than fresh, unknowingly complicated a prior clearer understanding of such systems.

Initially, LAK was perceived as an in vitro artefact of nonspecific effectors contaminating specific CTL populations and causing a major problem in interpretation of specificity results when tumors[5-11] or modified self targets[12-14] were employed. It is now realized that LAK activation can occur during any immune response in which the lymphokine cascade leads to abundant IL-2 production. LAK activity is undetected unless tumor or altered self target cells are employed as LAK do not lyse autologous or allogeneic normal targets (as can specifically sensitized CTL).

The current interest in the LAK system is due mainly to its tumor killing ability, but secondarily, to the current availability of purified recombinant interleukin-2 (rIL-2).[15] IL-2 is a 15,000 Dalton glycoprotein secreted by helper T lymphocytes in response to various immunologic stimuli such as bacteria, alloantigens, and mitogenic lectins.[16] The primary role for IL-2 is that of a growth factor[17] (IL-2 was originally designated T-cell growth factor or TCGF), and is the obligatory second signal responsible for clonal expansion of antigen primed lymphocytes.[18] Because we had found that human IL-2 would synergize with non-immunogenic antigen (U V - or heat-killed allogeneic stimulator cells) to produce optimally competent allospecific CTL in vitro, we tested whether IL-2 would augment the sensitization to autologous fresh tumor cells.[2,16] In these experiments, the negative control of human lymphocytes (PBL) plus IL-2 (in the absence of tumor stimulators) unexpectedly generated a very potent anti-tumor cytotoxic response. This cytotoxicity generated by culture of purified IL-2 and PBL alone in culture was hence named the lymphokine-activated killer cell (LAK) phenomenon.

As will be reviewed, LAK are distinct based on a variety of characteristics including kinetics of activation, target cell specificity, stimulus responsible for activation, phenotype of precursor and effector cells, and specifity of lysis directed toward fresh autologous and allogeneic tumor cells (sarcoma, melanoma, adenocarcinoma, glioma, lymphoma) and for modified self (TNP-PBL) in short term 51-chromium release assays. Murine adoptive immunotherapy models have proven that injection of LAK alone[19-21] or LAK with extra IL-2[21-25] substantially reduce or eliminate established tumors. Based on those findings, a number of clinical trials designed to test the safety and eventual efficacy of human LAK are in progress.

The purpose of this chapter is to briefly review pertinent aspects of the human LAK system, and to summarize new data concerning the potential biological role in the treatment of cancer and other human diseases.

II. METHODS EMPLOYED ARE DESIGNED TO APPROXIMATE IN VIVO CONDITIONS

The laboratory methods used to generate and to test LAK activity are critical to interpretation of results. Although our methods have been described in detail previously,[1,2,26,27] the salient aspects are reviewed. LAK can be generated from any sample of lymphoid tissue, including PBL from either normal or cancer patients, thoracic duct lymphocytes, cord blood lymphocytes, lymph node, spleen, thymus, bone marrow, and tumor infiltrating lymphocytes. Neither macrophages, mature T cells, NK cells, nor B cells appear to be required in the precursor population. By current criteria, LAK can develop from immature null cells which are found in the bone marrow. The responding cells are suspended in RPMI 1640 culture medium containing either human AB serum, autologous serum, or serum free substitutes. Optimal activation occurs when lymphocytes are cultured at 1 to 2×10^6 per mℓ. The only required culture additive is IL-2, with purified IL-2 being preferable. Our recent work has used IL-2 derived from delectinated TCGF (Cellular Products Inc., Buffalo, NY) or recombinant IL-2 (Cetus Corporation, Emeryville, CA).

Incubation of the lymphocytes and IL-2 is required for at least 48 hr at 37°C for LAK to develop. The culture contents are then harvested, washed, and used as effectors in a 4 hr 51-chromium release assay. Human LAK kill NK sensitive and resistant human and murine tumor cells. Fresh tumor target cells are obtained either by gentle mechanical dissociation (for glioma tumors) or by digestion in a mixture of enzymes (collagenase, hyaluronidase, and DNase) designed to dissociate the intercellular matrix. The resulting viable tumor cells are then washed, purified from infiltrating contaminants such as adherent lymphoid or myloid cells, and cryopreserved in human serum containing 10% DMSO until needed. For LAK target testing, an aliquot of freshly thawed tumor is labeled with chromium and used immediately. Either fresh sarcoma, glioma, or the NK resistant Daudi line were used as targets for experiments reported in this review. While the methods for production and testing of LAK are relatively simple, they are critical. The use of cultured tumor cells is to be avoided unless thoroughly characterized as to NK sensitivity. Additionally, we believe that the use of human serum and fresh (noncultured) tumor aids in viewing the potential application of LAK in vivo.

III. LAK ACTIVATION AND MAINTENANCE CHARACTERISTICS

A. IL-2 Alone Directly Activates LAK

From the viewpoint of classical immunology, the characteristics of LAK activation are enigmatic. Naive lymphocytes respond directly to IL-2 in the absence of any known antigenic exposure.[4] As will be shown, activation can be performed in serum-free medium and using lymphocytes from human cord blood or bone marrow. Activation is relatively rapid, requiring only 2 to 3 days in vitro, but it is clearly the result of differentiation and proliferation because of its sensitivity to either mitomycin C pretreatment or irradiation of the responder cells.[2,14] LAK do not derive from previously primed (memory) CTL as shown by a different serologic phenotype.[3] Purified recombinant IL-2 is sufficient for LAK activation; however, under some circumstances interferon gamma can augment this activation.[28] The precursors do not appear to express high affinity receptors for IL-2 by either direct binding experiments or as evidenced by their lack of expression of the Tac antigen.[2] The current evidence suggests an interaction with the newly described p75, or alpha chain of the receptor complex.[59-62] Thus, p75 is expressed alone on fresh PBL (see ''Additional References'' for details), and alone is responsible for LAK activation.[59-63] As reported previously,[2] IL-2 receptors as identified by the Tac antigen do appear later during LAK activation in parallel with the expression of cytotoxic activity. Our current hypothesis is that the hydrophobic IL-2 molecule causes a perturbation of the responder lymphocyte membrane which activates secondary signals leading to the expression of the cytotoxic activity.

The quantity of IL-2 needed for LAK activation is in the nanomolar range.[14] Titrations of the Cetus recombinant IL-2 consistently showed that 100 units per mℓ was optimal, with

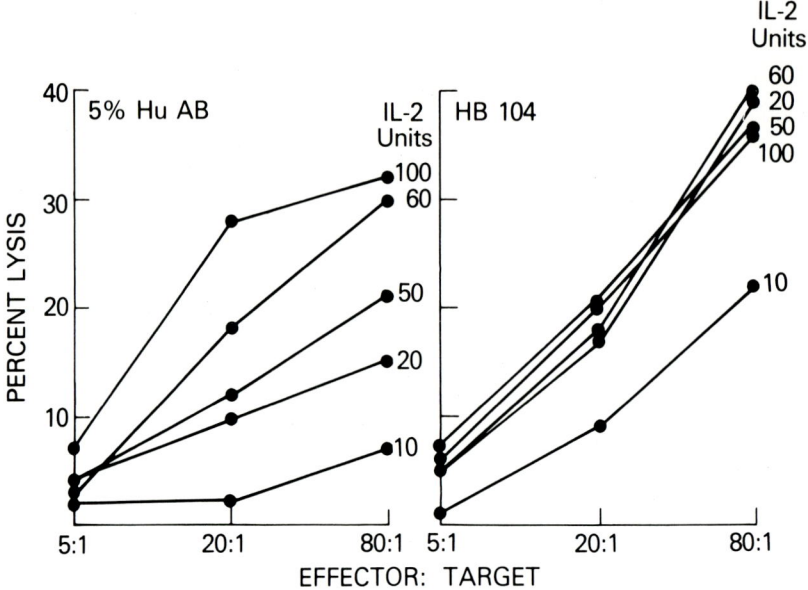

FIGURE 1. LAK activation occurs optimally using serum free medium. PBL were cultured in either standard CM containing 5% human AB serum or in the serum substitute medium, HB104, with varying concentrations of IL-2. Four days later, the culture contents from each flask were harvested and tested for lysis of a fresh sarcoma target.

no further increase nor any decrease of LAK activity at higher concentrations. This unitage is equivalent to 6.7 nanamolar using standard 5% serum supplemented medium, or 5 BRMP interim standard units.

The actual quantity of IL-2 needed to directly interact with the LAK precursors appears to be at least 5-fold less than described above. Recently we identified a serum-free medium substitute (HB104, Hana Biologicals, Inc., New England Nuclear, Boston, MA) which supports both activation and long term maintenance of the LAK. When IL-2 units were titrated using the HB104 medium, in comparison to our standard 5% serum-containing medium, it was consistently found that at least 5-fold less IL-2 was optimal (Figure 1). Therefore, 1 or 2 nanomolar is probably saturating for LAK precursor activation. The proven ability to use serum substitutes will be a great help in future clinical studies in which serum components are best avoided.

B. No Accessory Requirements are Obvious for LAK Activation

There is no known requirement for cell-cell interaction during LAK activation. Neither T helper cells nor adherent cells have been found to be necessary.[3] Additionally, the rapid kinetics of activation would argue against secondary interactions. Because we and others have been unable to detect LAK in PBL after injection of IL-2 i.v.(it has been reported that LAK can be found in other lymphoid organs after Il-2 exposure[31,32]), a series of studies to approximate conditions that might occur in the peripheral blood were performed. One consistent observation is that movement of the culture flask contents by rocking had a significant inhibitory effect (Figure 2). Our current interpretation of these results is that the cell movement probably disrupts the IL-2 and membrane interaction. There is no obligatory role for plastic, as LAK can be activated on agarose, glass, siliconized glass, or fibronectin equally well (unpublished).

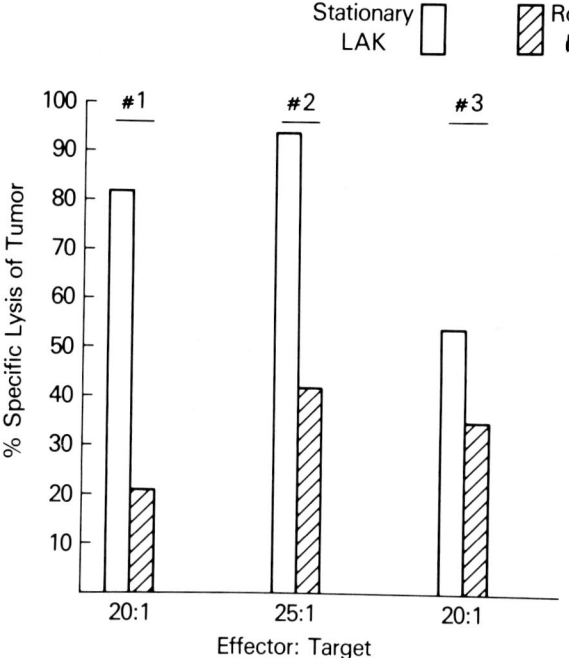

FIGURE 2. Rocking of cultures inhibits LAK activation. In 3 of 3 experiments shown, LAK activation cultures were prepared in duplicate, with one set stationary and the second set placed vertically on a rocker platform (10 to 30 revs/min). The flasks were maintained in either the stationary or rocking conditions for 3 days, after which contents were harvested and tested for lysis of tumor.

C. Presence of Tumor During Activation Can Be Inhibitory

Injection of IL-2 directly into tumor sites has been shown in animal models to be successful to reducing tumor[33] and resulting in a state of immunity.[1,34] To determine whether LAK could be generated in such a milieu, we tested the effects of tumor presence on LAK activation as a function of IL-2 concentration. Table 1 indicates that with either cultured glioma or fresh human sarcoma tumors, LAK activation was considerably suppressed. Many human tumors are known to secrete immunosuppressive factors, which can inhibit LAK activation.[35-37] Even at 500 units per mℓ of IL-2, we were unable to generate optimal LAK at a 100 to 1 lymphocyte to tumor ratio with either type of tumor cell included in the culture. If LAK activation in vivo at the tumor site is to be considered as a therapeutic option, then the lymphocytes and IL-2 must be available in excessive quantities in relation to the number of tumor cells, or tumors must not be as immunosuppressive as those we tested. However, once activated, these LAK can be maintained in the presence of activation-suppressive tumor cells at very high tumor to LAK ratios as reported previously.[37]

D. LAK Activation is Inhibited by Hydrocortisone, but Not Cyclosporine

Because we have been successful in activating patients' PBL even after extensive chemotherapy, it was of interest to us to define what effect known immunosuppressive drugs would cause. Our recent results showed that LAK activation is exquisitely sensitive to hydrocortisone, even at doses that have little or no effect on CTL activation (10^{-5} to 10^{-6} M).[38] Interestingly, cyclosporine A (CsA, Sandoz Pharmaceuticals) had no effect on LAK activation but totally prevented the activation of CTL (Figure 3).

Table 1
LAK ACTIVATION IS INHIBITED BY TUMOR PRESENCE — % LYSIS OF FRESH TUMOR AFTER 6 DAYS OF CULTURE

Cultured glioma cells/mℓ × 10^{-4}	Units of IL-2 per mℓ					
	500	250	100	50	25	0
0	63	64	65	45	35	0
1	29	23	28	24	3	1
10	12	13	6	10	6	3
50	5	17	9	8	2	0
100	0	1	0	0	0	0
200	0	0	0	0	0	0
Fresh sarcoma cells/mℓ × 10^{-4}						
0	35	36	32	23	19	0
1	18	17	27	18	12	0
10	13	11	9	7	3	0
50	4	15	7	11	6	0
100	0	6	0	0	0	0
200	0	0	0	0	0	0

Note: Tissue cultured glioma cells[27] or fresh sarcoma[14] were co-cultured with allogeneic normal PBL and IL-2 at the concentrations shown. After 6 days the culture contents were tested for LAK activity toward either the glioma or sarcoma.

IV. SPECIFICITY OF LAK LYSIS IS BROAD AND NOT LIMITED TO TUMORS

A. Autologous and Allogeneic Tumors are Lysed Comparably by LAK and LAK Clones

The hallmark of the LAK system is its extremely efficient and rapid ability to kill fresh tumor cells. It is generally accepted that classical NK cells do not kill fresh solid tumors to any significant degree, and that CTL generation to autologous human tumors is irreproducible. While some fresh human tumors may be NK sensitive (leukemias or blood-borne metastases) and others may be antigenic and lacking immunosuppressive factors so that they stimulate CTL production (melanoma), these are also rare and probably do not become clinically detectable. Because of an as-yet-undefined lytic potential, LAK kill all types of NK resistant tumors (Table 2), but do not require any tumor present for activation. All fresh normal cells for which we could obtain single cell suspensions in vitro were all LAK resistant.[1,2,39,40] Because LAK have been infused i.v. or injected in various organs directly with no obvious deleterious effects, we conclude that LAK recognize aspects of tumors that are absent on normal tissue.

In order to ascertain whether LAK represents a population of effectors, each with unique specificity, or whether all LAK cells kill multiple targets, LAK clones and subclones were generated from one to three cells per well in limiting dilution cultures.[39,40] All clones were observed to significantly kill the same panel of tumor targets in 58/61 combinations. An autologous sarcoma was lysed by clones from 33 to 53%, and 6 allogeneic tumors up to 68% at an effector to target ratio of 40:1. In our experiments, autologous PBL were included as target cells and were not lysed. From two of the original clones, a total of nine subclones were derived and also found to kill multiple targets in an HLA unrestricted fashion.[40] After several months, these clones gradually lost cytolytic activity and subsequently ceased growth, although the cultures were regularly supplemented with PHA and killer cells.[40] To date, no continuous LAK clone has been generated.

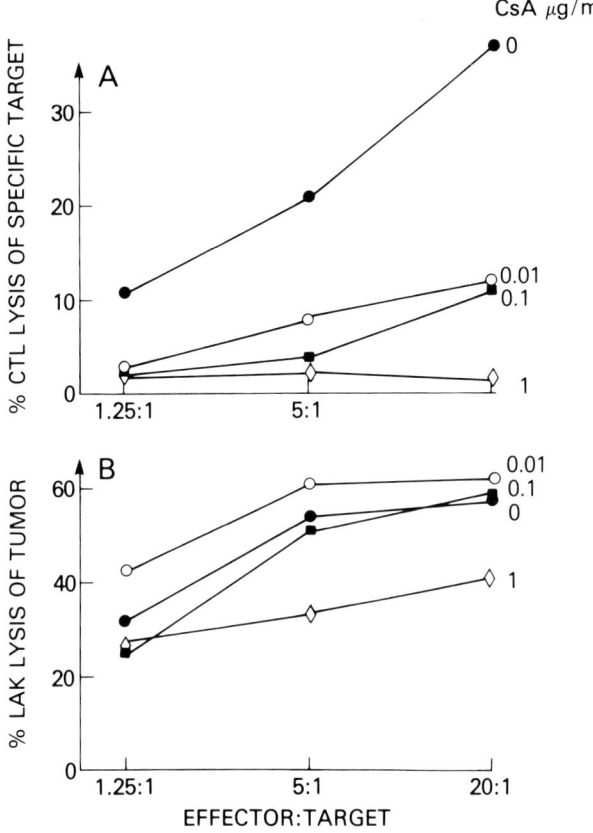

FIGURE 3. Sensitivity of CTL activation and resistance of LAK activation to cyclosporine A. CTL in vitro sensitivation cultures (A) and LAK activation cultures (B) were initiated in the presence of CsA at the μg/mℓ as designated. Cultures were incubated for 6 days after which CTL were tested for lysis of the specific priming cells, and LAK cultures tested for lysis of fresh sarcoma cells. The CTL and LAK recoveries from the cultures from which 2.5 μ/mℓ CSA was added for less than 10% of control, and therefore were insufficient for testing. Cell recovery from lower doses was greated than 70%. No differences in recoveries from either CTL or LAK cultures were significant.

It is unknown whether LAK recognize a single epitope common to all susceptible targets. It could be that LAK have multiple receptors and the targets have variable expression if ligands recogized by such receptors. Because of our lack of understanding of this phenomenon, we have called the specificity of LAK "polyspecific." Polyspecificity of LAK was also confirmed at the population level in cold target inhibition experiments in which HLA-typed allogeneic indivuduals' tumors totally inhibited the lysis of autologous tumor cells.[14,41]

B. Human Oncogene-Transfected 3T3 Cells are Lysed by LAK

Oncogenes are DNA sequences responsible for the transforming activity of the acute transforming retroviruses. Homologous sequences are present in human tumors and normal cells. Transfection studies have demonstrated the transforming potential of the human sequences. The mechanisms causing transformation are under investigation, but include mutation of the tumor-derived oncogene and amplified expression of the oncogene product. When oncogenes are transfected into nontransformed cells, the resultant transfectants have many of the growth and phenotypic characteristics of human tumors. The immunological characterization of oncogene transfected normal cells is being studied. Therefore, to determine the pattern of cytolysis of human oncogene transfected cells by LAK, we performed

Table 2A
CELLS SENSITIVE TO LYSIS BY HUMAN LAK

Fresh Tumors (Autologous and Allogeneic)
    Melanoma
    Sarcoma, osteo and soft tissue
    Carcinoma
    Glioma
    Benign Schwannoma
Cultured tumors

Table 2B
CELLS NOT LYSED BY HUMAN LAK

LAK
    Bowel, fresh normal
    Colon, fresh normal
    Kidney, fresh normal
    Liver, fresh normal
    Pancreas, fresh normal
    Con A Lymphoblasts

Data for results summarized above are in References 1-4, 14, 27, 37, 39-41.

a series of experiments in which we found that ras transfectants were totally NK resistant but did show susceptibility to murine and human LAK.[37,43] These transfectants were derived in vitro but grown in vivo prior to use as target cells in our assays.

C. Hapten Modification Confers LAK Sensitivity on Resistant PBL

It has previously been reported that partially purified IL-2 would activate mouse spleen cells into cytolytic lymphocytes that lysed autologous lymphocytes modified with TNBS, to express cell surface TNP moieties.[43] To determine whether human LAK represents an analogous system, we tested in parallel the lysis of autologous-TNP-PBL and that of tumor.[14] Figure 4 displays the results of one of eleven consistent experiments in which TNP-PBL were efficiently lysed by autologous LAK. As reported in cold-target inhibition experiments, autologous LAK also inhibited lysis of autologous tumor and vice versa.[14] The cross-reactivity of TNP-PBL with tumor is puzzling, and suggests that the masking or the absence of a normal controlling determinant may be operable in LAk recognition. The ability of TNBS reagent to perturb proteins suggests that a protein is somehow involved in LAK recognition, and that neither membrane lipid composition nor characteristics unique to rapidly dividing cells are primary candidates for LAK target structures.

D. LAK Recognition of Target Cells Requires a Trypsin-Sensitive Protein

The susceptibility of human tumor cells to killing by LAK was found to be abrogated by treating tumor cells with proteolytic enzymes. Treatment of human glioma with either trypsin or chymotrypsin eliminated the ability of these tumor cells to be killed, but they did remain completely viable and regained their LAK sensitivity after culture for 24 hr under standard

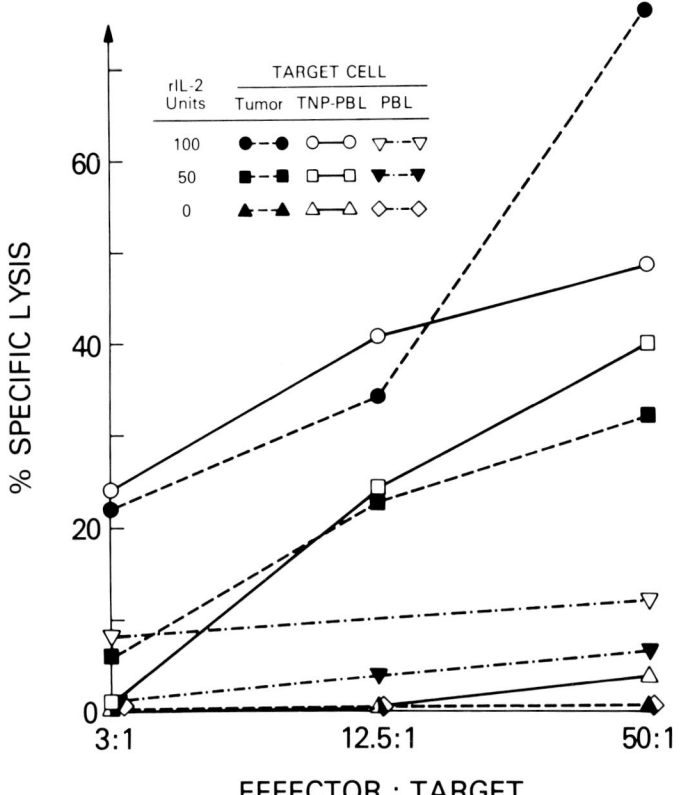

FIGURE 4. LAK lysis of autochthonous tumor and TNP-PBL. LAK were generated at the IL-2 concentrations shown and tested simultaneously for lysis of fresh TNBS treated PBL or tumor.

tissue culture conditions.[45,46] Neither glycosidases, neuraminidase, nor periodate treatment of tumors had any effect. Using either fresh sarcoma or cultured NK resistant Daudi tumors, identical results were found with nonspecific pronase treatment (Figure 5) or trypsin treatment (Figure 6). These results further indicate a role for a protein determinant in LAK recognition of tumor target cells, and provide the basis for our studies of LAK recognition currently in progress.

V. RELATIONSHIP OF LAK TO OTHER CYTOLYTIC LYMPHOCYTE SYSTEMS

A. The LAK Phenomenon is Unique

The LAK system can be distinguished from the classical NK and CTL cells by a variety of characteristics (Table 3). It has been shown that some of these major characteristics are common with NK cells, but others with CTL, thus complicating a complete separation of the LAK system from the others. A most likely explanation is that a continuum of various cytolytic cell types exists overlapping with one another to a certain degree, with each endowed with an inherent biologic role yet to be defined. Clear interpretation of experimental results is further complicated by the finding that high concentrations of IL-2 modulate the specificity of cloned CTL to acquire a broader specificity of lysis, including

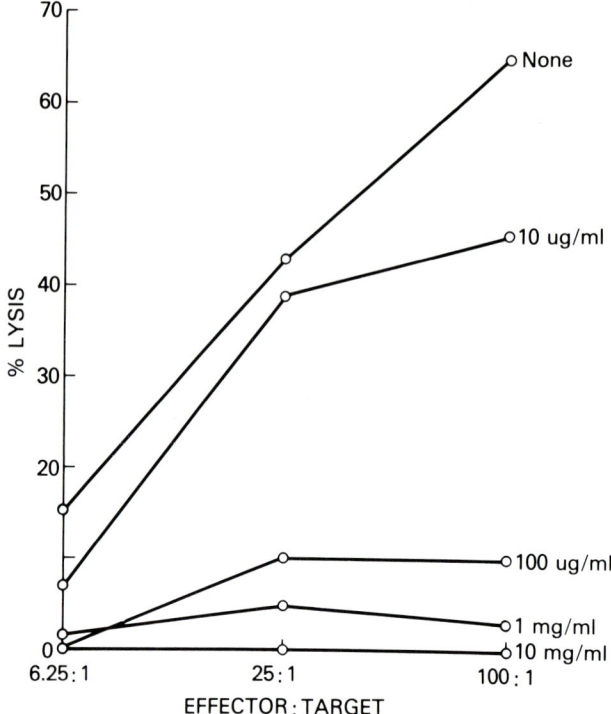

FIGURE 5. Pronase treatment of fresh tumors reduces LAK susceptibility. Non-specific Protense (Sigma Corporation, St. Louis, MO) was used to treat chromium-labeled fresh sarcoma cells for 10 min at 37°C. The tumors were then washed and used immediately as targets.

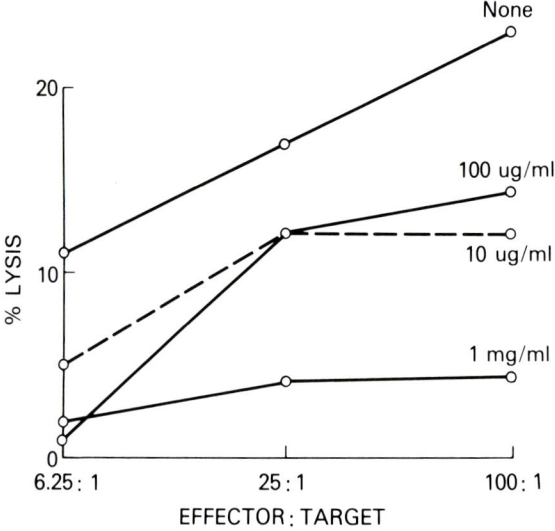

FIGURE 6. Trypsin treatment of fresh tumor reduces LAK susceptibility. Fresh chromium-labeled tumor cells were treated with trypsin (100 μg to 1 mg/mℓ for 10 min at 37°C), then washed and used immediately as targets for LAK lysis (Figure 7) LAK precursors cells are partially sensitive to Leu 11b and complement.

Table 3
COMPARISON OF NK, LAK, AND CTL

	Lytic activity		
Characteristic	NK	LAK	CTL
Development kinetics	Spontaneous	By day 2-3	By day 5-7
Stimulus	None, IFN augments	IL-2, ± IFN^{-8}	Specific antigen
Specificity of cytotoxicity	Bone marrow; leukemia cells K562	Fresh solid tumors, (plus all NK targets) TNP-PBL	Specific antigen expressing cells
Precursor location	Intestinal mucosa TDL− PBL+ Spleen+	TDL+, spleen+, PBL+, tumor+, BM+, cord blood+, intestinal mucosa+	TDL unknown PBL+
Serologic phenotype of effector	OKM1+ OKT3− OKT8− Leu 11+ Leu 7+	OKM1− OKT3+ OKT8+ Leu 1+ Leu 11± Tac+ 4F2+	OKM1− OKT3+ OKT8+ Leu 1+ Leu 11− Tac+ 4F2+
Serologic phenotype of precursor	Unknown	OKM1− OKT3− OKT11± Leu 1− OKT9− OKT10− TAC− Leu 11±	OKM1− OKT3+ Leu 1+

that of NK- and LAK-like activities.[46-48] Perhaps IL-2 is much more than just either the growth factor, as thought initially, or the LAK activation signal, but is also responsible for amplification of any cytolytic cell in the area. Such conditions might occur under circumstances of high IL-2 concentration, such as locally at a vigorous immune response. IL-2 would then be responsible for driving all cells with cytolytic machinery to acquire lytic capability directed toward any abnormal self or tumor cell. Much work is needed to clearly define the relationship among cytolytic lymphocytes. It would not be surprising if, as better molecular tools become available, we continue to define subpopulations of effector lymphocytes, as now are evident within the CTL population. Just as multiple isotypes of immunoglobulins exist, each intended for a unique role, it is likely that multiple types of cytolytic lymphocytes are available, perhaps overlapping in some characteristics and specificity. It is our current interest to help separate and define these multiple classes of lymphocytes.

B. LAK Precursor Cells are Not Well-Defined

LAK precursor cells are not always clearly distinguishable from monocytes, NK cells, B lymphocytes, CTL precursors, and CTL memory cells. Studies have included observations on the basis of adherence properties, serologic phenotypes, density gradient sedimentation, and tissue distribution.[1-4,14,16,38] The tissue distribution of LAK precursors is intriguing, because it appears that they exist in every lymphoid tissue available (Table 3). This tissue distribution of LAK precursors is one of the more compelling characteristics separating the LAK cells from the spontaneous NK cells which are usually limited to the peripheral blood circulation. Because of their large size, NK cells do not appear to infiltrate tissue as well

186 *Cytolytic Lymphocytes and Complement*

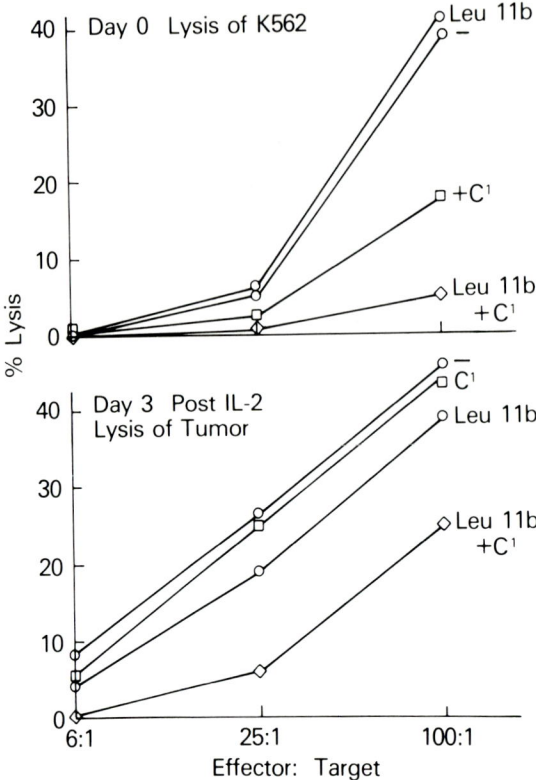

FIGURE 7. Nonadherent PBL were treated with the monoclonal antibody Leu 11b (Becton-Dickinson) and followed with or without complement. One aliquot of cells was tested immediately on day 0 for lysis of K562 as a measure of NK activity. The second aliquot of each treatment group was cultured for 3 days with IL-2 and tested for lysis of a fresh sarcoma tumor.

as do LAK, and have no apparent need for IL-2 to maintain their spontaneous lytic ability. The role of NK cells in the peripheral blood may be one of surveillance against extra bone marrow hematopoiesis and control of certain types of blood-borne metastases. In the peripheral blood LAK precursors appear to have the greatest overlap with NK cells. Our recent results as well as these of others[49] have shown that treatment of fresh PBL with Leu 11 B, a monoclonal antibody recognizing the Fc-Gamma receptor, is present on most NK cells and some LAK precursors (Figure 7). It is not yet known whether some NK cells directly differentiate into LAK, or merely share this marker in common. Other laboratories also distinguish LAK precursors from NK cells.[50] Further studies of ours (LeuOMe) have indicated that the lysosomotropic chemical, 1-leucine methyl ester, can be used to differentiate between NK and LAK precursors in the PBL, with NK being eliminated completely and LAK precursor activity retained after exposure to LeuOMe.[51]

C. LAK Effectors are Heterogeneous

As reported previously, some LAK effectors are often serologically indistinguishable from alloimmune CTL in that they may express OKT-3, OKT-8, Leu-1, and 4F2.[2,3] Our data concluding that Leu-11 can be negative on LAK effectors is shown in Figure 8, in which NK activity was greatly reduced by treatment with Leu-11 plus complement and that LAK effector activity to either K-562 or to Daudi was unaffected.

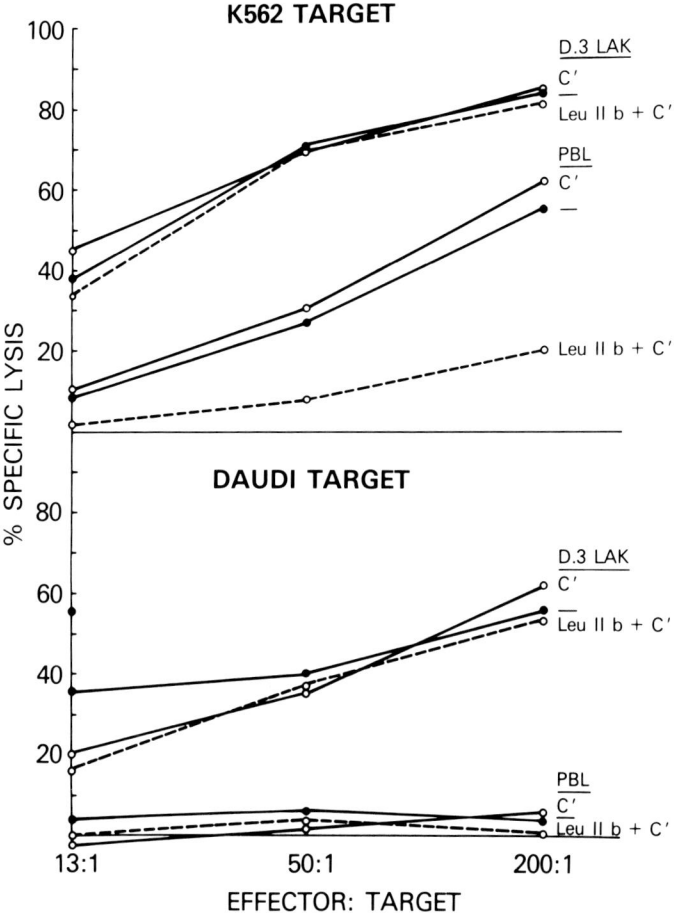

FIGURE 8. LAK effectors do not necessarily express Leu 11b. Day three LAK or fresh PBL were tested for sensitivity to Leu 11b and complement. The fresh PBL were significantly depleted of NK activity as measured by lysis of K562. No reduction in LAK population killing of either K562 or Daudi was observed.

VI. THERAPEUTIC POTENTIAL OF LAK

A. Studies in Progress

The unusual attributes of the LAK system point toward a unique antitumor effector mechanism that may well have application in cancer immunotherapy.

In many respects, the most elegant and controlled approach to adoptive immunotherapy is the activation in vitro of lymphocytes from cancer patients by culture with IL-2 and then adoptively transferring these back to the cell donor. Initial studies have shown that such autochthonous infusion is feasible, both via intravenous and intratumor injection, without untoward effects.[52-56] Murine studies employing adoptive transfer have affirmed that large numbers of cells are essential for effecting tumor regression, often with extra IL-2 given in conjunction. Preparation of relatively comparable quantities (10^{11} to 10^{12}) of activated human lymphocytes presents logistic problems, which have been overcome by several laboratories, including our own. Infusion of activated cytotoxic lymphocytes has proven safe, with some resulting stabilization and temporary regression of disease noted.[52-56] Other studies in which IL-2 was administered alone or in conjunction with lymphocytes established the toxicity of

IL-2 at high doses that clearly defined the safe limits when given systemically.[29,30] In contrast to the systemic toxicity of IL-2, we have found that no toxicity was apparent when escalating doses were administered intracerebrally into the peritumor area of glioma patients during surgery.[55,56] In our view, IL-2 may be meant to act locally in tissue at sites of immune responses, where it is not perceived as toxic, while in the peripheral blood mechanisms exist to rapidly eliminate the IL-2. We have administered IL-2 and/or LAK cells in a total of 10 patients as a preliminary part of our phase I trial. The absence of adverse side effects in our first 9 patients permitted us to continue into the potentially therapeutic part of this trial in which autochthonous LAK ($\geq 10^{10}$) suspended in IL-2 (10^6 units) are injected intraoperatively after removal of the bulk of glioma tumor.[54-56] To date, one patient has received this combined therapy with no adverse effects. A follow-up period of at least several more months is required before we can estimate any therapeutic effect of this treatment.

B. Advantages and Disadvantages of the Current Approach

Therapeutic attributes of LAK include the rapid and complete tumor killing, as observed in vitro, while sparing all normal tissue. No tumor is needed for LAK induction, and PBL from patients receiving other therapies may be used. The process of LAK activation in vitro provides a setting whereby it can be manipulated either by adding other factors, nutrients, or performing cell selection procedures to result in the most therapeutic cell from the LAK population. Subsequent injection of these cells either intravenously or into the tumor site permits a degree of localization depending on the mode of administration. In vitro activation also provides that cells may be cryopreserved until later times, perhaps when occult metastases arise and further treatment may be desired.

Several disadvantages of the current approach are quite obvious. The extremely tedious technical aspects of handling large numbers of cells with sterile technique is significant. The possibility of contamination is always present, and LAK cells must be tested thoroughly prior to infusion. LAK has a continuous dependence on IL-2 for prolonged killing function. If the tumor burden is massive and LAK are required to act for more than one day in vivo, then IL-2 must be administered and be able to reach the LAK cells in sufficient concentration to maintain them. LAK cells are rather large (often greater than 20 μm), and they appear to have great difficulty exiting the vasculature after intravenous infusion. No tumor specific homing of LAK has yet been apparent (unpublished), therefore we continue to suggest that intralesional therapy be strongly considered.

C. Future Prospects

Many attempts are in progress to make the LAK activation and administration procedure more efficient and safe. Our own results with serum-free medium substitutes is one method by which a number of contaminants could be avoided and activation optimized. Because tumor infiltrating lymphocytes have been reported to contain LAK precursor activity, it might be feasible to inject IL-2 directly into the tumor site and activate LAK locally. In animal studies, this has looked promising. However, as mentioned in this report, some human tumors are greatly immunosuppressive and, combined with the short half-life of IL-2, would present several difficulties to such an approach. Much research is being continued in the application of other immunotherapeutic biologicals, especially bacterial extracts, such as OK-432, which is known to activate IL-2 secretion and cause LAK generation,[57] and which has been used successfully for therapy of human peritoneal ascites.[58]

VII. SUMMARY AND CONCLUSIONS

Lymphokine-activated killer cells (LAK) are cytolytic lymphocytes with the unique capacity of killing NK-resistant fresh human tumor cells in short-term assays. LAK kill au-

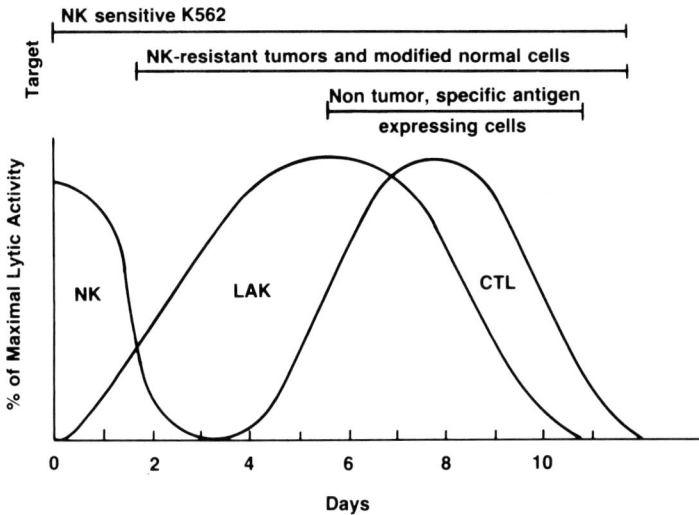

FIGURE 9. Putative relationship and overlap between NK, LAK, and CTL.

tologous as well as TNP-modified self and allogeneic tumors with complete cross-reactivity, both at the population and clonal level. Initial studies on the classification of LAK conclude that LAK are distinct from the classical NK and T-lymphocyte systems based on a number of criteria including surface phenotype, activation conditions, and spectrum of susceptible target cells (Figure 9). LAK kill ras oncogene transfected fibroblasts in a manner similar to fresh tumors. As yet, the target cell determinant responsible for susceptibility to LAK lysis is unknown, but cell surface proteins are prime candidates.

Activation of LAK requires only IL-2, and is most efficient using serum free conditions. Because only interleukin-2 alone is sufficient for LAK activation, we have tested in vitro whether fresh PBL could be activated in the presence of tumor, as might be desired in vivo. LAK activation was greatly suppressed by tumor presence. LAK activation is also suppressed by hydrocortisone, but not cyclosporine A.

Because of the above and other findings, we have initiated a clinical protocol to test whether LAK made from brain tumor patients' PBL could eliminate residual glioma tumor cells. Autochthonous LAK, plus rIL-2 to maintain lytic ability, are injected during surgery. Preclinical studies in a rat glioma model have shown this approach to be safe. Ten glioma patients have been injected intracerebrally with IL-2 and/or LAK with no immediate or long-term (6 months) adverse effects. Much work is needed to understand the LAK phenomenon and to resolve its potential usefulness in cancer therapy as well as its inherent biologic role.

REFERENCES

1. **Grimm, E. A., Mazumder, A., Zhang, H. Z., and Rosenberg, S. A.,** Lymphokine-activated killer cell phenomenon. Lysis of natural-killer resistant fresh solid tumor cells by Interleukin-2 activated autologous human peripheral blood lymphocytes, *J. Exp. Med.*, 155, 1823, 1982.
2. **Grimm, E. A. and Rosenberg, S. A.,** The human lymphokine-activated killer cell phenomenon, in *Lymphokines*, Vol. 9, Pick, E., Ed., Academic Press, New York, 1984, 279.

3. **Grimm, E. A., Ramsey, K., Mazumder, A., Wilson, D. J., Djeu, J., and Rosenberg, S. A.,** Lymphokine-activated killer cell phenomenon: II. The precursor phenotype is serologically distinct from peripheral T lympocytes, memory CTL, and NK cells, *J. Exp. Med.,* 157, 884, 1983.
4. **Grimm, E. A., Robb, R. J., Roth, J. A., Neckers, L. M., Lachman, L., Wilson, D. J., and Rosenberg, S. A.,** The lymphokine activated killer cell phenomenon. III. Evidence that IL-2 alone is sufficient for direct activation of PBL into LAK, *J. Exp. Med.,* 158, 1356, 1983.
5. **Martin-Chandon, M. R., Vanky, F., Carnaud, C., and Klein, E.,** In vitro education on autologous human sarcoma generates non-specific killer cells, *Int. J. Cancer,* 15, 342, 1975.
6. **Seeley, J. K. and Golub, S. H.,** Studies on cytotoxicity generated in human mixed lymphocyte cultures. I. Time course and target spectrum of several distinct concomitant cytotoxic activities, *J. Immunol.,* 120, 1415, 1978.
7. **Zarling, J. M., Robins, H. I., Raich, P. C., Bach, F. H., and Bach, M. L.,** Generation of cytotoxic T lymphocytes to autologous human leukemia cells by sensitization to pooled allogeneic normal cells, *Nature (London),* 274, 269, 1978.
8. **Seeley, J. K., Mascucci, G., Poros, A., Klein, E., and Golub, S. H.,** Studies on cytotoxicity generated in human mixed lymphocyte cultures. II. Anti-K562 effectors are distinct from allospecific CTL and can be generated from NK-depleted T-Cells, *J. Immunol.,* 123, 1303, 1979.
9. **Mascucci, M. G., Klein, E., and Argov, S.,** Disappearance of the NK effect after explanation of lymphocytes and generation of similar nonspecific cytotoxicity correlated to the level of blastogenesis in activated cultures, *J. Immunol.,* 124, 2458, 1980.
10. **Strausser, J. L., Mazumder, A., Grimm, E. A., Lotze, M. T., and Rosenberg, S. A.,** Lysis of human solid tumors by autologous cells sensitized in vitro to alloantigens, *J. Immunol.,* 127, 266, 1981.
11. **Bolhuis, R. L. H. and Schellekens, H.,** Induction of natural killer cell activity and allocytotoxicity in human peripheral blood lymphocytes after mixed lymphocyte culture, *Scand. J. Immunol.,* 13, 401, 1981.
12. **Lemmonier, F., Burakoff, S. J., Germain, R. N., and Benacerral, B.,** *Proc. Natl. Acad. Sci. USA,* 44, 1229, 1977.
13. **Palacios, R., Moller, G., Claesson, L., and Peterson, P. A.,** *Immunogenetics,* 14, 367, 1981.
14. **Grimm, E. A. and Wilson, D. J.,** The human lymphokine activated killer cell system. V. Purified recombinant Interleukin-2 activates cytotoxic lympocytes which lyse both NK resistant autologous and allogeneic tumors and trinitrophenyl-modified autologous PBL, *Cell. Immunol.,* 94, 568, 1985.
15. **Rosenberg, S. A., Grimm, E. A., McGrogan, N., Doyle, M., Kawasaki, E., Koths, K., and Mark, D. F.,** Biologic activity of recombinant human Interleukin-2 produced in E. Coli., *Science,* 223, 1412, 1984.
16. **Grimm, E. A. and Rosenberg, S. A.,** Production and properties of human IL-2, in *Isolation, Characterization and Utilization of T Lymphocyte Clones,* Fathman, G. and Fitch, F., Eds., Academic Press, New York, 1982, 57.
17. **Morgan, D. A., Ruscetti, F. W., and Gallo, R. C.,** Selective *in vitro* growth of T lymphocytes from normal human bone marrows, *Science,* 193, 1007, 1976.
18. **Grimm, E. A., Mazumder, A., and Rosenberg, S. A.,** *In vitro* growth of cytotoxic human lymphocytes. V. Generation of allospecific cytotoxic lymphocytes to nonimmunogenic antigen by supplementation of *in vitro* sensitization with partially purified T cell growth factor (PP-TCGF), *Cell. Immunol.,* 70, 248, 1982.
19. **Kedar, E., Herberman, R. B., Gorelik, E., Sredni, B., Bonnard, G. O., and Navarro, N.,** Antitumor reactivity *in vitro* and *in vivo* of mouse and human lymphoid cells cultured with T cell growth factor, in *The Potential Role of T Cells in Cancer Therapy,* Fefer, A. and Goldstein, A., Eds., Raven Press, New York, 1982, 173.
20. **Grimm, E. A., Gorelik, E., Rosenstein, M. M., and Rosenberg, S. A.,** The lymphokine-activated killer cell phenomenon: in vitro and in vivo studies, in *Interleukins, Lymphokines, and Cytokines,* Cohen, S. and Oppenheim, J., Eds., Academic Press, New York, 1983, 739.
21. **Mazumder, A. and Rosenberg, S. A.,** Successful immunotherapy of NK-resistant established pulmonary melanola metastases by the intravenous adoptive transfer of syngeneic lymphocytes activated *in vitro* by interleukin-2, *J. Exp. Med.,* 159, 495, 1984.
22. **Mulé, J. J., Shu, S., Schwarz, S. L., et al.,** Adoptive immunotherapy of established pulmonary metastases with LAK cells and recombinant interleukin-2, *Science,* 225, 1487, 1984.
23. **Mulé, J. J., Shu, S., and Rosenberg, S. A.,** The anti-tumor efficacy of lymphokine-activated killer cells and recombinant interleukin-2 *in vivo*, *J. Immunol.,* 135, 646, 1985.
24. **Lafreniere, R. and Rosenberg, S. A.,** Successful immunotherapy of experimental hepatic metastases with lymphokine-activated killer cells and recombinant interleukin-2, *Cancer Res.,* 45, 3735, 1985.
25. **Rosenberg, S. A., Mulé, J. J., Spiess, P. J., et al.,** Regression of established pulmonary metastases and subcutaneous tumor mediated by the systemic administration of high dose recombinant IL-2, *J. Exp. Med.,* 161, 1169, 1985.
26. **Rong, G. H., Grimm, E. A., and Sindelar, W. F.,** An enxymatic method for the consistent production of monodispersed viable cell suspensions from human solid tumors, *J. Surg. Oncol.,* 28, 131, 1985.

27. **Jacobs, S. K., Kornblith, P. L., Wilson, D. J., and Grimm, E. A.**, *In vitro* killing of human glioblastoma by interleukin-2 activated autologous lymphocytes, *J. Neurosurg.*, in press.
28. **Itoh, K., Shiiba, K., Shimizo, Y., Suzuki, R., and Kumagai, K.**, Generation of activated killer cells by recombinant interleukin-2 in collaboration with interferon-2, *J. Immunol.*, 134, 3124, 1985.
29. **Lotze, M. T., Frana, L. W., Sharrow, S. O., Robb, R. J., and Rosenberg, S. A.**, *In vivo* administration of purified human interleukin-2. I. Half life and immunologic effects of the JURKAT cell line-derived IL-2, *J. Immunol.*, 134, 157, 1985.
30. **Lotze, M. T., Matory, Y. L., Ettinghausen, S. E., Raynor, A. A., Sharrow, S. O., Seipp, C. A., Custer, M. A., and Rosenberg, S. A.**, *In vivo* administration of purified human interleukin-2. II. Half life, immunologic effects and expansion of peripheral lymphoid cells *in vivo* with recombinant IL-2, *J. Immunol.*, 135, 2865, 1985.
31. **Chang, A. E., Hyatt, C. L., and Rosenberg, S. A.**, Systemic administration of recombinant IL-2 in mice, *J. Biol. Response Mod.*, 3, 561, 1984.
32. **Ettinghausen, S. E., Lipford, E. H., Mulé, J. J., and Rosenberg, S. A.**, Systemic administration of recombinant interleukin-2 stimulates *in vivo* lymphoid cell proliferation in tissues, *J. Immunol.*, 135, 1488, 1985.
33. **Rosenberg, S. A., Mulé, J. J., Spies, P. J., Reichert, C. M., and Schwarz, S. L.**, Regression of established pulmonary metastases and subcutaneous tumor mediated by systemic administration of high dose recombinant IL-2, *J. Exp. Med.*, 161, 1169, 1985.
34. **Forni, G., Giovarelli, M., and Santoni**, Lymphokine-activated tumor inhibition *in vivo*, *J. Immunol.*, 134, 1305, 1985.
35. **Roth, J. A., Grimm, E. A., Osborne, B. A., and Ames, R. S.**, Suppressive immunoregulatory factors produced by tumors, *Lymphokine Res.*, 2, 67, 1983.
36. **Fontana, A., Hengartner, H., deTribolet, N., et al.**, Glioblastoma cells release interleukin-1 and factors inhibiting interleukin-2-mediated effects, *J. Immunol.*, 132, 1837, 1984.
37. **Grimm, E. A., Jacobs, S. K., Lanza, L., Roth, J. A., and Wilson, D. J.**, The role for lymphokine-activated killer cells: IL-2 activated cytotoxic lymphocytes (LAK) in cancer therapy, *Immunology and Cancer*, Fast, P. and Kripke, M., Eds., University of Texas Press, Austin, 1986, 209.
38. **Grimm, E. A., Muul, L. M., and Wilson, D. J.**, Cyclosporine and hydrocortisone exert differential inhibitory effects on the activation of human cytotoxic lymphocytes by recombinant IL-2 versus allospecific CTL, *Transplantation*, 39, 537, 1985.
39. **Rayner, A. A., Grimm, E. A., Lotze, M. T., Chu, E. W., and Rosenberg, S. A.**, Lymphokine activated killer (LAK) cells. Analysis of factors relevant to immunotherapy of cancer, *Cancer*, 55, 1327, 1985.
40. **Rayner, A. A., Grimm, E. A., Lotze, M. T., Wilson, D. J., and Rosenberg, S. A.**, Clonal analysis of human lymphokine activated killer (LAK) cells: LAK cell clones lyse multiple fresh human tumors, *JNCI*, 75, 67, 1985.
41. **Grimm, E. A., Rayner, A. A., and Wilson, D. J.**, Human NK resistant tumor cell lysis is effected by IL-2 activated killer cells, *Mechanisms in Cell-Mediated Cytotoxicity II*, Henkart, P. and Martz, E., Eds., Plenum Press, New York, 1985, 161.
42. **Lanza, L., Roth, J. A., Wilson, D. J., and Grimm, E. A.**, Human oncogene transfected tumors are resistant to NK activity and susceptible to lymphokine-activated killer cell cytotoxicity, *J. Immunol.*, 137, 2716, 1986.
43. **Ballas, A. K. and Ahmann, G. B.**, *Cellular Immunol.*, 76, 81, 1983.
44. **Jacobs, S. K., Wilson, D. J., Melin, G., Parham, C. W., Holcomb, B., and Grimm, E. A.**, Clinical and experimental studies on IL-2 and IL-2 activated killer cells in the treatment of malignant glioma. Host defense mechanisms against cancer, *Excerpta Medica*, 1985, Urushizakit, T., Aki, T., and Tsubura, E., Eds., 1986, 36.
45. **Jacobs, S. K., Wilson, D. J., Melin, G., Parham, C. W., Holcomb, B., Kornblith, P. L., and Grimm, E. A.**, Interleukin-2 and lympholine activated killer (LAK) cells in the treatment of malignant glioma: clinical and experimental studies, *Neurolog. Res.*, 1985, Urushizakit, T., and Tsubura, E., Eds., 1986, 36.
46. **Brooks, C. G., Urdal, D. L., and Henney, C. S.**, Lympholine-driven ''differentiation'' of cytotoxic T-cell clones into cells with NK-like specificity: correlations with display of membrane macromolecules, *Immunol. Rev.*, 72, 43, 1983.
47. **Binz, H., Fenner, M., Frei, D., and Wigzell, H.**, Two independent receptors allow selective target lysis by T cell clones, *J. Exp. Med.*, 157, 1252, 1983.
48. **DeVries, J. E. and Sptis, H.**, Cloned human cytotoxic T lymphocyte (CTL) lines reactive with autologous melanoma cells. I. *In vitro* generation, isolation, and analysis to phenotype and specificity, *J. Immunol.*, 132, 510, 1984.
49. **Itoh, K., Tilden, A. B., Kumagai, K., and Balch, C. M.**, Leu-11 lymphocytes with natural killer (NK) activity are precursors of recombinant interleukin-2 (rIL-2)-induced activated killer cells, *J. Immunol.*, 134, 802, 1985.

50. **Burns, G. F., Triglia, T., and Werkmeister, J. A.**, *In vitro* generation of human activated lymphocyte killer cells. Separate precursors and modes of generation of NK-like cells and 'anomalous' killer cells, *J. Immunol.*, 133, 1656, 1984.
51. **Yagita, M., Louden, W. G., Abraham, S. R., and Grimm, E. A.**, The differential toxic effect of the lysosomotropic agent 1-leucine methyl ester on NK activity, LAK precursor and LAK and CTL effector function, submitted.
52. **Rosenberg, S. A., Rosenstein, M., Grimm, E. A., Lotze, M., and Mazumder, A.**, The use of lymphoid cells expanded in IL-2 for the adoptive immunotherapy of murine and human tumors, *Thymic Hormones and Lymphokines*, Goldstein, A. L., Ed., Plenum Press, New York, 1984, 191.
53. **Rosenberg, S. A.**, Immunotherapy of cancer by systemic administration of lymphoid cells plus interleukin-2, *J. Biol. Resp. Modif.*, 3, 501, 1984.
54. **Jacobs, S. K., Wilson, D. J., Kornblith, P. L., and Grimm, E. A.**, Studies on the immunotherapy of human gliomas using autologous lymphokine-activated killer cells, *Surgical Forum*, 36, 504, 1985.
55. **Jacobs, S. K., Wilson, D. J., Kronblith, P. L., and Grimm, E. A.**, Interleukin-2 or autologous lymphokine activated killer cell treatment of malignant glioma: Phase I trial, *Cancer Res.*, 44, 2101, 1986.
56. **Jacobs, S. K., Wilson, D. J., Kornblith, P. L., and Grimm, E. A.**, Interleukin-2 and autologous lymphokine activated killer (LAK) cells in the treatment of malignant glioma: preliminary report, *J. Neurosurg.*, 372, 386, 1986.
57. **Grimm, E. A., Roth, J. A., and Yagita, M.**, Effect of OK-432 activated cytolytic lymphocytes on NK resistant fresh tumor cells. Proceedings of the 14th International Chemotherapy Congress, in press.
58. **Hoshino, T. and Uchida, A., Eds.**, Clinical and experimental studies in immunotherapy, OK-432, *Excerpta Medica*, Tokyo, 1984, 1.

ADDITIONAL REFERENCES

59. **Tsudo, M., Goldman, C. K., Bongiovanni, F., Chan, W. C., Winton, E. F., Yagita, M., Grimm, E. A., and Waldmann, T. A.**, The p75 peptide is the receptor for interleukin 2 expressed on large granular lymphocytes and is responsible for the interleukin 2-activation of these cells, *Proc. Natl. Acad. Sci. U.S.A.*, 84, 5394, 1987.
60. **Owen-Schaub, L. B., Loudon, W. G., Yagita, M., and Grimm, E. A.**, Functional differentiation of human lymphokine activated killing is distinct from expansion and involves dissimilar interleukin-2 receptors, *Cell. Immunol.*, in press.
61. **Yagita, M., Owen-Schaub, L. B., Tsudom, M., Waldmann, T. A., and Grimm, E. A.**, 1987 Detection of a non-Tac IL-2 binding peptide (p75) on fresh peripheral blood lymphocytes as a receptor associated with induction of lymphokine activated killer activity, submitted.
62. **Wang, H. M. and Smith, K. A.**, The interleukin-2 receptor. Functional consequences of its bimolecular structure, *J. Exp. Med.*, 166, 1055, 1987.
63. **Lowenthal, J. W. and Greene, W. C.**, Contrasting interleukin-2 binding properties of the gamma (p55) and beta (p70) protein subunits of the human high-affinity interleukin receptor, *J. Exp. Med.*, 166, 1156, 1987.

Chapter 26

THE CONTRIBUTION OF NATURAL KILLER AND T-CELLS TO THE LYMPHOKINE-ACTIVATED KILLER CELL PHENOMENON

Joseph H. Phillips, Brett T. Gemlo, Warren W. Myers, Anthony A. Rayner, and Lewis L. Lanier

TABLE OF CONTENTS

I.	Introduction	194
II.	Classification of Human Lymphocytes	194
III.	Effectors of LAK — Experimental Studies	195
	A. Activity of IL-2 Activated Human Peripheral Blood Mononuclear Cells	195
	B. Phenotype of LAK Effectors	196
	C. Lectin-Dependent Cytotoxicity	196
	D. Non-MHC Restricted CTL	197
	E. Cytotoxicity Mediated by IL-2 Dependent Cloned Cell Lines	197
IV.	Precursors of LAK — Experimental Studies	197
	A. Phenotype	197
	B. Kinetics of Response	198
V.	Effectors of LAK — Clinical Studies	199
	A. Effects of In Vivo Administration of IL-2	199
	B. In Vitro Generated LAK Effectors	200
VI.	Tissue Source of LAK Effectors	202
VII.	Implications and Conclusions	202
References		203

I. INTRODUCTION

In vitro culture of lymphocytes in interleukin-2 (IL-2) results in the generation of cytotoxic cells that lyse a broad spectrum of solid tumors, as well as hematopoietic cell tumors, without deliberate immunization. These cytotoxic cells can lyse both autologous and allogeneic tumor cells without major histocompatibility complex (MHC) restriction. This has been referred to as the "lymphokine-activated killer" (LAK) phenomenon.[1-3] LAK activity has been demonstrated using both human and mouse lymphoid cells (reviewed in Reference 4). Furthermore, re-infusion of in vitro activated LAK effectors into tumor-bearing mice has resulted in tumor regression and, in some cases, successful elimination of the cancer.[4,5] Recently, treatment with human autologous peripheral blood mononuclear cells (PBMC), activated in vitro by culture in recombinant IL-2 (rIL-2) and in vivo administration of rIL-2 has produced regression of a variety of cancers, including melanoma, colon carcinoma, renal carcinoma, and lymphoma.[5]

Rosenberg and Lotze[5] have recently published a comprehensive review of the LAK phenomenon. In the present article, we will focus on more recent studies undertaken by our laboratories to dissect the LAK phenomenon and to identify the precursor cell, effector cell, and mechanism of activation. These studies have been conducted using lymphocytes from both normal individuals and cancer patients who received rIL-2 and LAK therapy.

II. CLASSIFICATION OF HUMAN LYMPHOCYTES

Three distinct types of lympocyte exist: T cells, B cells, and NK cells. Each type can be identified and distinguished by unique genotypic and phenotypic characteristics.

T lymphocytes rearrange and productively transcribe the T cell antigen receptor genes (reviewed in Reference 6). Mature, functional T lymphocytes express an antigen receptor on the plasma membrane. The T cell antigen receptor present on most T lymphocytes is a glycoprotein complex composed of a disulfide-linked heterodimer (Ti) with α and β subunits, that is noncovalently associated with an invariant protein complex, designated CD3 (reviewed in Reference 7). Monoclonal antibodies (MAbs) directed against CD3 can be used to positively identify all mature T lymphocytes. Within the T cell population, subsets of cells have been identified that preferentially mediate cytotoxicity, secrete lymphokines, and induce suppression of the immune system.

B lymphocytes rearrange and productively transcribe immunoglobulin genes, and mature B lymphocytes express immunoglobulin on the plasma membrane (reviewed in Reference 8). B lymphocytes are responsible for immunoglobulin secretion, as well as production of other lymphokines that regulate the immune response.

NK cells are the predominant lymphoid population that mediate non-MHC restricted cytotoxicity. Furthermore, NK cells have been shown to secrete lymphokines and regulate hematopoietic development (reviewed in Reference 9). NK cells express neither immunoglobulin nor T cell antigen receptor on the plasma membrane.[10] Furthermore, NK cells do not rearrange the T cell antigen receptor β or γ genes.[11,12] We have proposed that NK cells constitute an independent lineage of lymphocytes, distinct from both B and T cells (reviewed in Reference 13). Human NK cells can be positively identified by the presence of two cell surface antigens, CD16 and/or Leu 19 (NKH-1).[14] CD16 (Leu 11/B73.1) is an antigen associated with the Fc receptor for IgG expressed on NK cells.[10] Leu 19 (NKH-1) is an ~200 to 220 kDalton glycoprotein of unknown function.[14] The target recognition receptor of NK cells has not been identified.

In this review, the term "T cell" is defined as a lymphocyte expressing CD3 on the plasma membrane, "B cell" is a lymphocyte expressing immunoglobulin or the B cell specific

CD19 antigen on the plasma membrane, and "NK cell" is a lymphocyte that expresses CD16 and/or Leu 19 on the plasma membrane, but does not express CD3.

In human peripheral blood, >98% of lymphocytes can be classified as either T cells, B cells, or NK cells by the criteria that we have defined. We have approached the characterization of the LAK phenomenon based on the premise that this activity is mediated by one of the two distinct populations of lymphocytes known to possess the machinery necessary to mediate cytotoxicity, i.e., either cytotoxic T cells or NK cells. Separation of lymphocytes based on these criteria have resulted in an unambiguous identification of the precursor and effector cells responsible for the LAK phenomenon.

III. EFFECTORS OF LAK — EXPERIMENTAL STUDIES

A. Activity of IL-2 Activated Human Peripheral Blood Mononuclear Cells

Peripheral blood is the source for lymphocytes used in human LAK immunotherapy.[5] Grimm and colleagues[1-3] have demonstrated that culture of peripheral blood mononuclear cells (PBMC) in lectin-induced "conditioned medium" containing IL-2 results in the generation of cytotoxic cells that lyse autologous and allogeneic solid tumor cells. Since the original reports of LAK activity, there have been significant advances in the ability to identify and isolate distinct subpopulations of human lymphocytes using MAbs. Furthermore, since the IL-2 gene has been cloned, it is now possible to use pure, recombinant preparations of lymphokine, eliminating the problems inherent in the use of lectin-induced "conditioned medium" as the source of IL-2. We have therefore critically investigated the characteristics of the cytotoxic cells mediating the LAK phenomenon.

PBMC were isolated from human peripheral blood using Ficoll/Hypaque density gradients. Cells were assayed for cytotoxicity against the "NK sensitive" erythroleukemia cell line, K562, as well as an "NK-insensitive" colon carcinoma cell line, COLO-205, and a panel of "NK insensitive" fresh (noncultured) human solid tumors including carcinomas, sarcomas, melanoma, and Wilm's tumor. Fresh PBMC killed K562, but not "NK insensitive" COLO-205 or fresh solid tumors. PBMC were activated by culture in rIL-2 (1000 U/mℓ) for 7 days. These rIL-2 activated PBMC were able to lyse "NK insensitive" fresh solid tumors and COLO-205, as well as K562. The LAK phenomenon, i.e., the generation by IL-2 of activated cells that kill "NK insensitive" fresh tumor targets, was reproducibly demonstrated in all donors tested.

The viable lymphocytes recovered after culture of PBMC in IL-2 were predominantly T cells (~70 to 80%); NK cells generally comprised 10 to 20%. The unseparated population of IL-2 activated lymphocytes demonstrated significant lysis against both the "NK-insensitive" COLO-205 and the "NK-sensitive" K562 cell lines.[15] The cytotoxic effector cells within the population were identified by positive selection of the T cells and NK cells using a fluorescence activated cell sorter (FACS). Activated NK cells (CD3−, Leu 19+), isolated to >98% purity using the FACS, mediated essentially all cytotoxicity against COLO-205, as well as most of the activity against K562.[15] In contrast, T lymphocytes (CD3+), which were the most abundant cell type in the cultures, failed to mediate significant lysis against COLO-205, although low levels of cytotoxicity against K562 were observed.[15]

Further experiments used freshly isolated tumor cells as targets. A representative experiment is presented in Figure 1. Activated NK cells demonstrated essentially all cytotoxicity mediated against fresh melanoma, sarcoma, and Wilm's tumor cells. None of the fresh tumors were susceptible to lysis by NK cells that had not been activated by culture in IL-2. IL-2 cultured T lymphocytes demonstrated no significant lytic activity against these solid tumors. Although only a single effector-to-target ratio is shown for the experiments presented in this review, we have demonstrated that NK cells were responsible for essentially all lysis of solid tumor targets over a broad range of effector-to-target ratios.[15] Additionally, NK

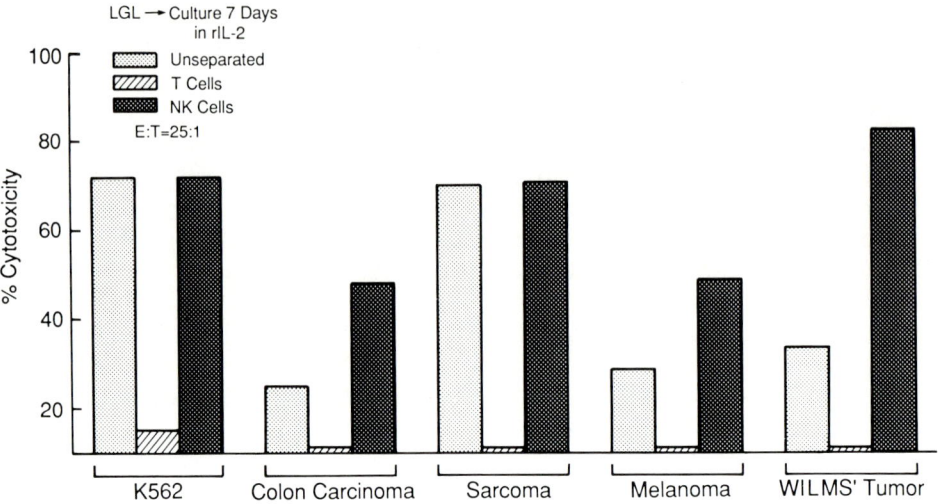

FIGURE 1. LAK Effectors are NK cells. Low buoyant density lymphocytes were isolated from normal human peripheral blood and were cultured in 1000 U/ml rIL-2 for 7 days.[15] Cells were harvested, stained with fluorescein conjugated (FITC) anti-Leu 1 (CD5) and phycoerythrin (PE) conjugated anti-Leu 19 monoclonal antibodies. NK cells (CD5−, Leu 19+) and T cells (CD5+) lymphocytes were isolated to >98% purity using a FACS.[15] Lymphocytes were assayed for cytotoxicity against the indicated ^{51}Cr-labeled tumor cells using a 4 hr radioisotope release assay.[15]

cells mediated detectable cytolytic activity at effector-to-target ratios of less than 1:1. With recognition of this very potent cytolytic activity of NK cells, it follows that contamination of the T cell population by even small numbers of NK cells can lead to the incorrect conclusion that T cells significantly contribute to lysis of fresh solid tumors. For this reason, we recommend positive selection, rather than negative selection, as a more reliable method to assess the functional capabilities of a particular lymphocyte subset. We conclude that the effector of LAK activity in peripheral blood is an IL-2 activated NK cell.

B. Phenotype of LAK Effectors

The predominant effectors of LAK activity in peripheral blood are NK cells, as defined by cells expressing CD16 and/or Leu 19, but lacking expression of CD3. Several additional characteristics of IL-2 cultured NK cells require consideration. Culture of NK cells in IL-2, under certain conditions, results in a significant decrease in the amount of CD16 on the cell surface. Under these circumstance, it is inappropriate to use antibodies against CD16 to enumerate or isolate NK cells. Fortunately, the amount of Leu 19 antigen is rapidly increased upon IL-2 induced activation of NK cells. Thus, activated NK cells are more readily identified by the phenotype, CD3 negative, Leu 19 positive.

The use of antibodies against several other "NK-cell associated" antigens has resulted in the incorrect conclusion that NK cells are not responsible for LAK activity. For example, although the CR_3 (OKM1, Leu 15) antigen is expressed on most freshly isolated NK cells, expression of this structure is lost upon activation of NK cells, under certain culture conditions. It was also observed that the Leu 7 antigen is only expressed on approximately half of freshly isolated NK cells.[10] Moreover, the NK cells expressing this antigen were less cytotoxic and less responsive to IL-2 activation than Leu 7 negative NK cells.[10,16,17]

C. Lectin-Dependent Cytotoxicity

The availability of purified, recombinant IL-2 has provided the opportunity to unequiocally demonstrate that IL-2 is necessary and sufficient to induce LAK activity. Furthermore, use of purified, recombinant lymphokine has circumvented the artifacts inherent in the use of lectin-containing conditioned medium as the source of IL-2. This is particularly important since it has been demonstrated that antigen-specific, MHC restricted cytotoxic T lymphocyte (CTL) clones can lyse inappropriate targets in the presence of mitogenic lectins, such as Con A, PHA, and pokeweed mitogen.[18] Recently, we have shown that T lymphocytes which co-migrate with NK cells in Percoll gradients were capable of mediating cytotoxicity in the presence, but not in the absence, of lectin.[19] In contrast, cytotoxicity mediated by NK cells was unaffected, or inhibited, by these lectins.[19] These results suggest that many of the early reports attributing LAK activity to T lymphocytes may have be an artifact of lectin-dependent cytotoxicity resulting from the use of lectin-containing conditioned medium.

D. Non-MHC Restricted CTL

Although most CTL recognize specific antigen in the context of a polymorphic MHC structure, we and other investigators have recently demonstrated that a unique subset of T lymphocytes can also mediate non-MHC restricted cytotoxicity.[14,20] In vivo these lymphocytes can be distinguished from other T lymphocytes by expression of the Leu 19 (NKH-1) antigen.[14,20] These Leu 19+ T lymphocytes lyse K562, and their cytotoxicity against K562 is augmented by culture in IL-2. However, we have shown that although IL-2 activated Leu 19+ cells can lyse "NK-insensitive" hematopoietic tumor cell targets (including Daudi), peripheral blood Leu 19+ T cells mediate only very low levels of cytotoxicity against solid tumors.[15] These unique non-MHC restricted CTL constitute a minor proportion of PBL (usually <5%), and contribute only a small fraction to the total cytotoxicity against K562.[14,15,20] As noted above, they did not significantly contribute to the LAK activity generated using peripheral blood.

E. Cytotoxicity Mediated by IL-2 Dependent Cloned Cell Lines

The ability of NK cells to mediate lysis of solid tumor targets has been confirmed using cloned, IL-2 dependent NK cell lines. These NK cell clones were established by limiting dilution and culture of CD16 or Leu 19 positive cells in IL-2. All clones expressed Leu 19 and CD16, but not CD3. The amount of CD16 antigen on the clones was less than the amount of CD16 present on fresh NK cells. Longevity of the clones in culture was limited, ranging from 2 to 6 months, depending on culture constituents and the rapidity of proliferation. Clones were capable of 50 to 60 doublings prior to senescence.

These IL-2 cultured NK cell clones were assayed for cytotoxicity against K562 and a panel of seven fresh solid tumor cell targets. All NK cell clones lysed K562. However, when tested against the solid tumor cell targets, some NK cells clones demonstrated an individual repertoire of cytotoxic activity. Other NK cell clones lysed K562, but not the other tumor cell targets. These results and prior studies using NK cell and non-MHC restricted CTL clones[21-24] support the concept that NK cells have a degree of clonal specificity or a limited diversity in cytotoxic potential.

IV. PRECURSORS OF LAK — EXPERIMENTAL STUDIES

A. Phenotype

T cells (comprising ~70% of PBL) and NK cells (~10 to 15% of PBL) have been isolated directly from peripheral blood using the FACS, and cultured in rIL-2. The NK cells, but not the T cells, acquired the ability to lyse solid tumors after culture in IL-2, indicating that the precursor of the peripheral blood LAK effector is an NK cell (Figure 2). Most in vivo NK cells express the phenotype CD3−, CD16+, Leu 19+.[14] A minor subset of NK cells lack CD16 (i.e., CD3−, CD16−, Leu 19+) (comprising <1% of peripheral blood).[14] Both CD16− and CD16+ NK cells can kill solid tumors after activation with IL-2.[15] It should

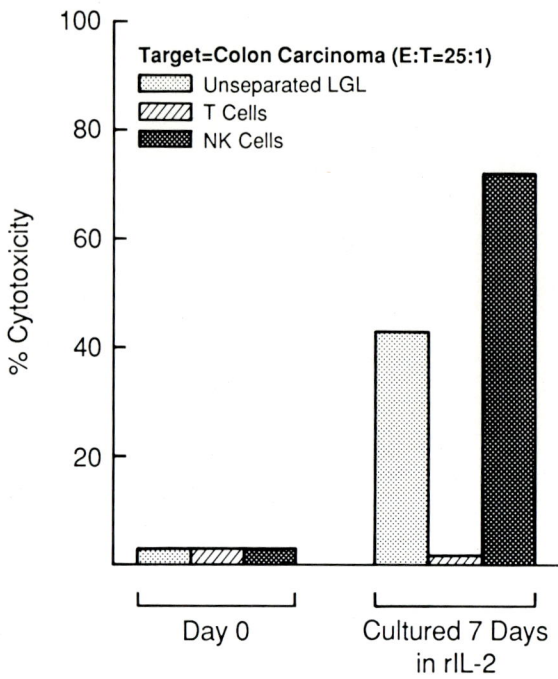

FIGURE 2. Precursors of LAK Effectors are NK Cells. Peripheral blood mononuclear cells were stained with FITC anti-Leu 1 (CD5) and PE anti-Leu 19, and the NK cells (CD5−, Leu 19+) and T cells (CD5+) were isolated to >98% purity using a FACS.[15] Cells were assayed immediately after culture for cytotoxicity against radiolabeled colon carcinoma cells (day 0) or were cultured for 7 days in 1000 U/mℓ rIL-2, and then assayed for cytotoxicity.

be noted that we have *never* observed the induction of CD3 on an NK cell population as a consequence of in vitro culture.[15] Prior reports of this phenomenon have now been attributed to outgrowth of contaminating T cells, since T cells possess a faster growth rate than NK cells. In summary, the precursors of peripheral blood LAK effectors present the phenotype of NK cells. Finally, these experiments demonstrate that purified NK cells can respond directly to rIL-2, without a requirement for accessory cells or T cells to initiate the response.

B. Kinetics of Response

We have examined the kinetics of the generation of LAK activity using purified populations of peripheral blood T cells and NK cells cultured in 1000 U/mℓ rIL-2. As shown in Figure 3, maximal NK cell-mediated cytotoxicity against a solid tumor, as well as K562, was observed within 18 hr.[15] Cytotoxicity was not further increased when tested at 3, 5, and 7 days. T lymphocytes failed to kill the solid tumor even after culture for 7 days; however, maximal cytotoxicity against K562 was also evident in the T cell population after 18 hr.[15] Leu 19+ T cells were responsible for this T cell-mediated cytotoxicity against K562.[15]

The rapid acquisition of cytotoxicity in the purified NK population implies that replication is not required for the generation of LAK activity. However, augmentation of NK cell-mediated cytotoxicity by IL-2 does require protein synthesis.[16] These studies conflict with prior reports by Grimm and colleagues[1] indicating that several days of culture and DNA replication were required for the generation of LAK activity. It seems likely that this discrepancy can be explained by the low concentrations of IL-2 used for activation, or presence of inhibitory cells. In the earlier reports,[1-3] <5 U/mℓ IL-2 were used for activation, whereas it has now been established that >500 U/mℓ IL-2 are required for optimal enhancement of cytotoxicity by NK cells.[16,25]

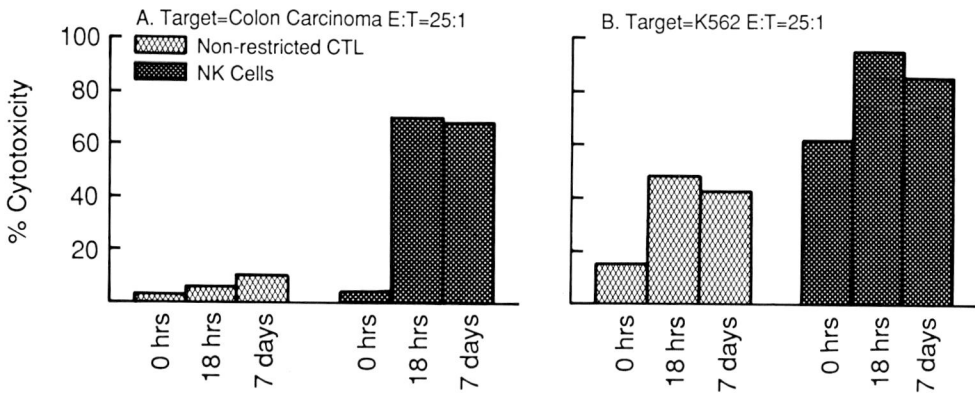

FIGURE 3. Kinetics or rIL-2 activation of NK cells and non-MHC restricted CTL. Low-buoyant-density lymphocytes were isolated from normal human peripheral blood and stained with fluorescein conjugated (FITC) anti-Leu 1 (CD5) and phycoerythrin (PE) conjugated anti-Leu 19 monoclonal antibodies. NK cells (CD5−, Leu 19+), Leu 19+ T cells (non-MHC restricted CTL, CD5+, Leu 19+) and Leu 19− T cells (CD5+, Leu 19−) were isolated to >98% purity using a FACS.[15] Lymphocytes were assayed for cytotoxicity against the indicated ^{51}Cr labeled tumor cells: (A) colon carcinoma (B) K562, immediately after isolation (0 hr), after 18 hr culture in 1000 U/mℓ rIL-2, or after 7 days culture in 1000 U/mℓ rIL-2. Leu 19− T cells failed to demonstrate cytotoxicity at all time points (not shown).

V. EFFECTORS OF LAK — CLINICAL STUDIES

During the past year, we have participated in a clinical therapeutic trial to assess the efficacy of rIL-2 and LAK therapy in cancer patients with renal-cell carcinoma, melanoma, and colon cancer. This has provided us with the opportunity to determine whether or not LAK precursor and effector cells from cancer patients are NK cells, as we have previously shown using lymphocytes from normal donors.

The therapeutic protocol consisted of: (1) in vivo administration of rIL-2, (2) in vitro activation by rIL-2 of autologous PBMC obtained by leukapheresis, (3) re-infusion of the activated cells, and (4) additional in vivo treatment with IL-2 (a modified protocol of the regimen described by Rosenberg et al.[4]). Although our findings are preliminary, the results have clearly substantiated the conclusions derived from experiments using normal individuals. Additionally, these clinical experiments have provided us with valuable insight into the cytotoxic potential of NK cells activated in vivo by IL-2.

A. Effects of In Vivo Administration of IL-2

We found that in vivo treatment with IL-2 resulted in a rapid disappearance (within 30 min) of most circulating lymphocytes in peripheral blood, including T cells, B cells, and NK cells. This disappearance of lymphocytes was paralleled by a substantial loss in cytotoxicity against K562, due to the absence of effectors. These findings confirm and extend the description of this phenomenon initially reported by Lotze et al.[26] After discontinuation of IL-2 administration, lymphocytes and cytotoxic activity against K562 returned within 1 to 3 days. Of particular interest was our observation that circulating LAK effectors were detected in vivo after this initial IL-2 treatment. Cytotoxicity against fresh solid tumors was detected using PBMC isolated from these patients. These findings indicate that rIL-2 is effective in vivo in the generation of cytotoxic cells that lyse fresh solid tumors. It further demonstrates that the IL-2 induced cytotoxic cells must not be directed against normal tissues; otherwise we would be unable to detect cytotoxicity due to "cold target inhibition" by normal tissues.

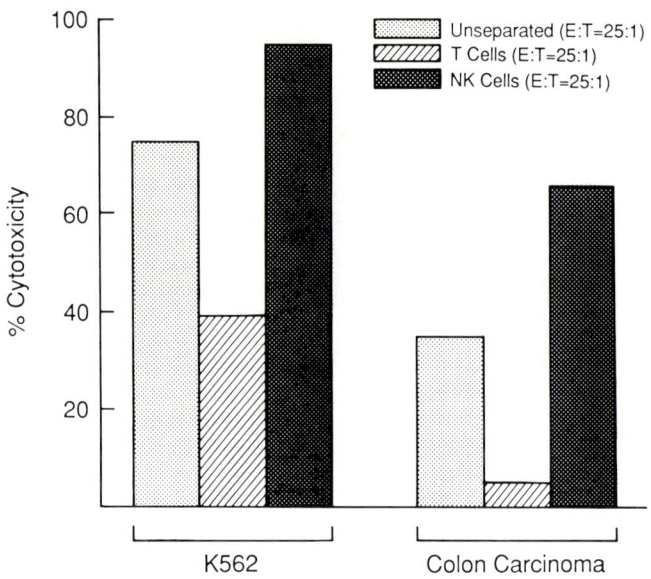

FIGURE 4. LAK patient studies. As described in the text, patients were treated in vivo with rIL-2. Three days after the last treatment with rIL-2, patients were leukapheresed. PBMC were isolated by density gradient centrifugation and were cultured in RPMI-1640 medium containing 2% human AB serum, antibiotics, and 1000 U/mℓ rIL-2.[4] After 3 to 5 days of in vitro culture, activated cells were reinfused into the patient. Patients were given a final in vivo treatment with rIL-2. After the final in vivo treatment with rIL-2, peripheral blood was obtained and the PBMC isolated by density gradient centrifugation. PBMC were strained with FITC anti-Leu 1 (CD5) and PE anti-Leu 19. NK cells (CD5−, Leu 19+) and T cells (CD5+) were assayed for cytotoxic activity against K562 and COLO.

In order to establish the cell type responsible for this in vivo generated cytotoxicity, we isolated peripheral blood T cells and NK cells from a patient that had been infused with autologous IL-2 activated PBL, followed by in vivo administration of rIL-2. As demonstrated in Figure 4, essentially all cytotoxicity against a colon carcinoma, as well as K562, was mediated by activated NK cells. A comprehensive investigation of the kinetics of this response, the antigenic phenotype of the responsive cells, and further functional analysis of the in vivo effector cells is currently under way.

B. In Vitro Generated LAK Effectors

Two to three days after discontinuation of in vivo administration of IL-2, lymphocytes returned to the circulation and the patients were leukopheresed to obtain large number of lymphocytes for in vitro activation with rIL-2. PBMC were isolated by density gradient centrifugation, and were cultured in 2.5-liter roller bottles containing RPMI-1640, 2% human AB serum, antibiotics, and 1000 U/mℓ rIL-2.[4] After 3 to 5 days of in vitro culture, approximately half of the original number of cells were recovered and re-infused into the patient. At the time when in vitro activated lymphocytes were harvested from the roller bottles, the cultures were assayed for the presence of LAK effectors. Furthermore, we isolated NK and T lymphocytes to high purity (>98%) by positive selection, using a FACS to determine which cell population was responsible for the cytotoxic activity. Representative data from one patient are presented in Figure 5. Identical to our prior results using normal donors, NK cells mediated essentially all cytotoxicity against solid tumors, including both cultured and freshly isolated solid tumors. T lymphocytes contributed little to the total cytotoxic activity. Thus, we conclude that the peripheral blood LAK effectors being reinfused into these patients were predominantly NK cells.

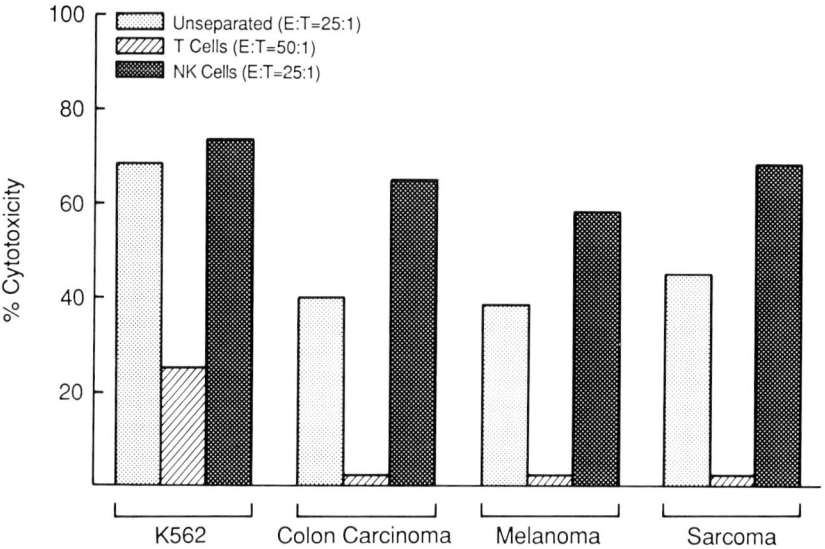

FIGURE 5. LAK patient studies: Cytotoxic effector cells generated in vitro. As described in the text, patients were treated in vivo with rIL-2. Three days after the last treatment with rIL-2, patients were leukapheresed. PBMC were isolated by density gradient centrifugation and were cultured in RPMI-1640 medium containing 2% human AB serum, antibiotics, and 1000 U/mℓ rIL-2.[4] After 3 to 5 days of in vitro culture, approximately half of the original number of cells were recovered and reinfused into the patient. An aliquot of the activated cells were strained with FITC anti-Leu 1 (CD5) and PE anti-Leu 19. NK cells (CD5−, Leu 19+) and T cells (CD5+) were assayed for cytotoxic activity against the indicated fresh and cultured tumor cell lines.

By sequentially monitoring the antigenic phenotype of the in vivo and in vitro activated lymphocytes several potentially important facts were determined. First, it was clear that in vivo administration of rIL-2 resulted in a dramatic disappearance of circulating lymphocytes almost immediately. However, 2 to 3 days after rIL-2 treatment, we observed a relative increase in the proportion of NK cells within the lymphocyte population. Whereas NK cells generally constitute ~10 to 15% of total lymphocytes, after in vivo rIL-2 therapy ~30% of lymphocytes were NK cells. This increase was reflected in the absolute number of cells, as well as the percentage. The second observation was that both in vivo and in vitro activation of NK cells with rIL-2 resulted in the induction of HLA-DR antigens on the cell surface of a significant proportion of NK cells.[27] We have previously reported that NK cells activated in mixed lymphocyte cultures acquire HLA-DR expression. Furthermore, HLA-DR positive NK cells were more efficient cytolytic effectors than HLA-DR negative NK cells in the mixed lymphocyte culture.[27] A final important observation was that the CD16 antigen expressed on NK cells was rapidly lost or masked during in vitro culture, using the culture conditions defined for the clinical protocol. Nonetheless, NK cells were readily identified by the phenotype, CD3−, Leu 19+. As mentioned previously, the amount of Leu 19 antigen present on the surface of IL-2 activated NK cells is significantly increased. However, since the Leu 19 antigen can be expressed on some T cells, as well as NK cells, it is necessary to monitor the phenotype by two-color immunofluorescence using both anti-CD3 (e.g., Leu 4) and anti-Leu 19 antibodies to discriminate CD3+, Leu 19+ T lymphocytes from CD3−, Leu 19+ NK cells. Further studies are underway to determine the kinetics and functional significance of the antigenic changes that result from in vivo and in vitro activation of NK cells.

VI. TISSUE SOURCE OF LAK EFFECTORS

All of the experimental and clinical results discussed in this review relate to studies of the LAK phenomenon using human peripheral blood as the tissue source for lymphoid cells. This is appropriate, since autologous peripheral blood is the exclusive source of lymphocytes in the clinical applications of LAK therapy. However, this implies neither that blood is the only source of LAK effectors, nor that T cells from other lymphoid tissues are incapable of mediating lysis of solid tumors.

Several years ago, Torten and colleagues[28] reported that culture of human thymocytes in conditioned medium containing IL-2 resulted in the generation of cytotoxic lymphocytes that lysed tumor targets without deliberate immunization or MHC-restriction. Grimm and colleagues[2] confirmed these finding using solid fresh tumors as targets. Recently, we have reinvestigated this phenomenon. We have also observed that culture of normal human thymocytes in rIL-2 for 1 to 2 weeks resulted in the generation of cytotoxic cells that killed cultured and freshly isolated solid tumors.[29] However, in striking contrast to results obtained using peripheral blood, the predominant cytotoxic effectors in these cultures were CD3+ T lymphocytes, as determined by positive selection of this population using a FACS.[29] Furthermore, within the T cell population, cytotoxic activity was restricted to T cells expressing the Leu 19 antigen (i.e., CD3+, Leu 19+).[29] Studies directed at determining the thymic precursor population revealed that these non-MHC restricted cytotoxic thymocytes were generated from CD3+ T lymphocytes that lacked detectable Leu 19 antigen expression. We are presently pursuing the question of how these thymic cytotoxic T lymphocytes differ from circulating peripheral T lymphocytes. However, we have established that these cytotoxic effectors can be generated from CD1 (Leu 6/T6) positive and CD4+, CD8+ immature thymocytes, excluding the possibility that these cells represent pre-existing mature T lymphocytes.[30] It should be mentioned that in addition to the CD3+ cytotoxic T cells that were generated from IL-2 activated thymocytes, we have also identified a CD3 negative cytolytic effector cell.[30] Whether these CD3 negative lymphocytes represent immature thymocytes, or alternatively, NK cells, perhaps due to blood contamination, is under investigation.

VII. IMPLICATIONS AND CONCLUSIONS

Based on experimental and clinical research, the following general points have been established:

1. Using peripheral blood as the tissue source for lymphocytes, NK cells were both the precursors and effectors of LAK activity. This was clearly demonstrated using peripheral blood lymphocytes obtained from both normal donors and cancer patients undergoing rIL-2 and LAK therapy. rIL-2 was apparently necessary and sufficient for direct activation of purified NK cell. Using optimal concentrations of rIL-2, maximal cytotoxicity was induced within 18 hr of culture; accessory cells or T cells were not required for induction of cytotoxicity. These findings suggest that short-term activation of purified NK cells may be a preferable method for therapeutic applications.
2. IL-2 cultured peripheral blood T lymphocytes contribute little to the cytotoxic activity against fresh solid tumors. However, a unique subset of peripheral blood T lymphocytes, i.e., T cells expressing the Leu 19 antigen, lyse certain hematopoietic tumor targets without deliberate immunization or MHC restriction. We have designated these cells "non-MHC" restricted CTL.[10,12,13,15] Based on studies of cloned, IL-2 dependent T cell lines, some non-MHC restricted CTL can kill solid tumors; however, these cells are quite rare in cultures of IL-2 activated peripheral blood lymphocytes and contribute little to the total cytolytic activity.

3. IL-2 activated NK cells with LAK activity are present in vivo in patients receiving rIL-2 therapy. These finding indicate that rIL-2 efficiently activates NK cells in vivo. Moreover, the ability to detect LAK activity in vivo indicates that normal tissues are not optimal targets for activated NK cells, otherwise we would have been unable to detect cytotoxicity in the presence of normal tissue "cold targets".
4. Human NK cells can be identified by expression of the CD16 (Leu 11/B73.1) antigen and/or Leu 19 (NKH-1) antigen, and by the absence of CD3/Ti. Since some T cells can express CD16[31] or Leu 19,[13,15,20] it is necessary to determine the phenotype of NK cells by the combined use of antibodies against CD3 and CD16 or Leu 19, preferably by direct two-color immunofluorescence. Caution should also be exercised in using antibodies against CD16 to detect IL-2 activated NK cells, since this antigen is apparently down-regulated or masked as a consequence of culture conditions or the activation process.
5. Finally, we have demonstrated that the tissue source of the lymphocytes determines the cell type responsible for LAK activity. Using human peripheral blood, clearly NK cells are the predominant precursors and effectors of IL-2 induced cytotoxicity against fresh solid tumors, whereas T lymphocytes contribute little to this activity. In contrast, culture of human thymocytes in rIL-2 results in cytotoxicity, mediated predominantly by T lymphocytes. Thus, we caution against direct extrapolation of results using animal models for the LAK phenomenon, where the effector cell populations are usually derived from the spleen, and not peripheral blood.

In conclusion, the potential for therapeutic application of IL-2 activated autologous lymphocytes has been clearly substantiated by recent clinical and experimental studies. Future research in this area will undoubtedly reveal the recognition and target structures involved in discriminating malignant from normal tissues and establish the mechanism of the cytotoxic process. We conclude this review with an optimistic view for the future of rIL-2 and LAK therapy.

REFERENCES

1. **Grimm, E. A., Mazumder, A., Zhang, H. Z., and Rosenberg, S. A,** Lymphokine-activated killer cell phenomenon. Lysis of natural killer-resistant fresh solid tumor cells by interleukin 2-activated autologous human peripheral blood lymphocytes, *J. Exp. Med.*, 155, 1823, 1982.
2. **Grimm, E. A., Ramsey, K. M., Mazumder, A., Wilson, D. J., Djeu, J. Y., and Rosenberg, S. A.,** Lymphokine-activated killer cell phenomenon. II. Precursor phenotype is serologically distinct from peripheral T lymphocytes, memory cytotoxic thymus-derived lymphocytes, and natural killer cells, *J. Exp. Med.*, 157, 884, 1983.
3. **Grimm, E. A., Robb, R. J., Roth, J. A., Neckers, L. M., Lachman, L. B., Wilson, D. J., and Rosenberg, S. A.,** Lymphokine-activated killer cell phenomenon. III. Evidence that IL-2 is sufficient for direct activation of peripheral blood lymphocytes into lymphokine-activated killer cells, *J. Exp. Med.*, 158, 1356, 1983.
4. **Rosenberg, S. A., Lotze, M. T., Muul, L. M., Leitman, S., Chang, A. E., Ettinghausen, S. E., Matory, Y. L., Skibber, J. M., Shiloni, E., Vetto, J. T., Seipp, C. A., Simpson, C., and Reichert, C. M.,** Observations on the systemic administration of autologous lymphokine-activated killer cells and recombinant interleukin-2 to patients with metastatic cancer, *N. Eng. J. Med.*, 313, 1485, 1985.
5. **Rosenberg, S. A. and Lotze, M. T.,** Cancer immunotherapy using interleukin-2 and interleukin-2 activated lymphocytes, *Ann. Rev. Immunol.*, 4, 681, 1986.
6. **Kronenberg, M., Siu, G., Hood, L. E., and Shastri, N.,** The molecular genetics of the T-cell antigen receptor and T-cell antigen recognition, *Ann. Rev. Immunol.*, 4, 529, 1986.
7. **Allison, J. A. and Lanier, L. L.,** The T cell antigen receptor: Structure, serology, and function, *Ann. Rev. Immunol.*, 5, 503, 1987.
8. **Honjo, T.,** Immunoglobulin genes, *Ann. Rev. Immunol.*, 1, 499, 1983.

9. **Trinchieri, G. and Perussia, B.,** Human natural killer cells: Biologic and pathologic aspects, *Lab. Invest.*, 50, 489, 1984.
10. **Lanier, L. L., Le, A. M., Phillips, J. H., Warner, N. L., and Babcock, G. F.,** Subpopulations of human natural killer cells defined by expression of Leu 7 (HNK-1) and Leu 11 (NK-15) antigens, *J. Immunol.*, 131, 1789, 1983.
11. **Lanier, L. L., Cwirla, S., Federspiel, N., and Phillips, J. H.,** Human natural killer cells isolated from peripheral blood do not rearrange T cell antigen receptor β chain genes, *J. Exp. Med.*, 163, 209. 1986.
12. **Lanier, L. L., Cwirla, S., and Phillips, J. H.,** Genomic organization of T-cell γ genes in human peripheral blood natural killer cells, *J. Immunol.*, 137, 3375, 1986.
13. **Lanier, L. L., Phillips, J. H., Hackett, J., Tutt, M., and Kumar, V.,** Natural killer cells: definition of a cell type rather than a function, *J. Immunol.*, 137, 2735, 1986.
14. **Lanier, L. L., Le, A. M., Civin, C. I., Loken, M. R., and Phillips, J. H.,** The relatioship of CD16 (Leu 11) and Leu 19 (NKH-1) antigen expression on human peripheral blood NK cells and cytotoxic T lymphocytes, *J. Immunol.*, 136, 4480, 1986.
15. **Phillips, J. H. and Lanier, L. L.,** Dissection of the lymphokine-activated killer phenomenon. Relative contribution of peripheral blood natural killer cells and T lymphocytes to cytolysis, *J. Exp. Med.*, 164, 814, 1986.
16. **Lanier, L. L., Benike, C. J., Phillips, J. H., and Engleman, E. G.,** Recombinant interleukin 2 enhanced natural killer cell-mediated cytotoxicity in human lymphocyte subpopulations expressing the Leu 7 and Leu 11 antigens, *J. Immunol.*, 134, 794, 1985.
17. **Itoh, K., Tilden, A. B., Kumagai, K., and Balch, C. M.,** Leu 11+ lymphocytes with natural killer (NK) activity are precursors of recombinant interleukin 2 (rIL-2) induced activated killer (AK) cells, *J. Immunol.*, 134, 802, 1985.
18. **Spits, H., Borst, J., Terhorst, C., and de Vries, J. E.,** The role of T cell differentiation markers in antigen-specific and lectin-dependent cellular cytotoxicity mediated by T8+ and T4+ human cytotoxic T cell clones directed at class I and class II MHC antigens, *J. Immunol.*, 129, 1563, 1982.
19. **Phillips, J. H. and Lanier, L. L.,** Lectin-dependent and anti-CD3 induced cytotoxicity are preferentially mediated by peripheral blood cytotoxic T lymphocytes expressing Leu-7 antigen, *J. Immunol.*, 136, 1579, 1986.
20. **Schmidt, R. E., Murray, C., Daley, J. F., Schlossman, S. F., and Ritz, J.,** A subset of natural killer cells in peripheral blood displays a mature T cell phenotype, *J. Exp. Med.*, 164, 351, 1986.
21. **van de Griend, R. J., van Krimpen, B. A., Ronteltap, C. P. M., and Bolhuis, R. L. H.,** Rapidly expanded activated human natural killer cell clones have strong antitumor cell activity and have the surface phenotype of either Tγ, T-non-γ or null cells, *J. Immunol.*, 132, 3185, 1984.
22. **Allavena, P. and Ortaldo, J. R.,** Characteristics of human NK clones: target specificity and phenotype, *J. Immunol.*, 132, 2363, 1984.
23. **Hercend, T., Reinherz, E. L., Meuer, S., Schlossman, S. F., and Ritz, J.,** Phenotypic and functional heterogeneity of human cloned natural killer cell lines, *Nature*, 301, 158, 1983.
24. **Rayner, A. A., Grimm, E. A., Lotze, M. T., Wilson, D. J., and Rosenberg, S. A.,** Lymphokine-activated killer (LAK) cell phenomenon. IV. Lysis by LAK cell clones of fresh human tumor cells from autologous and multiple allogeneic tumors, *J. Natl. Cancer Inst.*, 75, 67, 1985.
25. **Trinchieri, G., Matsumoto-Lobayashi, M., Clark, S. C., Seehra, J., London, L., and Perussia, B.,** Response of resting human peripheral blood natural killer cells to interleukin 2, *J. Exp. Med.*, 160, 1147, 1984.
26. **Lotze, M., Matory, Y. L., Ettinghausen, S. E., Rayner, A. A., Sharrow, S. O., Seipp, C. A. Y., Custer, M. C., and Rosenberg, S. A.,** In vivo administration of purified human interleukin 2 II. Half life, immunologic effects, and expansion of peripheral lymphoid cells in vivo with recombinant IL 2, *J. Immunol.*, 135, 2865, 1985.
27. **Phillips, J. H., Le, A. M., and Lanier, L. L.,** Natural killer cells activated in a human mixed lymphocyte response culture identified by expression of Leu 11 and class II histocompatibility antigens, *J. Exp. Med.*, 159, 993, 1984.
28. **Torten, M., Sidell, N., and Golub, S. H.,** Interleukin 2 and stimulator lymphoblastoid cells will induce human thymocytes to bind and kill K562 targets, *J. Exp. Med.*, 156, 1545, 1982.
29. **Lanier, L. L. and Phillips, J. H.,** Human thymic and peripheral blood non-MHC restricted cytotoxic lymphocytes, *Med. Oncol. Tumor Pharmacother.*, 3, 247, 1987.
30. **Phillips, J. H. and Lanier, L. L.,** *J. Immunol.*, 139, 683, 1987.
31. **Lanier, L. L., Kipps, T. J., and Phillips, J. H.,** Functional properties of a unique subset of cytotoxic CD3+ T lymphocytes that express Fc receptors for IgG (CD16/Leu-11 antigen), *J. Exp. Med.*, 162, 2089, 1985.

Chapter 27

TARGETING FOR T-LYMPHOCYTE-MEDIATED LYSIS BY HYBRID ANTIBODIES

Uwe D. Staerz, Leo Lefrancois, and Michael J. Bevan

TABLE OF CONTENTS

I. Introduction 206

II. Results 207
    A. Monoclonal Antibodies Covalently Coupled to the Target Cell Surface 207
    B. Monoclonal Antibodies Bound to the Fc Receptor of the Target Cell 209
    C. Heteroconjugates of Monoclonal Antibodies as Targeting Agents 210
    D. Hybrid Antibodies as Targeting Agents 211

III. Summary and Discussion 214

References 216

I. INTRODUCTION

The effector phase of the immune response is carried out by either humoral or cell-mediated mechanisms in which antibodies or T lymphocytes, respectively, confer specific recognition of antigen. With the advent of the B cell hybridoma technology,[1] monoclonal antibodies, because of their unique characteristics, have been exploited as important tools in all facets of biomedical research. Besides possessing high specificity, monoclonal antibodies can easily be produced in large quantities and are therefore a highly reproducible agent. Cloned T cell lines and T cell hybridomas represent defined populations in the cellular compartment of the immune response, but in contrast to monoclonal antibodies, T lymphocytes do not recognize antigens alone, but only in the context of major histocompatibility complex (MHC)-encoded molecules located on the surface of the target or stimulator cell. Moreover, T lymphocytes express MHC molecules, which make them a prime target for rejection. For these reasons, it appears inconceivable, at the momemt, to transplant antigen-specific effector T cells in vivo. In the case of certain diseases, however, it would be desirable to focus a strong T cell response at a chosen target. Such examples would involve treatment of tumors or infections that have escaped the normal host response.

In recent years, the T cell antigen receptor has been defined as a disulphide-bonded heterodimer of 80,000 to 90,000 mol wt.[2-8] The gene structure of both the α and β chains of the receptor has been determined and shows striking homology with the genetic organization of the immunoglobulin heavy and light chains.[9-19] A number of low-molecular-weight surface proteins are noncovalently associated with the T cell receptor heterodimer, which in the human are referred to as the T3 complex.[3,20,21]

Monoclonal antibodies which react with components of the T cell receptor complex and identify various fractions of T lymphocytes have been described. Anti-idiotypic (clonotypic) antibodies recognize the T cell receptor of a specific clone of cytotoxic T lymphocyte (CTL) or helper T cell lineage.[3,5-8] A second generation of monoclonal antibodies, like the antibody KJ16 which is specific for an allotypic determinant on the β chain, reacts with 25% of peripheral T cells in most common mouse strains independent of their phenotype.[22,23] In our laboratory, monoclonal antibodies of both classes have been established and are used in the present study. For example, F9 is a clonotypic antibody which reacts uniquely with the CTL clone G4 ($H-2^b$ anti $H-2^d$),[8] and F23.1 is an anti-allotypic antibody with a reactivity pattern similar to KJ16.[23]

Similar to anti-T3 antibodies,[24-26] anti-idiotypic (clonotypic) or anti-allotypic antibodies can not only block the effector function of both T cell subsets,[3,5-8] but in some circumstances can substitute for antigen-plus-MHC recognition. Clonotypic antibodies against the T cell receptor can induce both proliferation of the specific T cell clone and the release of interleukins such as Interleukin 2 (IL-2) or γ-interferon.[5,8,27] Antibodies reactive with either an allotypic determinant on the T cell receptor (F23.1) or with T3 can activate naive, peripheral T cells to express IL-2 receptors and to proliferate.[28-32] Furthermore, monoclonal antibodies reactive with components of the T cell receptor can act as target structures for T cell-mediated lysis. Recent evidence indicates that CTL clones can lyse B cell hybridomas, producing clonotypic antibodies reactive with the specific T cell clone.[33] A later report also demonstrated that B cell hybridomas producing anti-T3 antibodies are lysed by all human cytotoxic T cells.[34] In different approaches, the same antibodies have been linked to the surface of target cells, thus rendering those cells susceptible to T cell-mediated lysis. Monoclonal antibodies against the T cell receptor or components of the T3 complex could by either covalently fixed to the surface or could attach to the target cell via its Fc receptors. Both protocols resulted in effective T cell-mediated lysis.[35-38]

Here we define some of the properties of monoclonal antibodies as T cell targets. This information led us to develop a technology which combines the power of T lymphocytes to

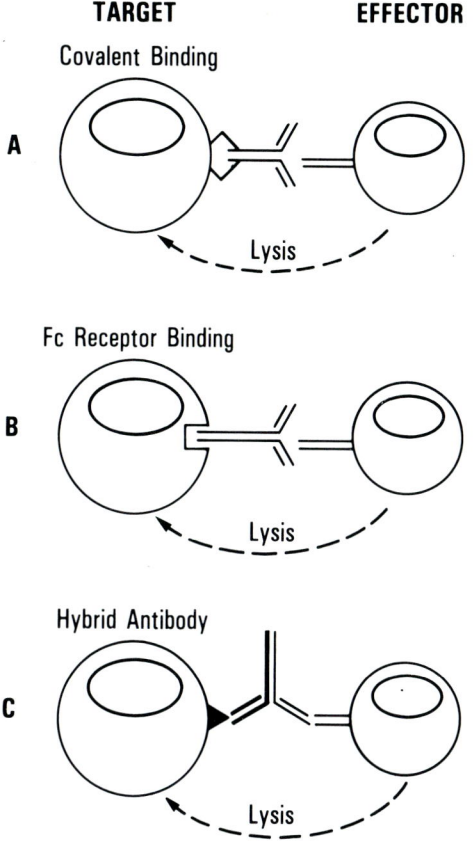

FIGURE 1. Schematic representation of different targeting strategies. Monoclonal antibodies reactive with the T cell antigen receptor were covalently bound to the surface of the target cells (A) or were used to coat the target cell via its Fc receptor (B). Heteroconjugated or hybrid antibodies, in which one binding site is anti-T cell receptor and the other binding site is directed against a target antigen, can focus the T cell effector function (C).

eliminate unwanted cells and cause beneficial inflammatory reactions with the great advantages of monoclonal antibodies, i.e., their specificity and availability. We show that hybrid antibodies, in which one of the component binding sites is anti-T cell receptor and the other component binding site is directed against any chosen target antigen, can focus T cells to act at the targeted site, thus circumventing the limits imposed on T cell immunity by MHC-restricted recognition.

II. RESULTS

A. Monoclonal Antibodies Covalently Coupled to the Target Cell Surface

Previous published work has shown that when monoclonal antibodies reactive with idiotypic or allotypic determinants of the T cell receptor are chemically fixed to a nucleated cell, they render that cell a sensitive target for an effector CTL which is recognized by the antibody (Figure 1A).[35,36] We wished to examine what were the *minimal* requirements for CTL lysis by asking whether MHC Class I-negative lymphoma cells and mammalian erythrocytes could be lysed by T cells in this antibody-directed system.

We had produced B cell hybridoma lines producing two kinds of monoclonal antibodies reactive with the T cell receptor, the clonotypic antibody F9 (IgG1,k) and the allotypic

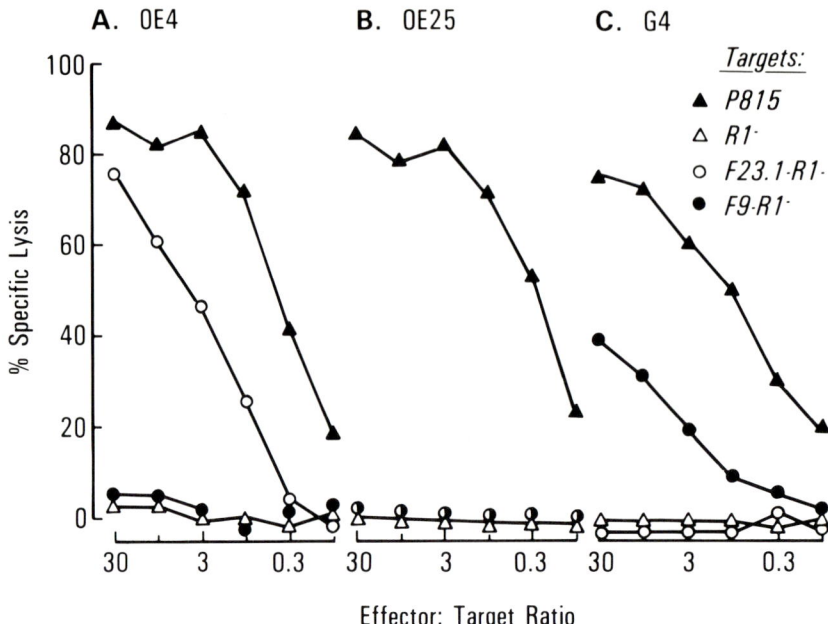

FIGURE 2. Anti-receptor monoclonal antibodies coupled to the target cell surface render tumors susceptible to lysis by CTL clones. The H-2^d reactive CTL clones, OE4 (F23.1$^+$, F9$^-$) (A), OE25 (F23.1$^-$, F9$^-$) (B), and G4 (F23.1$^-$, F9$^+$) (C), were tested for lytic ability on their specific target, P815 (DBA/2 derived mastocytoma, H-2^d) (▲), or unmodified R1(TL$^-$) (△), on F23.1-modified (○), and on F9-modified R1(TL$^-$) (●). The protein A-purified antibodies against the T cell receptor, the allotypic antibody F23.1, and the clonotypic antibody F9, were reacted with a three-fold excess of the heterobifunctional cross-linker SPDP. The modified antibody was then reacted with R1(TL$^-$) cells which had been pretreated with 0.5 mM dithiothreitol to introduce free sulphydryl groups at the cell surface. After washing, 1 × 10^4 ^{51}Cr-labeled target cells were incubated at 37°C with three-fold serial dilutions of the CTL clones for 4 hr. Percent specific lysis of these targets cells and of P815 (DBA/2, H-2^d) targets was calculated as described elsewhere.

antibody F23.1 (IgG2a,k). As effectors, we chose three cloned CTL lines with similar reactivity, but different T cell receptor phenotypes: G4 (BALB.B anti BALB/c, F9$^+$, F23.1$^-$), OE4 (C57BL/6 anti DBA/2, F9$^-$, F23.1$^+$), and OE25 (C57BL/6) anti DBA/2, F9$^-$, F23.1$^-$). As the nonspecific target, we selected R1(TL$^-$), a lymphoma of C58 origin, which cannot be killed by any of the effector cells, presumably due to the lack of expression of MHC Class I molecules on its cell surface (Figure 1).[39] To examine whether the monoclonal antibodies, F9 and F23.1, could render R1(TL$^-$) susceptible to CTL lysis directed by the T cell receptor antibody, we bound F9 and F23.1 covalently to the surface of the target cell.[36] The purified 7s antibodies were reacted with a three-fold excess of the heterobifunctional cross-linker N-succinimydyl-3-(1-pyridyldithio) propionate (SPDP; Sigma). The modified antibodies were then reacted with R1(TL$^-$) cells, which had been pretreated with dithiothreitol to introduce free sulphydryl groups at the cell surface. As demonstrated in Figure 2, the antibody-coated target cells are specifically recognized and lysed by the appropriate cloned effector cells: OE4 (F9$^-$, F23.1$^+$) only lyses the F23.1-modified targets, and G4 (F9$^+$, F23.1$^-$) only the F9-modified targets, whereas OE25 (F9$^-$, F23.1$^-$) cannot react with the altered R1(Tl$^-$) cells. Other experiments had already shown that the ligation of the effector to the target cell must engage components of the T cell receptor to result in lysis.[35,36] For example, anti-H-2^b antibodies on the target cell surface cause approximation of the two cell types, but no lethal hit occurs. In other experiments, we found that sheep

Table 1
TARGETING MAMMALIAN ERYTHROCYTES FOR LYSIS BY THE CTL CLONE OE4

Target cell[a]	% Specific lysis at 2:1 E:T ratio[b]
SRBC	0
SRBC-F23.1	34
HRBC	0
HRBC-F23.1	47

[a] The monoclonal antibody F23.1 was reacted with the heterobifunctional cross-linker SPDP and then covalently bound to ^{51}Cr-labeled sheep and human red blood cells (SRBC and HRBC) which had been pretreated with 0.5 mM dithiothreitol to introduce free sulphydyl groups at the cell surface.
[b] 1×10^5 F23.1 coated or uncoated erythrocyte targets ere incubated with 2×10^5 cells of the CTL clone OE4 at 37°C for 4hr. Percent specific lysis of the targets was calculated as described in the legend to Figure 1.

and human erythrocytes can be lysed by OE4 when they are coated with F23.1 (Table 1), although they do not carry MHC molecules on their surface and have quite different membranes from the normal nucleated CTL target cells.

At this point in our work, we were convinced that we could target cells for T lymphocyte effector function independent of influences of MHC molecules via antibodies against the T cell receptor. But on the side of the target cell, covalent binding does not permit any specificity. A first step in the direction of specific targeting was explored in the following approach.

B. Monoclonal Antibodies Bound to the Fc Receptor of the Target Cell

In this system, CTL populations were coated with F23.1 and tested for lysis of a P815 subline that expresses Fc receptors capable of binding to antibodies of the IgG2a subclass (Figure 1B). For this protocol, it was necessary to demonstrate that such killing was induced via the T cell receptor of the effector cell, in contrast to the mechanism of antibody-dependent cell-mediated cytotoxicity (ADCC) where the effector cell is armed by antibodies bound to its Fc receptors. For this purpose, Con A-induced blasts from BALB/c and C57L/J (F23.1$^+$ or F23.1$^-$ mouse strains, respectively) were tested for their lytic activity in lectin-mediated and F23.1 antibody-mediated killing assays. As shown in Table 2, Con A blasts from both mouse strains lyse ^{51}Cr-labeled P815 targets in the presence of the lectin PHA. However, only Con A blasts derived from BALB/c mice could kill P815 after precoating with F23.1. Assuming that the only relevant difference in this system between Con A blasts derived from a C57L/J mouse and those from a BALB/c mouse is in the expression of an F23.1-reactive epitope on a fraction of the T cell receptors, we conclude that in the F23.1-mediated lysis, the antibody cross-bridging between the effector and target cell engages to the T cell receptor on the effector cell. To determine whether the binding site of F23.1 on the target cell is really the Fc receptor for IgG2a, we tested F(ab')$_2$ fragments of this monoclonal antibody that showed unimpaired ability to react with T cell receptors. BALB/c Con A blasts were coated with different concentrations of either purified (7s) F23.1 antibody of F(ab')$_2$ fragments. Confirming our assumption, two different concentrations of a purified F(ab')$_2$ preparation of F23.1 could not induce any lysis of P815 targets, while 7s antibody was able to mediate lysis over a wide concentration range (Figure 3). Together with IgG2a competition studies at the target level, these experimental data strongly suggest that F23.1 has to bind to the Fc receptor on the target cell. Thus, F23.1 cross-bridges the effector and target cells

Table 2
F23.1-MEDIATED LYSIS BY T CELLS VIA THE Fc RECEPTOR OF TARGET CELLS[a]

Origin of Con A blasts	Mediator	% Specific lysis of P815 at 60:1 E:T
C57L/J	—	4
C57L/J	PHA	55
C57L/J	F23.1	5
BALB/c	—	6
BALB/c	PHA	52
BALB/c	F23.1	23

[a] Nylon wool-enriched T lymphocytes, together with anti-Thy-1 plus C-treated, irradiated spleen cells (accessory cells), were incubated with medium containing a mitogenic dose of concanavalin A. On day 3 of culture, effector cells were harvested, washed with α-methyl-D-mannoside, and a portion coated with F23.1 antibody. 6×10^5 antibody coated or uncoated Con A blasts and 1×10^4 ^{51}Cr-labeled P815 were incubated for 4hr. For lectin-mediated lysis, phytohemagglutinin (PHA) was introduced into the 4hr assay at a final concentration of 10 μg/mℓ.

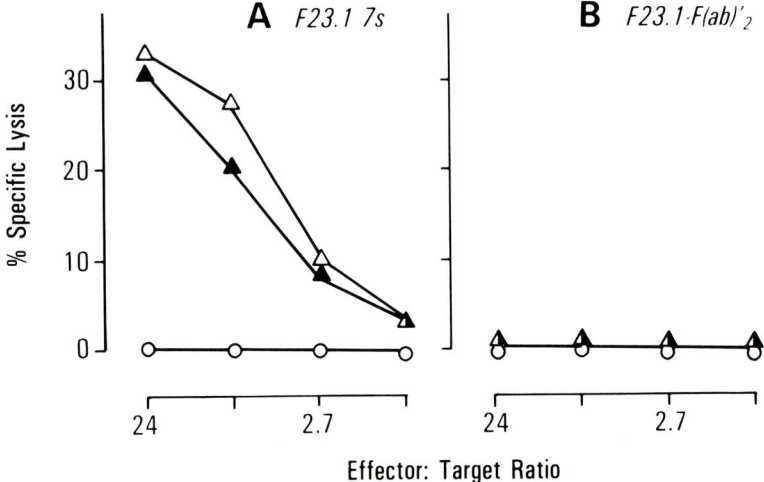

FIGURE 3. The Fc portion of the anti-receptor antibody F23.1 is required to reveal Fc receptor guided cytotoxicity. Four-day Con A blasts were precoated with medium alone (○) or with 0.26 μg/mℓ of the antibody (▲) or with 26 μg/mℓ antibody (△). 7s antibody was used in (A) and a purified F(ab')$_2$ preparation in (B). The protocol was similar to the experiment described in Table 2.

via the T cell receptor and the Fc receptor, respectively, resulting in specific targeting via the Fc receptor.

C. Heteroconjugates of Monoclonal Antibodies as Targeting Agents

To widen the scope of possible targets beyond Fc receptor-bearing cells, we attempted to specifically bind antibodies against the T cell receptor to target cells. Heteroconjugates of monoclonal antibodies were constructed in which one antibody reacts with the T cell receptor (anti-idiotype or anti-allotype), and the other antibody binds to a chosen surface antigen on any target cell, but not on the CTL (Figure 1C). Two experimental systems were

Table 3
ANTIGEN-SPECIFIC TARGETING BY HETEROCONJUGATED MONOCLONAL ANTIBODIES

		% Lysis at 6:1 E:T ratio[c]	
Target cell[a]	Heteroconjugates[b]	G4 (F9+, H-2b, anti H-2d)	OE4 (F23.1+, H-2b, anti H-2d)
P815 (H-2d)	—	83	79
EL4 (H-2b, Thy 1.2)	—	1	1
S.AKR (H-2k, Thy 1.1)	—	3	2
EL4	19E12/F9	9	1
EL4	19E12/F23.1	2	4
S.AKR	19E12/F9	65	1
S.AKR	19E12/F23.1	1	61

[a] Prelabeled target cells were incubated with heteroconjugated antibody for 20 min, where indicated, and introduced into the killing assay.
[b] Protein A-purified monoclonal antibodies, 19E12, F9, and F23.1, were modified with SPDP and cross-linked according to the manufacturer's handbook on SPDP (Pharmacia).
[c] The coated and uncoated target cells were assayed for lysis by the CTL clones, G4 and OE4, at an E:T of 6:1 at 37°C for 4 hr.

explored. As a model for tumor antigen recognition, we chose as the targeting monoclonal antibody, 19E12, which is specific for the Thy 1.1 alloantigen that is found on AKR/J (H-2k)-derived T lymphomas, but not on the CTL clones G4 and OE4. We produced two heteroconjugates of monoclonal antibodies, (19E12/F9) and (19E12/F23.1), using the crosslinker SPDP. Both heteroconjugates worked efficiently and specifically, as shown in Table 3. The construct (19E12/F9) targeted only S.AKR cells for lysis by G4 effector cells, while (19E12/F23.1) targeted S.AKR cells for lysis by OE4 effectors only. Neither construct rendered EL4 (H-2b, Thy 1.2) susceptible to lysis.

A second model tested the ability of similar heteroconjugates to specifically eliminate virus-infected cells. The G protein of vesicular stomatitis virus (VSV) is expressed on the surface of infected murine cells such as EL4.[40] This antigen is bound by the monoclonal antibody 8E11, which was incorporated into two heteroconjugates, (8E11/F9) and (8E11/F23.1). The results, depicted in Figure 4, demonstrate the efficiency of this targeting. While uninfected EL4 are not lysed via the heteroconjugates, infected cells are killed by the appropriate CTLs. The construct (8E11/F9) specifically enables G4 to lyse VSV-infected EL4, where (8E11/F23.1) only mediates attack by OE4. Thus, targeting via heteroconjugated antibodies works extremely well both for tumor targets and for virus-infected cells, possessing a high degree of specificity both for the binding to the CTL and to the target cell.

D. Hybrid Antibodies as Targeting Agents

Our final goal was to recruit T lymphocytes as effectors at tumor sites or sites of infection in vivo. Heteroconjugated bispecific antibodies had demonstrated the targeting efficiency of these agents. Heteroconjugates of 7s monoclonal antibodies, however, may be quickly removed from circulation in vivo and may not readily access certain target sites. Chemical synthesis of recombinant F(ab')$_2$ bispecific fragments was successful, but the procedure proved rather cumbersome.[41] Therefore, we established a B cell hybrid hybridoma line, H1.10.1.6, which produced a 7s hybrid monoclonal antibody.[42] We fused a F23.1-producing line that is HAT-sensitive, ouabain-resistant, with a 19E12-producing line that is HAT-

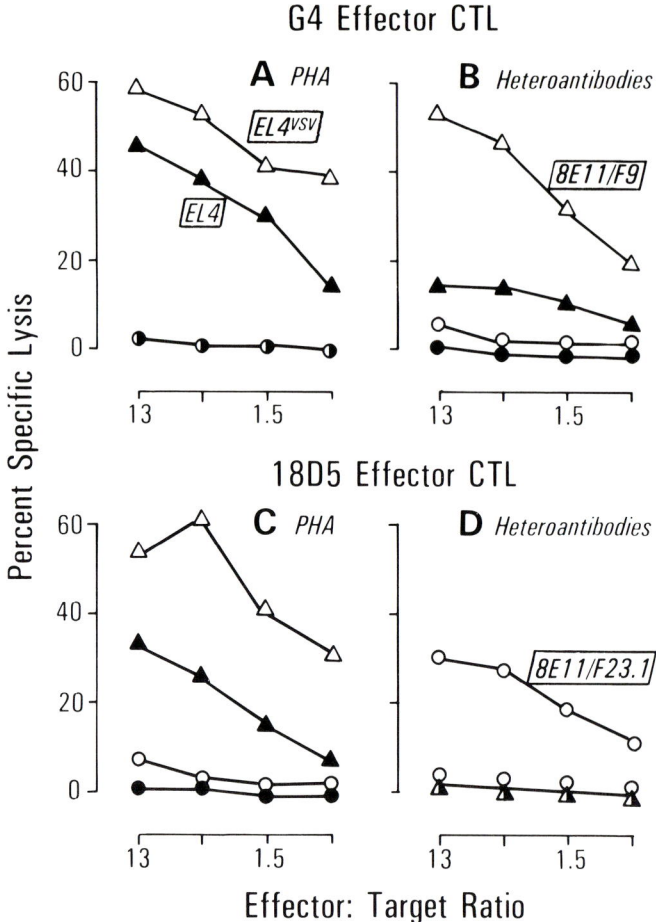

FIGURE 4. Heteroconjugates of monoclonal antibodies can specifically target virus infected cells for lysis by CTL. The CTL clones G4 (A and B) (BALB.B (H-2^b) anti BALB/c (H-2^d), F9$^+$, F23.1$^-$) and 18D5 (C and D) (BALB.B (H-2^b) anti BALB/c (H-2^d), F9$^-$, F23.1$^+$) were assessed for the lytic ability for normal (●, ▲) and vesicular stomatitis virus (VSV) infected EL4 (○,△) in the presence (△,▲) or absence (○,●) of the lectin PHA (A and C). In panels B and D, the heteroconjugates 8E11/F9 (△,▲) and 8E11/F23.1 (○,●) were tested for their targeting potential. The monoclonal antibody 8E11, which reacts with the G protein of VSV, was cross-linked to the T cell receptor antibodies F9 and F23.1, as described in the text. The antibody constructs were used to coat normal and VSV infected ^{51}Cr-labeled EL4 by incubation at 37°C for 20 min followed by washing. These target cells were assayed for lysis by serial three-fold dilutions of the CTL G4 and 18D5 at 37°C for 4 hr.

resistant, ouabain-sensitive. The resulting double-resistant B cell hybrid hybridoma, H1.10.1.6, secretes both anti-T cell receptor and anti-Thy 1.1 reactive antibodies, together with hybrid antibodies capable of focusing T cell activity (Figure 1C). This was determined with antibody enriched by fractionation of ascites preparation on Protein A columns.[43] The experiment reported in Figure 5A shows that OE4 (F23.1$^+$) effector cells, but not OE25 (F23.1$^-$) effectors, are induced to lyse S.AKR (Thy 1.1) targets by the H1.10.1.6 immunoglobulin. Both CTL clones are able to lyse S.AKR targets in the presence of a mitogenic lectin such as PHA. The antibody secreted by H1.10.1.6 does not target EL4 cells for lysis by OE4 effector cells presumably because EL4 expresses Thy 1.2 rather than Thy 1.1 (Figure 5B). Both lymphoma targets are lysed by OE4 CTL in the presence of PHA.

In order to further characterize the putative 19E12/F23.1 hybrid antibody secreted by H1.10.1.6, it was necessary to fractionate the Protein A-Sepharose-purified immunoglobulins

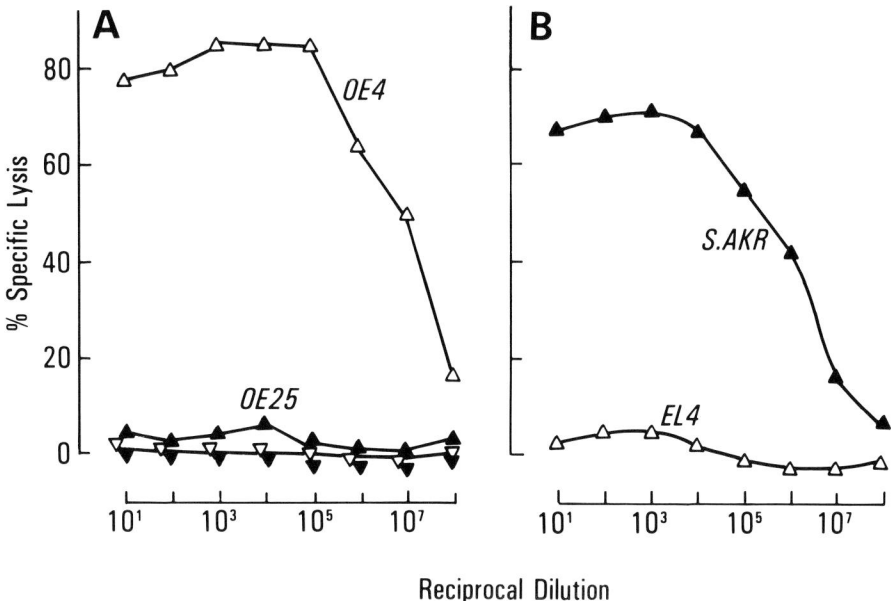

FIGURE 5. Specific targeting of Thy 1.1⁺ tumor cells for lysis by F23.1⁺ CTL by the hybrid antibody secreted by the hybrid hybridoma cell line H1.10.1.6. (A) S.AKR (H-2^k, Thy 1.1) target cells were incubated with serial dilutions of H1.10.1.6 immunoglobulin starting at 2 mg/mℓ with the CTL clones OE4 (△, H-2^b anti H-2^d, F23.1⁺) or OE25 (▲, H-2^b anti H-2^d, F23.1⁻), or with control immunoglobulin (▽,▼). (B) OE4 effector cells were incubated with ⁵¹Cr-labeled S.AKR targets (▲) or EL4 targets (△, H-2^b, Thy 1.2) in the presence of serial dilutions of H1.10.1.6 antibody.

on hydroxylapatite HPLC. An elution profile of the Protein A-Sepharose-purified secretory products of H1.10.1.6 is shown in Figure 6. Pools of the three major peaks of the first run were made as indicated and rechromatographed under the same conditions. Peak I corresponds in elution position to the F23.1 monoclonal antibody, and Peak III coincides with 19E12 monoclonal antibody. Peak II thus contains the putative hybrid antibody. Functional evidence consistent with this suggestion is shown in Figure 7. Peak I demonstrates little activity in inducing lysis of S.AKR targets by OE4 CTL; Peak III has some activity, but on a weight basis is less than 1% as active as Peak II. In accord with this, the hydroxylapatite chromatography shows that Peak III is likely to be contaminated with the material in Peak II (Figure 6). Chemical characterization of the putative hybrid antibody peak from the hydroxylapatite column on isoelectric focusing shows that the hybrid antibody is distinct from the two parent antibodies and is comprised of all the components of both F23.1 and 19E12. Thus, by functional and chemical criteria, it appears that H1.10.1.6 secretes approximately one-third of its total immunoglobulin output as an F23.1/19E12 hybrid antibody. This hybrid can efficiently target Thy 1.1⁺ cells for lysis of CTL clones that express the allotypic determinant recognized by F23.1.

We have not been able to determine the actual yield of the desired bispecific hybrid antibody secreted by H1.10.1.6. As discussed in Reference 44, under the assumption that the rate of production of the two pairs of H and L chains is equal, that there is no preference of the HL pairs for homologous or heterologous pairing (i.e., L_1H_1, L_2H_2, L_1H_2, and L_2H_2 form with equal probability), and that H-H pairing occurs randomly, the yield of the desired bispecific hybrid antibody, L_1H_1-L_2H_2, amounts to 12.5% of the total immunoglobulin output. Most likely, homologous LH pairing will occur preferentially,[44] which would drive the yield of the desired bispecific hybrid up to 50% if this preference were absolute. Although

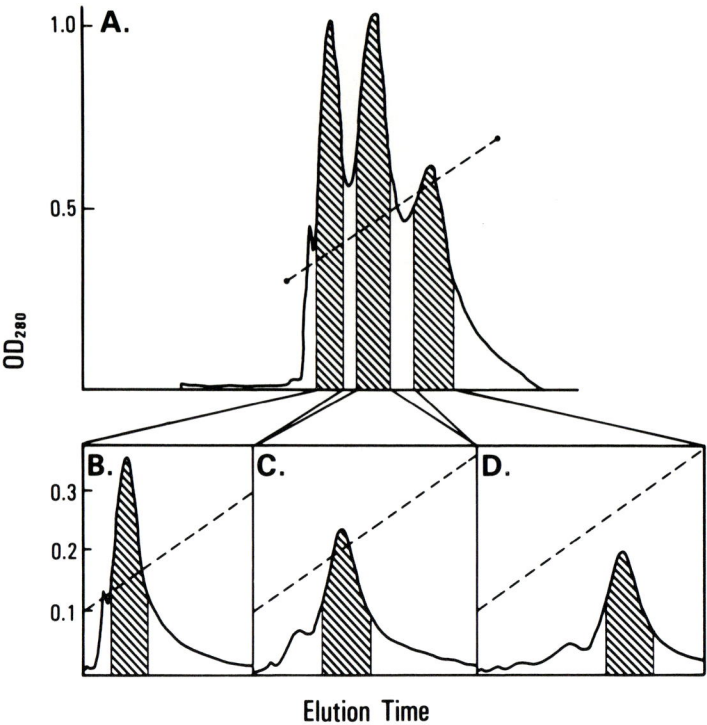

FIGURE 6. Fractionation of Protein-A-Sepharose purified immunoglobulin produced by the hybrid hybridoma H1.10.1.6. The hydroxylapatite HPLC column was loaded in 10 mM sodium phosphate, pH 6.8, and eluted with a gradient of 50 to 180 mM sodium phosphate, pH 6.8. The three shaded fractions indicated in (A) were pooled, concentrated, and run under the same conditions: (B) = Peak I, (C) = Peak II, (D) = Peak III.

our antibody preparation is to a certain extent enriched for the desired bispecific hybrid, a protein concentration as low as 2 ng/mℓ of Pool II is sufficient to cause significant lysis of the S.AKR targets by a three-fold excess of OE4 CTL (Figure 6).

III. SUMMARY AND DISCUSSION

The present report examines the possibility of specifically focusing the effector function of T lymphocytes without the limits usually imposed on T cell recognition. Previous studies had suggested that monoclonal antibodies can act as targets for T cells, thus mimicking the effects of MHC-plus-antigen recognition. To further define the mechanisms involved in this recognition function, we chose cells that do not express classical MHC Class I molecules as targets for typical cloned CTL lines. Both the β-2-microglobulin negative (R1(TL$^-$)) lymphoma line and erythrocytes from two different sources could be rendered susceptible to T lymphocyte-mediated lysis after antibodies that are reactive with the T cell receptor were covalently attached to their cell surface. Evidently, neither Class I nor Class II MHC molecules are important for the antibody-induced lysis, excluding the participation of these molecules in the lytic process. These studies clearly demonstrate that antibodies reactive with the T cell receptor can entirely substitute for recognition of antigen and MHC in the effector phase of the cellular immune response.

In a more sophisticated approach, we tried to exploit these findings by directing the

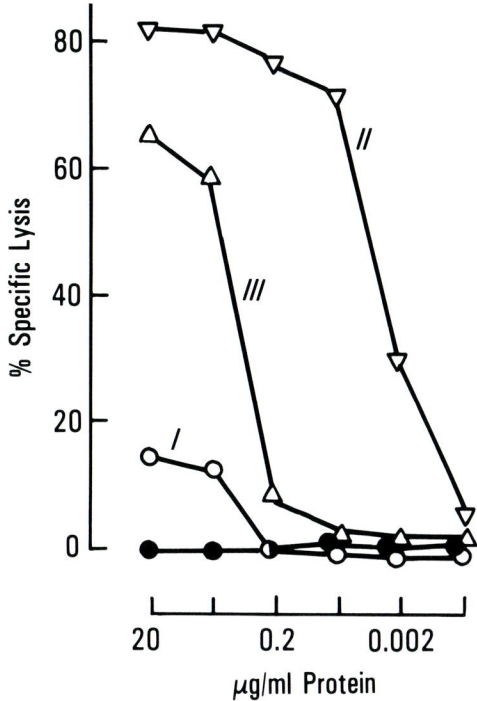

FIGURE 7. The three peaks of H1.10.1.6 immunoglobulin from HPLC were titrated for their ability to cause the OE4-mediated lysis of ^{51}Cr-labeled S.AKR target cells. 1×10^4 ^{51}Cr-labeled S.AKR and 3×10^4 OE4 were incubated together with different dilutions of the concentrated HPLC: Peak I (○), Peak II (▽), and Peak (△), or medium alone (●) at 37°C for 4 hr.

binding of the T cell receptor antibodies to different target cells. We should be able to discriminate between different targets on the basis of different structures on their surface. The first approach we took used the Fc receptor on the target cell as the attachment site for the T cell receptor antibody. We were thus able to specifically target Fc receptor-bearing cells, such as P815, for lysis by cytolytic T cells. This principle allows only for cells that can fix the Fc part of antibodies against the T cell receptor to serve as suitable targets. Since our final goal was to focus a strong T cell response to a wide variety of target cells, we constructed heteroconjugates of monoclonal antibodies that attach to the target cell via one monoclonal antibody binding site exposing antibodies against the T cell receptor on the cell surface. The results presented here demonstrate that these constructs are powerful tools for targeting tumor cells or viral infections for CTL-mediated lysis. This technique could gain clinical relevance if certain requirements are fulfilled. First, antibody against a chosen target, i.e., a tumor-associated or viral antigen, must be available. The second requirement is an antibody against the T cell receptor complex. This technique circumvents the failure of the patients' T cells to respond in an effective way to the antigenic challenge (if any) with a specific MHC-restricted response. Since we have established H1.10.1.6, a hybrid hybrodima line which secretes bivalent 7s antibodies that react both with a wide spectrum of T cell receptors and with Thy 1.1 as a surface marker of a tumor model, we are presently assessing the in vivo applications in a murine system. AKR/J (Thy 1.1) T lymphomas have been established in AKR/Cum (Thy 1.2) hosts; the hosts' own effector T cells, and H1.10.1.6, the 19E12/F23.1 hybrid, will be used in an attempt to eradicate the tumor cells. If it proves to be necessary, two protocols are available to expand and activate the effector CTL population. Effector cells can be induced in vivo either by skin-grafting or by immunization with cells of different MHC haplotypes. Alternatively, in vitro-activated CTL can be adoptively transferred to the host. Pilot studies with in vitro activated CTL have provided preliminary evidence that hybrid antibodies can be effective in targeting established tumors for destruction by T lymphocytes in vivo, resulting in significantly prolonged survival of the animal. Further studies are presently under way to confirm these results.

REFERENCES

1. **Kohler, G. and Milstein, C.**, Continuous cultures of fused cells secreting antibody of predefined specificity, *Nature*, 256, 495, 1975.
2. **Allison, J. P., McIntyre, B. W., and Block, D.**, Tumor-specific antigen of murine T-lymphoma defined with monoclonal antibody, *J. Immunol.*, 129, 2293, 1982.
3. **Meuer, S. C., Fitzgerald, K. A., Hussey, R. E., Hodgdon, J. C., Schlossman, S. F., and Reinherz, E. L.**, Clonotypic structures involved in antigen-specific human T cell function. Relationship to the T3 molecular complex, *J. Exp. Med.*, 157, 705, 1983.
4. **Reinherz, E. L., Meuer, S. C., Fitzgerald, K. A., Hussey, R. E., Hodgdon, J. C., Acuto, O., and Schlossman, S. F.**, Comparison of T3-associated 49-and 43-kilodalton cell surface molecules on individual human T-cell clones: Evidence for peptide variability in T-cell receptor structures, *Proc. Natl. Acad. Sci. USA*, 80, 4104, 1983.
5. **Haskins, K., Kubo, R., White, J., Pigeon, M., Kappler, J., and Marrack, P.**, The major histocompatibility complex-restricted antigen receptor on T cells. I. Isolation with a monoclonal antibody, *J. Exp. Med.*, 157, 1149, 1983.
6. **Lancki, D. W., Lorber, M. I., Loken, M. R., and Fitch, F. W.**, A clone-specific monoclonal antibody that inhibits cytolysis of a cytolytic T cell clone, *J. Exp. Med.*, 157, 921, 1983.
7. **Samelson, L. E., Germain, R. N., and Schwartz, R. H.**, Monoclonal antibodies against the antigen receptor on a cloned T-cell hybrid, *Proc. Natl. Acad. Sci. USA*, 80, 6972, 1983.
8. **Staerz, U. D., Pasternack, M. S., Klein, J. R., Benedetto, J. D., and Bevan, M. J.**, Monoclonal antibodies specific for a murine cytotoxic T-lymphocyte clone, *Proc. Natl. Acad. Sci. USA*, 81, 1799, 1984.
9. **Hedrick, S. M., Cohen, D. I., Nielsen, E. A., and Davis, M. M.**, Isolation of cDNA clones encoding T cell-specific membrane-associated proteins, *Nature*, 308, 149, 1984.
10. **Yanagi, Y., Yoshikai, Y., Leggett, K., Clark, S. P., Alexander, J., and Mak, T. W.**, A human T cell-specific cDNA clone encodes a protein having extensive homology to immunoglobulin chains, *Nature*, 308, 145, 1984.
11. **Chien, Y., Becker, D. M., Lindsten, T., Okamura, M., Cohen, D. I., and Davis, M. M.**, A third type of murine T-cell receptor gene, *Nature*, 312, 31, 1984.
12. **Saito, H., Kranz, D. M., Takagaki, Y., Hayday, A. C., Eisen, H. N., and Tonegawa, S.**, A third rearranged and expressed gene in a clone of cytotoxic T lymphocytes, *Nature*, 312, 36, 1984.
13. **Sim, G. K., Yague, J., Nelson, J., Marrack, P., Palmer, E., Augustin, A., and Kappler, J.**, Primary structure of human T-cell receptor β-chain, *Nature*, 312, 771, 1984.
14. **Hedrick, S. M., Nielson, E. A., Kavaler, J., Cohen, D. I., and Davis, M. M.**, Sequence relationships between putative T-cell receptor polypeptides and immunoglobulins, *Nature*, 308, 153, 1984.
15. **Chien, Y.-H., Gascoigne, N., Kavaler, J., Lee, N. E., and Davis, M. M.**, Somatic recombination in a murine T-cell receptor gene, *Nature*, 309, 322, 1984.
16. **Malissen, M., Minard, K., Mjolsness, S., Kronenberg, M., Goverman, J., Hunkapiller, T., Pryslowsky, M. B., Yoshikai, Y., Fitch, F., Mak, T. W., and Hood, L.**, Mouse T cell antigen receptor: Structure and organization of constant and joining gene segments encoding the β polypeptide, *Cell*, 37, 1101, 1984.
17. **Gascoigne, N. R. J., Chien, Y.-H., Becker, D. M., Kavaler, J., and Davis, M. M.**, Genomic organization and sequence of T-cell receptor β-chain constant- and joining-region genes, *Nature*, 310, 387, 1984.
18. **Winoto, A., Mjolsness, S., and Hood, L.**, Genomic organization of the genes encoding mouse T-cell receptor α-chain, *Nature*, 316, 832, 1985.
19. **Kavaler, J., Davis, M. M., and Chien, Y.-H.**, Localization of a T-cell receptor diversity-region element, *Nature*, 310, 421, 1984.

20. **Bergman, Y., Stewart, S. J., Levy, S., and Levy, R.,** Biosynthesis, glycosylation, and in vitro translation of the human T cell antigen Leu-4, *J. Immunol.,* 131, 1876, 1983.
21. **Borst, J., Coligon, J. E., Oettgen, H., Pessano, S., Malin, R., and Terhorst, C.,** The δ- and ε-chains of the human T3/T cell receptor complex are distinct polypeptides, *Nature,* 312, 455, 1984.
22. **Haskins, K., Hannum, C., White, J., Roehm, N., Kubo, R., Kappler, J., and Marrack, P.,** The major histocompatibility complex-restricted antigen receptor on T cells. VI. An antibody to receptor allotype, *J. Exp. Med.,* 160, 452, 1984.
23. **Staerz, U. D., Rammensee, H.-G., Benedetto, J. D., and Bevan, M. J.,** Characterization of a murine monoclonal antibody specific for an allotypic determinant on the T cell antigen receptor, *J. Immunol.,* 134, 3994, 1985.
24. **Landegren, U., Ramstedt, U., Axberg, I., Ullberg, M., Jondal, M., and Wigzell, H.,** Selective inhibition of human T cell cytotoxicity at levels of target recognition or initiation of lysis by monoclonal OKT3 and Leu 2a antibodies, *J. Exp. Med.,* 155, 1579, 1982.
25. **Meuer, S. C., Hussey, R. E., Hodgdon, J. C., Hercend, T., Schlossman, S. F., and Reinherz, E. L.,** Surface structures involved in target recognition by human cytotoxic T lymphocytes, *Science,* 218, 471, 1982.
26. **Tsoukas, C. D., Carson, D. A., Fong, S., and Vaughan, J. H.,** Molecular interactions in human T cell-mediated cytotoxicity to EBV. II. Monoclonal antibody OKT3 inhibits a post-killer-target recognition/adhesion step, *J. Immunol.,* 129, 1421, 1983.
27. **Meuer, S. C., Hussey, R. E., Cantrell, D. A., Hodgdon, J. C., Schlossman, S. F., Smith, K. A., and Reinherz, E. L.,** Triggering of the T3-Ti antigen-receptor complex results in clonal T-cell proliferation through an interleukin 2-dependent autocrine pathway, *Proc. Natl. Acad. Sci. USA,* 81, 1509, 1984.
28. **von Wauve, F. B., DeMay, J. R., and Goossener, J. G.,** OKT3: A monoclonal anti-human T lymphocyte antibody with potent mitogenic properties, *J. Immunol.,* 124, 2708, 1980.
29. **Chang, T. W., Kung, P. C., Gingras, S. P., and Goldstein, G.,** Does OKT3 monoclonal antibody react with the antigen-recognition structure on human T cells?, *Proc. Natl. Acad. Sci. USA,* 78, 1805, 1981.
30. **Burns, G. F., Boyd, A. W., and Beverley, P. C. L.,** Two monoclonal anti-human T lymphocyte antibodies have similar biologic effects and recognize the same cell surface antigen, *J. Immunol.,* 129, 1451, 1982.
31. **Lancki, D. W., Ma, D. I., Havran, W. F., and Fitch, F. W.,** Cell surface structures involved in T cell activation, *Immunol. Rev.,* 81, 65, 1984.
32. **Crispe, I. N., Bevan, M. J., and Staerz, U. D.,** Selective activation of Lyt 2^+ precursor T cells by ligation of the antigen receptor, *Nature,* 317, 627, 1985.
33. **Lancki, D. W. and Fitch, F. W.,** A cloned CTL demonstrates different interaction requirements for lysis of two distinct target cells, *Fed. Proc.,* 43, 1659, 1984.
34. **Hoffman, R. W., Bluestone, J. A., Oberdan, L., and Shaw, S.,** Lysis of anti-T3-bearing murine hybridoma cells by human allospecific cytotoxic T cell clones and inhibition of that lysis by anti-T3 and anti-LFA-1 antibodies, *J. Immunol.,* 135, 5, 1985.
35. **Kranz, D. M., Tonegawa, S., and Eisen, H. N.,** Attachment of an anti-receptor antibody to non-target cells renders them susceptible to lysis by a clone of cytotoxic T lymphocytes, *Proc. Natl. Acad. Sci. USA,* 81, 7922, 1984.
36. **Staerz, U. D., Kanagawa, O., and Bevan, M. J.,** Hybrid antibodies can target sites for attack by T cells, *Nature,* 314, 628, 1985.
37. **Staerz, U. D. and Bevan, M. J.,** Cytotoxic T lymphocyte-mediated lysis via the Fc receptor of target cells, *Eur. J. Immunol.,* 1985, in press.
38. **Spits, H., Yssel, H., Leeuwenberg, J., and de Vries, J. E.,** Antigen-specific cytoxic T cell and antigen-specific proliferating T cell clones can be induced to cytolytic activity by monoclonal antibodies against T3, *Eur. J. Immunol.,* 15, 88, 1985.
39. **Hyman, R. and Stallings, V.,** Characterization of a TL$^-$ variant of a homozygous TL$^+$ mouse lymphoma, *Immunogenetics,* 3, 75, 1976.
40. **Lefrancois, L. and Lyles, D. S.,** The interaction of antibody with the major surface glycoprotein of vesicular stomatitis virus. I. Analysis of neutralizing epitopes with monoclonal antibodies, *Virology,* 121, 157, 1982.
41. **Nisonoff, A. and Rivers, M. M.,** Recombination of a mixture of univalent antibody fragments of different specificity, *Arch. Biochem. Biophys.,* 93, 460, 1961.
42. **Milstein, C. and Cuello, A. C.,** Hybrid hybridomas and their use in immunohistochemistry, *Nature,* 305, 537, 1983.
43. **Staerz, U. D. and Bevan, M. J.,** Hybrid hybridoma producing a bispecific monoclonal antibody which can focus effector T cell activity, *Proc. Natl. Sci. USA,* 1986, in press.
44. **Milstein, C. and Cuello, A. C.,** Hybrid hybridomas and the production of bispecific monoclonal antibodies, *Immunol. Today,* 5, 199, 1984.

Chapter 28

LONG-TERM GROWTH AND EXPANSION OF rIL-2 ACTIVATED NK-CELLS FOR CANCER THERAPY

Eckhard R. Podack, Kristin O. Penichet, Ben-Yao Lin, Jen Wei Chiao and Abraham Mittelman

TABLE OF CONTENTS

I.	Introduction	220
II.	Preparation and Culture of PMBL	220
III.	Increased Cytotoxic Activity in Long-Term rIL-2 Cultures	220
IV.	Increased CD 16 (Leu 11) Expression	221
V.	Summary	221
	Acknowledgments	222
	References	222

I. INTRODUCTION

Incubation of human peripheral mononuclear blood leucocytes (PMBL) with high levels of recombinant interleukin-2 (rIL-2) results in the generation of cells cytotoxic for fresh tumors and cultured tumor cell lines. These cells, termed lymphokine activated killer cells (LAK) by Grimm et al.,[1-3] are detectable within 24 hr of addition of rIL-2 and increase in activity during the following 5 to 7 days of culture. LAK cells and rIL-2 have been shown to be effective for cancer therapy.[4] Although LAK cells were originally postulated to represent a cell population distinct from cytotoxic T-cells and NK-cells,[1-3] more recent evidence attributes the activity to CD16+ (Leu 11+), CD3 negative NK-cells, and to minor populations of CD16+, CD3+ type II cytotoxic T-cells.[5,6] Both types of cytotoxic cells recognize and preferentially lyse tumor cells in an MHC-unrestricted fashion.

Prolonged culture of human PMBL with IL-2 for up to 16 days, as described in this study, results in the increase of the CD16+ (Leu 11+) population of up to 60% while maintaining tumoricidal activity to NK-resistant tumor target cells. This preferential expansion of the apparent killer cell population in vitro may be important for cancer therapy.

II. PREPARATION AND CULTURE OF PMBL

Patients with metastatic cancer received 3 daily doses of 10^5 to 10^6 U/mℓ^2 rIL-2 and two days later were leukophoresed to obtain the lymphocyte-rich fraction of blood. PMBL were isolated from 500 mℓ of lymphocyte-enriched blood by standard Ficoll Hypaque gradient separation, using 50 mℓ conical centrifuge tubes. The PMBL layer was harvested and washed three times with Ca-free Hank's balanced salt solution (HBSS). An aliquot of the cells was tested immediately for cytotoxicity and surface markers, and the remaining cells cultured at 1.5×10^6 cells/mℓ in Iscove's modified Dulbeccos minimum essential medium containing 10% blood-group-compatible human serum, 40 µg/mℓ gentamycin, and 1000 U/mℓ rIL-2.

As culture containers, Nunc cell factories were used, holding up to 21 culture media and providing a surface area of 6000 cm^2. Incubation was at 37°C in 5% CO_2, 95% air. On the third day of culture one third of the original volume of activation medium was added. On the fifth day, one half of the cell culture, after resuspension, was harvested and replaced with the same volume of culture medium containing 1000 U/mℓ rIL-2 (Hoffmann-LaRoche). From then on, cells were harvested in the same manner every second day up to day 16 or, occasionally, to day 21. The harvested cells were washed three times in HBSS with Ca, containing 0.5% human albumin and 1000 U/mℓ rIL-2, resuspended in the same medium, and subjected to analysis for cytotoxicity towards K562 (NK-sensitive), Colo 38 (NK-resistant), and Raji (NK-resistant).

III. INCREASED CYTOTOXIC ACTIVITY IN LONG-TERM rIL-2 CULTURES

Figure 1A-D shows the results of cytotoxicity assays at three killer target ratios. Each symbol represents cells obtained from one patient and tested on day 0 prior to culture with rIL-2 and at various days after incubation in rIL-2-containing medium. Before exposure to rIL-2, the PMBL had low cytotoxic activity towards K562 and no or very low cytotoxicity towards Colo 38 and Raji. This base-line level of K562 cytotoxicity is attributed to the NK-population contained in the PMBL. After 5 to 6 days culture in rIL-2, the cells show strong cytotoxicity to both NK-sensitive and NK-resistant targets. The cells are equally cytotoxic to Daudi (not shown), another NK-resistant tumor line. Cytotoxicity increases to a maximal level on day 12 of culture and then tends to decrease. Cytotoxicity is 3 to 4 times higher on day 12 (mean of all cultures) for all targets compared to day 5 (Figure 1).

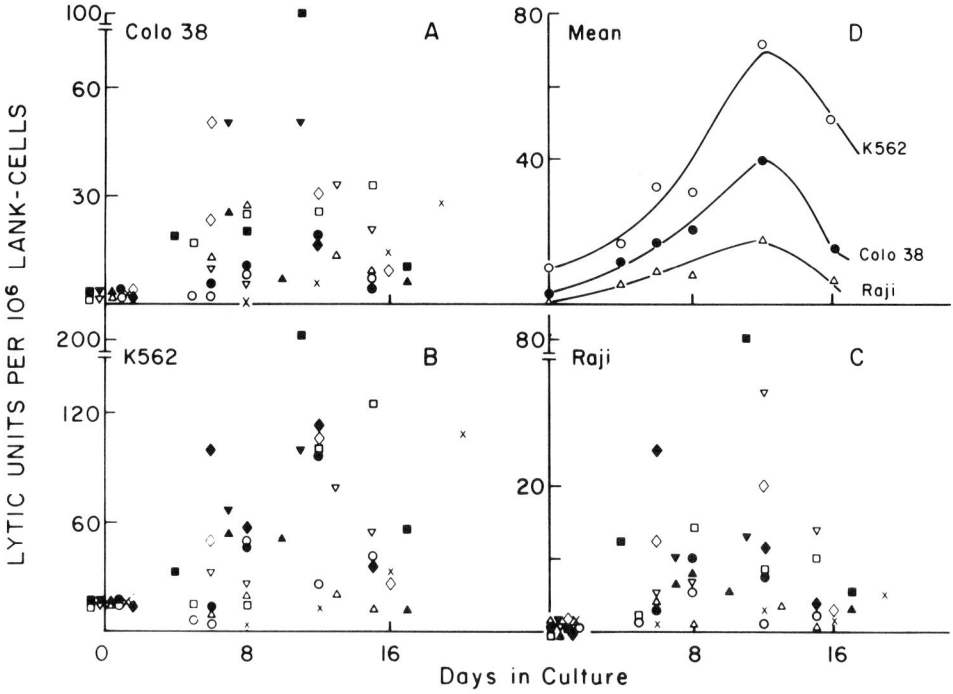

FIGURE 1. Increase in cytotoxicity of Il2 activated killer cells. One lytic unit is defined as the activity causing 30% ^{51}Cr release from 10^4 target cells in 4 hr at 37°. 100 lytic units per 10^6 cells thus will cause 30% ^{51}Cr release at 1:1 killer target ratio.

IV. INCREASED CD 16 (LEU 11) EXPRESSION

The same cell populations analyzed in Figure 1 for cytotoxicity were also subjected to surface marker analysis, using the fluorescent-activated cell sorter. The surface molecules studied were CD16 (Leu 11), CD3, CD4, and CD8. Only the results for CD16 and CD3 are shown in Figure 2. PMBL on day 0 contained on the average 5% to 10% of Leu 11 positive cells. The number of Leu 11$^+$ cells doubled in the first five days of culture and then continuously increased to up to 60% within the 16-day culture period. The increase of Leu 11 positive cells was fairly linear within this period.

The frequency of CD3 positive cells was high on day 0 and generally showed a declining tendency during the culture period. However, considerable variability in the decrease of CD3 was observed from patient to patient. The CD8-positive cells (not shown) increased in parallel with Leu 11, whereas CD4-positive cells generally behaved similar to CD3.

V. SUMMARY

CD16 (Leu 11) positive cells are believed to be the effector cells for the so-called LAK phenomenon. Current evidence suggests that this cell population is comprised predominately of IL-2 activated CD3 negative Leu 11$^+$ NK cells and a minor proportion of Leu 11$^+$ CD3$^+$ MHC unrestricted type II cytotoxic T-cells.[4,5] The current study demonstrates a continuous increase in the frequency of Leu 11$^+$ (and CD8$^+$) cells and a decline of CD3 and CD4 positive cells during prolonged culture of human PMBL with high levels of rIL-2. Cytotoxicity also increases in this time period parallel with Leu 11 to a maximum of activity on the 12th day of culture. This correlation suggests that the long-term activated killer cells generated in this period are Leu 11$^+$, CD8$^+$, CD3$^-$, and CD4$^-$ activated NK-cells.

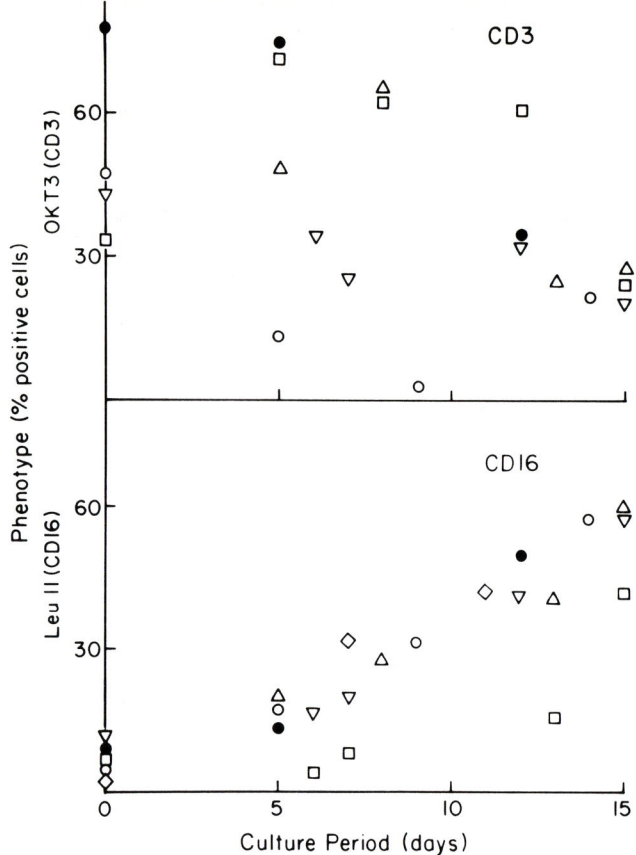

FIGURE 2. Increase in frequency of Leu 11 and decrease of CD3 on I12 activated killer cells. The same cultures analyzed for cytotoxicity in Figure 1 were subjected to surface marker analysis using Leu 11, Okt3, Okt4, and Okt8. Each symbol represents 1 culture analyzed on succeeding days for up to 16 days.

With regard to tumor therapy, the long-term culture of PMBL in rIL-2 may be of advantage over short-term activation protocols. If the Leu 11$^+$ cells are in fact the mediators of the therapeutic response, the long-term culture generates up to 6 times more effector cells. In addition, this method allows significant savings in the expense for leukophoresis, cell culture, and laboratory personnel. The efficacy of long-term, cultured IL-2 activated, Leu 11$^+$ cells for tumor therapy is currently being investigated in clinical trials.

ACKNOWLEDGMENTS

This study was supported in part by funds of the Dr. I. Fund Foundation and by Hoffmann-LaRoche.

REFERENCES

1. **Grimm, E. A., Mazumder, A., Zhang, H. Z., and Rosenberg, S. A.,** Lymphokine-activated killer cell phenomenon. Lysis of natural killer-resistant fresh solid tumor cells by interleukin 2-activated autologous human peripheral blood lymphocytes, *J. Exp. Med.*, 155, 1823, 1982.

2. **Grimm, E. A., Ramsey, K. M., Mazumder, A., Wilson, D. J., Djeu, J. Y., and Rosenberg, S. A.**, Lymphokine-activated killer cell phenomenon. II Precursor phenotype is serologically distinct from peripheral T-lymphocytes, memory cytotoxic thymus-derived lymphocytes and natural killer cells, *J. Exp. Med.*, 157, 884, 1983.
3. **Grimm, E. A., Robb, R. J., Roth, J. A., Nekers, L. M., Lachman, L. B., Wilson, D. J., and Rosenberg, S. A.**, Lymphokine-activated killer cell phenomenon. III. Evidence that Il2 is sufficient for direct activation of peripheral blood lymphocytes into lymphokine activated killer cells, *J. Exp. Med.*, 158, 1356, 1983.
4. **Rosenberg, S. A., Lotze, M. T., Muul, L. M., Leitman, S., Chang, A. E., Ettinghausen, S. E., Matory, Y. L., Skibber, J. M., Shiloni, E., Vetto, J. T., Seipp, C. A., Simpson, C., and Reicher, C. M.**, Observations of the systemic administration of autologus lumphokine-activated killer cells with recombinant interleukin 2 to patients with metastatic cancer, *N. Engl. J. Med.*, 313, 1485, 1985.
5. **Phillips, J. H. and Lanier, L. L.**, Dissection of the lymphokine activated killer phenomenon. Relative contribution of peripheral blood natural killer cells and T-lymphocytes to cytolysis, *J. Exp. Med.*, 164, 814, 1986.
6. **Ortaldo, J. R., Mason, A., and Overton, J. R.**, Lymphokine activated killer cells. Analysis of progenitors and effectors, *J. Exp. Med.*, 164, 1193, 1986.

Index

INDEX

A

Aclacinomycin A, 108
Actinomycin D, 108, 122
Activated protein C, 118
ADCC, see Antibody-dependent cell cytotoxicity
Adriamycin, 108, 147
Agarose gel electrophoresis, 71
AIDS, 101
Amino acids carboxyl to cysteins, 77
Amino acid sequence of TNF, 112—113
Anaphylatoxins C3A and C5a, 136, 147
Antibodies
   anti-allotypic, 206
   anti-idiotypic, 206
   anti-T3, 206
   bivalent 7s, 215
   bone marrow graft rejection by, 156—159
   CTL, 206
   H-2 specific monoclonal, 157—158
   hybrid, 206—207, 211—214
   of IgG, 136—141, 158
   monoclonal
      9.2.27, 141, 145
      in biomedical research, 206
      bound to Fc receptor, 209—210
      conjugating CVF to, 136
      covalently coupled to TC, 207—209
      heteroconjugates of, 210—212
      IgG3, 144
   R24, 145
Antibody-CF conjugates
   cytotoxic activity of, 145
   dimeric and trimeric, 139
   electron microscopy of, 140
   immunotherapeutic potential of, 146
   in vivo stability of, 148
   in vivo studies of, 146—148
   plasma half-times of, 147
   ratios of, 137
   reaction mixture of, 138
   synthesis of, 136—141
Antibody-dependent cell cytotoxicity (ADCC)
   involvement of pore formation in, 20
   mechanism of, 209
   NK-mediated, 158
   PMN-mediated, 117—118
   specificity of serum in, 157
Antibody-ricin conjugates, 148
Antigen activation requirements, 64—65
Antigen-positive target cells, 138
Antigen-specific effector T cells, 206
Antigen-specific, MHC restricted CTL clones, 197
Antigen-specific targeting, 211
Antigens
   CD19, 195
   CR_3, 196
   Leu 19, 197
   MHC, 123
   protein, 119
   surface, 136
   tumor-specific, 123, 211
   viral, 166—168
Antitumor action of TNF, 123
Anti-viral effector activity, 167—168
Apoptosis, 36
   changes in nuclear structure as, 48
   compared to necrosis, 39
   morphology of, 38, 47

B

Ba, 136
Bacillus Calmette-Guerrin (BCG), 114
Bb, 136
B cells
   characteristics of, 194
   hybridoma line, 207, 211—212
   lipopolysaccharide activated, 63
   lymphocytes as, 195
BCG, see Bacillus Calmette-Guerrin
Nα-Benzyloxycarbonyl-1-lysine-thiobenzylester (BLT), 10
B lymphocytes, 194
Bone marrow allograft rejection, 153—159
   by antibody, 156—158
   NK-mediated, 154—155
Bone marrow transplantation model, 154
Bone remodeling, 119
Bone resorption, 118—120
Brain tumor patients, 189
Bystander cells, 141
Bystander killing, 66—67

C

C3, 136
C3b, 136
C3b, Bb, 136
C3bi receptor/adherence glycoprotein CD11, 118
C3c, 136
C3/C5 convertase, 136, 147
C5 convertase, 144
C5b-6 formation, 144
C5b-8, 8
C9, 7, 10, 28
21C11 helper T cell clone, 69
Cachectin, 83, 108, see also tumor necrosis factor
Cachectin/TNF-α, 117
Cachexia, 82
cAMP/cGMP pathway, 122
Cancer, 145, 187, 219—222
Carcinoma, colon, 196, 198—201
CD3

classification of, 194
decrease of, in patients, 221—222
expression of, 194—196
phenotype of, 197, 201
plus T lymphocytes, 202
type II cytotoxic T-cells, 220
use of antibodies against, 203
CD4, 221
CD8, 221
CD16
   in cancer therapy, 220
   classification of, 194
   culture of, 197, 201
   cytotoxicity of, 221
   expression of, 195—196, 203
CD19 antigen, 195
cDNA, 10, 63, 77, 106, 112, 114
CDW18 neutrophil membrane protein complex, 118
Cell death, programmed, 47, 48, 51—52
Cell differentiation, hematopoietic, 118
Cells, 144, see also Melanoma target cells
Channels, 23, 28, 30
Chondroitinsulfate A, 12—13, 15
Chromatin, 3, 47
Chromatography, 25—26, 110—111, 138
Chromium release, 65—66, see also ^{51}Cr release
Chymotrypsin, 183
Cobra venom factor (CVF)
   conjugates of, 141—145, see also Antibody-CVF conjugates
   cytotoxic activity of, 141—146
   derivation and conjugation of, 141
   description of, 136
   in vivo studies of, 146
   secondary structures of, 141
   synthesis and biochemical characterization of, 136—141
Coley's toxins, 106, 115
Collagenase stimulation, 120
Colon carcinoma, 196, 198—201
Complement component C9, 8
Complement-mediated cytolysis, 37—38
Con A, see Concanavalin A
Concanavalin A-induced blasts, 209—210
Concanavalin A-Sepharose, 110
Concanavalin A stimulation
   autodestruction by, 68—69
   of cytotoxic T cells, 65—66
   of NK cells, 96, 101
   of NKCF, 93
Controlled pore glass (CPG), 110
Corynebacterium Parvum (CP), 114
CR_3 antigen, 196
^{51}Cr-labelled target cells, 39—40, 209
^{51}Cr release
   cytoplasmic, 69
   effect of antigen on, 64
   4 hr peak, 67
   microtoxicity of, 94
   peak levels of killing measured by, 70
   rapid, 63—64

   relation to DNA fragmentation, 44—46
   target cell death measured by, 49
   target cell lysis measured by, 37—38
CTL, see Cytolytic T lymphocytes, Cytotoxic T lymphocytes
CTLL-20, 48
CTLMC, see Cytotoxic T lymphocyte-mediated cytolysis
CVF, see Cobra venom factor
Cycloheximide, 116, 122
Cyclosporine A, 179, 181
Cysteine, 77, 112
Cytokines, 119—120
Cytolysin, see Perforin 1
Cytolysis, 4, 5, 37—38, see also Cytotoxic T lymphocyte-mediated cytolysis
Cytolytic granules
   activity of, 5
   in cell-mediated cytolysis, 4
   composition of, 4, 6—15
      complement component 9 in, 8
      granule-associated factors in, 10—14
      perforin 1 in, 6—8
      perforin 2 in, 9—10
Cytolytic T cell killing, 63—64
Cytolytic T lymphocytes (CTL)
   class I MHC restricted, 162—163
   class II MHC restricted, 168—169
   cloned
      anti-viral effector activity of, 166—167
      effector activity of, 165—166
      H-2 restriction of recovery mediated by, 165
      IFN release by, 169
      IL-2 dependent, 166
      influenza virus specificity of, 163
      prophylactic use of, 166
      pulmonary virus reduction by, 165, 171
      recognition of influenza polypeptides by, 166—167
   uncloned and, 4—5
      viral antigenic specificity of, 164
   comparison to NK and LAK, 185
   identification of, 162
   in vivo action of, 169—170
   relationship of LAK to, 183—187
   -target cell interaction, 6
Cytoplasm, granules in, 21
Cytotoxic activity in rIL-2 cultures, 220—221
Cytotoxicity
   of antibody-CVF conjugates, 145
   of CVF, 141—146
   lectin-dependent, 196—197
   mediated by IL-2 dependent cloned cells, 197
   monitoring, 108
   NK CMC mediated, see Natural killer cell mediated cytotoxicity
   of TNF, 82
   variant targets in, 100
Cytotoxic reaction, NK-mediated, 92
Cytotoxic T cell clones, 70, 92
Cytotoxic T lymphocyte-mediated cytolysis

(CTLMC)
  changes in nuclear structure during, 38—39
  characteristics of, 36—39
  compared to complement-mediated cytolysis, 37—38
  DNA fragmentation induced during, 39—44
    assay, 39—40
    induction in target cells, 40—44
  effector cell phases of, 37
  importance of PI in, 15
  killer cell-independent, 37, 45—46
  mechanism of, 36
  model of, 49—50
  stages of, 37
Cytotoxic T lymphocytes (CTL)
  active principle from, 20
  antigen and MHC activation requirements of, 64—65
  antigen-specific, MHC restricted clones of, 197
  autodestruction of, 67—68
  bystander killing in presence of, 66—67
  coated with F23.1, 209
  differentiation from LAK cells, 176
  generation of, from IL-2, 202
  granules in, 22, 68—69
  in vitro activated, 216
  killing by, 21, 30—31, 67—68
  non-MHC restricted, 197, 202
  role of LT in, 64
  target cell DNA fragmentation induction by, 69—70
  -target cell interaction, 50—52
  TNP-specific, 65
Cytotoxins, 99—100, 108

D

DEAE, 110
Dedgranulation, 118
Delayed type hypersensitivity (DTH) reactions, 169—170
DFP treatment, 10
DNA
  detergent-soluble, 39, 44
  electrophoresis of, 42
  -nucleoprotein interactions, 43, 51—52
  oligonucleosome-sized, 51
  target-cell, 119
DNA degradation in target cells, 12
DNA fragmentation
  double-stranded, 52
  effect on lysis, 47—48
  enzymes, 51
  induced during CTLMC, 39—44
    assay of, 39—40
    early, 41
    oligonucleosomes production in, 41—43
    in target cells, 40—44
  mechanism of, 50—52
  patterns of, 52
  relation to target ^{51}Cr release, 44

relation to target cell lysis, 44—48
target cell, 69—70
DTH, see Delayed type hypersensitivity

E

E14 target cells, 12
E. coli, 106, 114
EDTA, 37—38, 46
Effector activity, 166—168
Effector cells
  antigen-specific, 206
  LAK, 186—187
    clinical studies on, 199—200
    experimental studies on, 195—197
    in vitro generated, 200—201
    phenotype of, 196
  lytic granules isolated from, 21—22
  phases of CTLMC, 37
  polyacrylamide gel, 78
  pore-formatin mediated by, 20—21
  T lymphocyte, 211
EGTA, 23
Electrophoresis, 25, 42, 71, 78, 111
Encephalomyocarditis virus (EMCV), 117
Endonuclease, 41—42, 51
Endothelial cells, 116, 118
Endotoxin, 76, 78—80
Entamoeba histolytica, 31
Enzymes, DNA fragmentation-inducing, 51
Eosinophil cytotoxicity enhancing factor, 117
Erthrocytes, mammalian, 209
Erysipelas, 106, 110
Esterase 1 (granzyme 1), 10, 15
Esterase 2 (granzyme 2), 10, 15
Esterases, granule-associated, 10—11

F

F9, 206—207
F23.1, 209—213
FACS, see Fluorescence activated cell sorter
Factor B, 136
Factor D, 136
Factor H, 136
Factor I, 136
Fast protein liquid chromatography (FPLC), 111
Fc receptors, 206, 209—210, 215
Fibroblasts, 62, 117, 119—120
Fluorescence activated cell sorter, 195, 197, 202
FMX-MET II melanoma cells, 142
FPLC, see Fast protein liquid chromatography

G

Gel filtration chromatography, 110
Gel permeation chromatography, 138
Genentec, see rTNFα
B-Glucoronidase, 22
Granule-associated factors, 10—14
  chemotactic, 13—14

mediating Pl independent L-cell killing, 11—12
proteins as, 14—15
proteoglycans as, 12—13
responsible for DNA degradation in target cells, 12
in target lysis, 14
Granules
  in CTL, 68—69
  cytolytic, see Cytolytic granules
  in cytoplasm, 21
  isolated by Percoll gradient, 22
  kinetics of formation of, 69
  lesions produced by, 22—25
  lymphocyte, 4, 5
  lytic, 21—22
  of NK cells, 24
  PFP isolated from, 25—30
Granulocyte, 118
Granzyme 1, see Esterase 1
Granzyme 2, see Esterase 2
6 M Guanidine thiocyanate

H

H1.10.1.6, immunoglobulin, 215
H-2 specific monoclonal antibody, 157—158, 165
Hapten modification, 182
Hematopoietic cell differentiation, 118
Hemopoietic histocompatibility (Hh), 154
Hemorrhagic necrosis, 106, 115, 118
Heparin-Sepharose, 13
Hepatocarcinoma, 145
HEP-2 cells, 117
Hh, see Hemopoietic histocompatibility
High performance liquid chromatography (HPLC), 25, 26, 79, 110—111, 213
Histadine, 112
HL-60 (myeloid), 110—112
HLA-A,B antigens, 118
Holotoxin/necrosin, 108
HPLC, see High performance liquid chromatography
Hydrocortisone, 179, 181
Hypersensitivity, 168—170
Hypotension, 80

I

IAHS, see Iodoacetyl-N-hydroxysuccinimide ester
IFN, see Interferon
IFN-β_2, 116
IFN-β antibodies, 117
IFNγ, see Interferon gamma
IgG antibodies, 136—141, 158
IgG2a,k, 208
IgG3 monoclonal antibody, 144
IL-1, see Interleukin 1
IL-2, see Interleukin 2
IL-2 activated NK-cells, 219—222
IL-2 dependent CTL clones, 166, 197
IL-2-dependent CTLL-20 cells, 48
IL-2 dependent NK cells, 197
Immunoconjugates, 136

Immunoglobulin-depleted serum, 156
Immunoglobulin, H1.10.1.6, 216
Immunoglobulins, protein A-Sepharose-purified, 212—214
Immunotoxins, 147
Influenza polypeptides, 166—167
Influenza virus recognition, 162—163
Interferon (IFN)
  release of, by CTL clones, 169
  suppression of lipoprotein activity by, 117
  synergism with TNF, 120
  target cells pretreated with, 96
  therapeutic use of, 102
Interferon gamma (IFNγ)
  augmentation of LAK activation by, 177
  DNA fragmentation by, 70
  effect on bone resorption, 119
  effect on neutrophils, 83
  effect on TNF, 78—79, 109, 122
  production of, 169
  release of, 206
  secretion by lymphocytes, 116
Interleukin 1 (IL-1)
  biologic activity of, 80
  bone resorption promotion by, 119
  from endothelial cells, 118
  modulation of LPL activity by, 83
  molecule of, 80
  mRNA of, 77
  secretion of, 116
  similarities with TNF, 119—120
  suppression of lipoprotein activity by, 117
Interleukin-2 (IL-2)
  activation of LAK by, 177—178, 189
  activity of, 195
  in CTL culture, 163—164
  effect on AIDS, 101
  generation of CTL by, 202
  incubation of, 177
  injection into tumor sites, 179
  in vivo administration of, 199—200
  lymphocyte cultures in, 196
  primary role of, 176
  production of TNF by, 109
  release of, 206
  removal of, 47
  T cell lines maintained by, 62—63
  therapeutic use of, 101—102
  TNF induction by, 78
  toxicity of, 187—188
Iodoacetyl-N-hydroxysuccinimide ester (IAHS), 146
Ion exchange chromatography, 110
Ionophores, 97
^{125}IUdR-labeled E14, 12
^{125}IUdR-labeled target cells, 39—41, 69—71

K

K562, 197, 199, 220
Killer cell-independent CTLMC, 37, 45—46
Killer cells, 4, 11, see also Natural killer cells

Killing mechanisms, 4
Klebsiella pneumoniae, 117

L

L3T4 cell, 168
L-929 cells
 in vitro cytotoxicity method on, 111
 murine, 106—108
 as target, 62
LAK, see Lymphokine-activated killer
Large granular lymphocyte lines (LGL), 21
L-cells, 11—12
LDL, receptor, 8
Leaky patch, 7
Lectin affinity chromatography, 110
Lectins, 78, 93, 110, 197
Lesions, 22—25, 27—28
Lethal hit, 49—51
Leu 7 antigen, 196
Leu 11b antigen, 196
Leu 19 antigen, 194—197, 201—203
Leucotaxin, 76
Leukemia, myeloic, 145
Leukoregulin, 108
LGL, see Large granular lymphocyte lines
LH pairing, 213
Lipid depletion in 3T3-L1 cells, 84—85
Lipid vesicles, 28
Lipopolysaccharides (LPS), 106
Lipoprotein lipase (LPL), 82, 83, 117, 120
Liposomes, 98
Listeria monocytogens, 117
LPL, see Lipoprotein lipase
LPS, see Lipopolysaccharides
LT, see Lymphotoxin
Lymphocyte-enriched blood, 220
Lymphocyte granules, 4, 5
Lymphocytes
 B, 194
 cytolytic, see Cytolytic lymphocytes
 cytotoxic, see Cytotoxic lymphocytes
 genes for, 114
 human, classification of, 194—195
 IFN-γ secretion by, 116
 incubation of, 177
 in vitro culture of, 194—195, 201
 large granular, 4
 low buoyant density, 196
 T, 194
Lymphoid, see RMPI 1788
Lymphokine, 7, 169, 172, 195, 197
Lymphokine-activated killer (LAK) cells
 activation of, 177—181
 activity of, test for, 176—177
 clones of, 180—181
 comparison with NK and CTL, 183, 185
 definition of, 176
 detection of, 220
 effect of NK cells on, 202—203
 effectors of
 clinical studies on, 199—200
 experimental studies with, 195—197
 heterogeneity of, 186
 in vitro generated, 200—201
 leu 11b expression of, 187
 phenotype of, 196
 tissue source of, 202
 granules in, 4
 lysis of, 180—183
 precursors of, 185—186, 197—199
 recognition of TC by, 182—183
 relationship to other CTL systems, 183—187, 189
 sensitivity of, 182
 susceptibility of, 184
 therapeutic potential of, 187—188, 199—200
 uniqueness of, 183—185
Lymphokine-activated killer (LAK) phenomenon, 194, 198—199
Lymphokine-producing cells, 64, 109
Lymphokine research, 76
Lymphomas, 62—63, 207
Lymphotoxin (LT)
 assay for, 62
 cloning gene for, 63
 cytotoxicity of, 108
 description and definition of, 62
 effect on neutrophils, 83
 genes encoding, 77
 induction of chromium release by, 65—66
 -producing cells, 64—65, 67—68
 properties of, 63
 rapid killing by, 62—63, 65—66
 relationship to NKCF, 99
 role in CTL killing, 64
 secretion of, 65
 targets for, 11
Lysis
 colloid osmotic, 37—38
 by CTL, 212
 effect of DNA fragmentation on, 47—48
 F23.1-mediated, 210
 LAK, 180—183
 by macrophages, 92
 by NKCF, 98
 of NK-resistant target cells, 98
 by OE4 clone, 209
 target cell, see Target cell lysis
Lytic process, 36
Lyt phenotype, 64—65

M

Macrophages, 92, 109, 116, 118
Major histocompatibility complex (MHC)
 activation requirements of, 64—65
 antigens of, 123
 antigen-specific clones, 197
 class I-negative lymphoma cells, 207
 class I-restricted CTL, 162—164, 169, 170
 class II-restricted CTL, 168—170
 encoded molecules, 206

restriction by, 194
m-Maleimidobenzoylhydroxysuccinimide ester (MBS), 146
Mammalian erythrocytes, 209
Manganes, 46
Mast cell protease type III, 10
MBS, see *m*-Maleimidobenzoylhydroxysuccinimide ester
Melanoma, 201
Melanoma cells, 141—144
Membrane attack complex, 147
Membrane curent, 25
Membrane damage, 36, 49—50
Meth A cells, 63, 122—123
Meth A sarcoma, 106, 108, 115
Mg-EGTA, 145—146
MHC, see Major histocompatibility complex
Mitogens, 93
Mitomycin C, 108
Monoclonal antibodies, see Antibodies, monoclonal
Monocytes, 108, 114, 116
mRNA, 77, 117
Muramyl dipeptide derivatives, 110
Myeloic leukemia, 145
Myeloid, see HL-60

N

Naja naja, 145
Natural killer cellmediated cytotoxity (NK CMC), 92, 93, 95—98
Natural killer (NK) cells
  activated, 200
  active principle from, 20
  bone marrow allograft rejection by, 153—159
  classification of, 194—195
  cloned/uncloned, 4, 154
  comparison with LAK and CTL, 183, 185
  cultured, 195—196, 201
  defective, effector function of, 100—101
  distinction from LAK cells, 176
  effect on LAK activity, 202—203
  granules from, 22, 24
  identification of, 194
  IL-2 activated, 219—222
  IL-2 dependent, 197
  isolated from peripheral blood, 197
  killing by, 21, 30—31
  lysis of tumor cells by, 20
  lytic activity of, 92
  phenotype of, 197—198
  recognition and binding of, 95
  relationship with LAK and CTL, 189
  role in peripheral blood, 186
Natural killer cell sensitive membranes, 98
Natural killer cytoxic factors (NKCF)
  activation of release mechanism for, 95—96
  assay of, 94
  biochemical characterization of, 99
  cytotoxicity of, 108
  diagnostic and clinical implications of, 100—103

mechanism of action of, 98—99
mechanism of release of, 96—98
as mediators of NK CMC mechanism, 95
production of, 92—95
relationship to other cytotoxins, 99—100
Natural killer-resistant target cells, 98, 220
Necrosil, 76
Neoplastic tissue, 123
Neuramindase, 99, 183
Neutrophils, 92, 117
NK, see Natural killer
NKCF, see Natural killer cytoxic factors
NK CMC, see Natural killer cell mediated cytotoxicity
Nuclear damage, 49
Nuclear structure changes, 47, 50
Nucleoprotein-DNA interactions, 43, 51—52

O

OAF, see Osteoclast activating factor
OE4 phenotype, 208—209, 214
OE25 phenotype, 208
OK-432, 110
Oligonucleosomes, 39, 41, 47
Oligonucleosome-sized DNA, 51
Oligo P, 15
Oncogenes, 181—182
Osteoclast activating factor (OAF), 118—119

P

P1, see Perforin 1
P815 cells, 63, 67
Parathyroid hormone, 119
Patch clamp recording of target cell, 27, 29
PBL, 182, 186
PBMC, see Peripheral blood mononuclear cells
Percoll gradients, 11, 21—22
Perforin, 11, 69, 99
Perforin 1 (P1, cytolysin), 6—8, see also Pore-forming protein
  binding to heparin-Sepharose by, 13
  channel-forming activity of, 7
  composition of, 15
  homology of, 8
  inhibition of, 13
  isolation of, 25
  murine, 10
  polymerization of, 7
Perforin 2, 9—10
Periodate, 183
Peripheral blood mononuclear cells (PBMC), 194—196, 199
Peripheral mononuclear blood leucocytes (PMBL), 220, 222
PFP, see Pore-forming protein
PGE_2, see Prostaglandin E_2
Phagocytosis, 117—118
Phenotypes, 197—198, 208
Phenylalanine, 112
Phorbol myristate acetate, 78

Planar bilayers, 23, 28
Plasmodium, 117
Platelets, 92
PMBL, see Peripheral mononuclear blood leucocytes
PMN, see Polymorphonuclear neutrophils
PMSF, 10
Polyacrylamide gel electrophoresis, 78, 111
Poly C9, 8
Polymerization of C9, 7—8
Polymorphonuclear neutrophils (PMN), 117, 123
Poly P1, 7, 9, 15
Poly P2, 9
Polypeptides, influenza, 167
Pore formation, 20—21, 31, 99
Pore-forming protein (PFP), see also Perforin
  assay of, 21
  channels produced by, 28, 30
  depolarization of muscle cells by, 28
  functional lesions produced by, 27—28
  immunological cross-reactivity between C9 and, 28
  mediation of tumor cell lysis by, 28
  in other cell types, 30
  polymerization of, 25—27
  production of, 20
  properties of, 25—30
  purification of, 26
  putative, 20—21, 25
Programmed cell death, 47, 48, 51—52
Pronase, 184
Prostaglandin E_2, 119
Proteases, 96
Protein antigens, 119
Protein A-Sepharose-purified immunoglobulins, 212—214
Protein C, activated, 118
Protein kinase C pathway, 97, 122
Proteins
  acute phase response, 78—79
  granule associated, 14—15, 23
  nucleocapsid, 166
  regulatory complement, 136
  trypsin-sensitive, 182—183
Protein synthesis mechanism, 51
Proteoglycans, 12—13
Pulmonary virus reduction by CTL, 165, 170—171

R

Raji cells, 144
^{86}Rb release, 37—38
Recombinant interleukin 2 (rIL-2), 220
  added to LAK, 189
  clinical trials of, 199—200
  culture of thymocytes in, 202—203
  induction of TNF secretion by, 119
  in vitro activation with, 200—201
  in vivo administration of, 194
  PBMC activated by culture in, 194—195
  purified, 176—177, 196
Recombinant interleukin 2 cultures, 220—221
Renal cancer, 145

Ricin, 147
rIL-2, see Recombinant interleukin 2
RPMI 1788 (lymphoid), 110

S

S.AKR cells, 211
Sarcoma, 63, 106, 108, 115, 201
Scatchard plot, 121—122
Schistosoma mansoni, 117
Schwartzman reaction, 80
SDS, 9
SDS-polyacrylamide gel electrophoresis, 25, 63
Sedimentation coefficients, 138—139
Sendai virus, 110
Serine esterase inhibitors, 10
Serum, 155—157
Sheep red blood cells (SRBC), 23, 110, 209
Shock, 79—80
SMCC, see Succinimidyl-4-(N-maleimidomethyl)cyclohexane-1-carboxylate
SMPM, see Succinimidyl-4-(*p*-maleimidophenyl)-butyrate
SPDP, see N-Succinimidyl-3-(2-pyridyldithio)-propionate
SRBC, see Sheep red blood cells
Streptococcus pyogenes, 110
Succinimidyl-4-(N-maleimidomethyl)cyclohexane-1-carboxylate (SMCC), 146
Succinimidyl-4-(*p*-maleimidophenyl)-butyrate (SMPM), 146
N-Succinimidyl-3-(2-pyridyldithio)-propionate (SPDP), 139, 141, 146, 208
Sulfhydryl groups, 136

T

3T3-L1 cells, 82, 84, 117, 181
Target cell binding, 36—38, 50—52
Target cell death, 49
Target cell DNA fragmentation, 69—70, 119
Target cell lysis
  granule components in, 14
  mechanism of, 50—52
  relation to DNA fragmentation, 44—48
  resistance of NK cells to, 101—102
  target structures for, 206
Target cell nuclear structures, 36
Target cells (TC)
  activation of cell death program in, 51—52
  antigen-positive, 138
  binding of NK cells to, 95
  complement-mediated killing of, 136
  conjugates of, 46
  ^{51}Cr release from, 65—66
  damage induced by CTL in, 49—50
  DNA degradation in, 12
  DNA fragmentation in, 40—44, 52
  DNA-nucleoprotein interactions in, 43
  E14, 12
  endonuclease in, 41—42

Fc receptor of, 209—210, 215
^{125}IUdkR-labelled, 39—41
LAK recognition of, 182—183
NKCF binding to, 97—98
patch clamp recording of, 27, 29
pretreated with INF, 96
resistance of, 101
stimulation of NKCF production by, 98
surface of, 207—209
TC receptors to, 215
tumor, 177
Targeting, 211, 213, 215
Targeting agents, 210—214
Targeting strategies, 207
TC, see Target cell
T cell receptor phenotypes, 208, 215
T cell recognition, 214
T cells
  antigen-specific effector, 206
  cloned, 206
  cytolytic, 4
  hybridomas, 206
  isolated from peripheral blood, 197
  lymphocytic, 194—195
  lysis by, 210
^{3}H-Tdr, 69
TGF-β, 116
Thy 1.1 tumor cells, 213, 215
^{3}H-Thymidine, 63—64
Thymosin alpha-1, 78
T lymphocytes
  activity of, 194
  antigen recognition by, 206
  cytotoxicity against K562, 197
  effector function of, 211, 214
  IL-2 cultured peripheral blood, 202
  influenza virus specific, 162
  role in viral infection, 163—166
  in TNF production, 109
TNF, see Tumor necrosis factor
TNF-α
  amino acid sequence of, 112
  antibodies to, 108
  bioassay for, 106
  cDNAs for, 114
  clinical trials with, 102
  collagenase stimulation by, 119
  effect on endothelial cells, 118
  human, 111, 113
  molecular characteristics of, 111
  from natural sources, 114
  production of, 99, 109
  protection against infections by, 117
  relationship to NKCF, 100
  relationship to TNF-β, 109
  sources for, 110
rTNFα (Genentec), 99, 118
TNF-β
  amino acid sequence of, 112
  antibodies to, 108
  bioassay for, 106
  clinical trials of, 102
  molecular characteristics of, 111
  from natural sources, 114
  production of, 109
  relationship to NKCF, 99
  relationship to TNF-α, 109
  sources for, 110
  suppression of lipoprotein activity by, 117
TNF-Luk II, 108
TNF-receptor complex, 122
TNP-PBL, 182—183
TNP-specific CTLs, 65
TNP-specific cytotoxic T cell clones, 70
TNS, see Tumor necrosis serum
TPA, 97
Triton X-100, 43
Trypan blue exclusion, 94
Trypsin, 99, 184
Trypsin-sensitive protein, 182—183
Tumor antigen, 211
Tumor cells, 28, 30—31, 213, 215
Tumor implant, 123
Tumor necrosis, 80—81, 106, 115
Tumor necrosis factor (TNF)
  amino acid composition of, 112—113
  antitumor action of, 123
  bioassays of, 106—108
  biologic activities of, 78—83, 116
    acute phase response protein, 78—79
    adipocyte differentiation/metabolism, 82—83
    cytotoxicity, 82
    induction of, 78—79
    in vitro properties, 80—83
    tumor necrosis, 80
  biological properties of, 114—122
    antipathogenic and antiviral, 117
    antitumor, 114—116
    bone resorption, 118—119
    cachectin/TNF-α, 117
    endothelial cell effects, 118
    hematopoietic cell differentiation, 118
    normal cell proliferation, 116
    PMN activation, 117—118
    receptors of, 120—122
    in relation to other cytokines, 119—120
  cellular receptor of, 83, 86
  effect on cells in vitro, 107
  gene structure of, 114
  history of, 76—77
  HPLC gel filtration of, 79
  isolation of, 106
  mechanism of action of, 83, 86, 122—124
  nomenclature for, 108
  physical properties of, 77—78
  physicochemical characterization of, 111—114
  purification of, 99, 110—111
  radiolabeled, 120—122

research on, 76
  sources of, 109—110
  targets for, 11
  therapy with, 115
Tumor necrosis serum (TNS), 117
Tumors
  autologous and allogenic, 180—181
  brain, 189
  effect on LAK activation, 179—181
  hemorrhagic necrosis of, 118
  NK-resistant, 220
  sites of, 211
  transplanted mouse, 115
  treatment of, 184, 206

Tumor target cells, 177

U

$U937_{NR}$, 100

V

Vesicular stomatitis virus (VSV), 117, 211
Viral antigen, 164—168
Viral infection, 163—166, 169—171
Vitamin D, 119
VSV, see Vesicular stomatitis virus

LIBRARY
UNIVERSITY OF TEXAS
SOUTHWESTERN MEDICAL SCHOOL
DALLAS, TEXAS